Update on Complex Infectious Diseases Issues in the Intensive Care Unit

Editors

SAMEER S. KADRI
NAOMI P. O'GRADY

INFECTIOUS DISEASE CLINICS OF NORTH AMERICA

www.id.theclinics.com

Consulting Editor
HELEN W. BOUCHER

December 2022 • Volume 36 • Number 4

ELSEVIER

1600 John F. Kennedy Boulevard ● Suite 1800 ● Philadelphia, Pennsylvania, 19103-2899.
http://www.theclinics.com

INFECTIOUS DISEASE CLINICS OF NORTH AMERICA Volume 36, Number 4
December 2022 ISSN 0891–5520, ISBN-13: 978-0-323-96087-8

Editor: Kerry Holland
Developmental Editor: Hannah Almira Lopez

Infectious Disease Clinics of North America (ISSN 0891–5520) is published in March, June, September, and December by Elsevier Inc., 360 Park Avenue South, New York, NY 10010-1710. Periodicals postage paid at New York, NY and additional mailing offices. Subscription prices are $357.00 per year for US individuals, $950.00 per year for US institutions, $100.00 per year for US students, $408.00 per year for Canadian individuals, $979.00 per year for Canadian institutions, $445.00 per year for international individuals, $979.00 per year for international institutions, $100.00 per year for Canadian students, and $200.00 per year for international students. To receive student rate, orders must be accompanied by name of affiliated institution, date of term, and the *signature* of program/residency coordinator on institution letterhead. Orders will be billed at individual rate until proof of status is received. Foreign air speed delivery is included in all *Clinics* subscription prices. All prices are subject to change without notice. **POSTMASTER:** Send address changes to *Infectious Disease Clinics of North America*, Elsevier Health Sciences Division, Subcription Customer Service, 3251 Riverport Lane, Maryland Heights, MO 63043. **Customer Service: 1-800-654-2452 (US). From outside of the US and Canada, call 1-314-447-8871. Fax: 1-314-447-8029. E-mail: JournalsCustomerService-usa@elsevier.com (print support) or JournalsOnlineSupport-usa@elsevier.com (online support).**

Infectious Disease Clinics of North America is also published in Spanish by Editorial Inter-Médica, Junin 917, 1er A 1113, Buenos Aires, Argentina.

Reprints. For copies of 100 or more, of articles in this publication, please contact the Commercial Reprints Department, Elsevier Inc., 360 Park Avenue South, New York, New York 10010-1710. Tel. 212-633-3874, Fax: 212-633-3820, E-mail: reprints@elsevier.com.

Infectious Disease Clinics of North America is covered in *MEDLINE/PubMed (Index Medicus), Current Contents/ Clinical Medicine, Science Citation Alert, SCISEARCH,* and *Research Alert.*

Contributors

CONSULTING EDITOR

HELEN W. BOUCHER, MD, FIDSA, FACP
Dean *ad interim* and Professor, Tufts University School of Medicine, and Chief Academic Officer, Tufts Medicine, Boston, Massachusetts

EDITORS

SAMEER S. KADRI, MD, MS, FIDSA
Tenure Track Investigator and Head, Clinical Epidemiology Section, Critical Care Medicine Department, National Institutes of Health Clinical Center, Bethesda, Maryland

NAOMI P. O'GRADY, MD
Chief, Internal Medicine Services, Senior Research Physician, National Institutes of Health Clinical Center, Bethesda, Maryland

AUTHORS

JANHAVI ATHALE, MD
Assistant Professor, Department of Critical Care Medicine, Division of Hematology and Oncology, Mayo Clinic, Phoenix, Arizona

STACI T. AUBRY, MD
Assistant Professor of Surgery, Division of Acute Care Surgery, Department of Surgery, University of Michigan Health System, Ann Arbor, Michigan

AHMED BABIKER, MBBS
Department of Medicine, Department of Laboratory Medicine and Pathology, Division of Infectious Diseases, Emory University School of Medicine, Atlanta, Georgia

STEPHANIE BUSBY, MD
Department of Surgery, Emory University School of Medicine, Atlanta, Georgia

LINDSAY M. BUSCH, MD
Assistant Professor, Division of Infectious Diseases, Emory University School of Medicine, Emory Critical Care Center, Department of Medicine, Emory University Hospital, Atlanta, Georgia

KELLY CAWCUTT, MD, MS
Associate Professor, Division of Infectious Diseases, Department of Internal Medicine, University of Nebraska Medical Center, Omaha, Nebraska

CORNELIUS J. CLANCY, MD
Professor, Department of Medicine, University of Pittsburgh, Pittsburgh, Pennsylvania

BROOKE K. DECKER, MD
Hospital Epidemiology Service, National Institutes of Health Clinical Center, Bethesda, Maryland

CHUKWUNYELU H. ENWEZOR, MD
Clinical Fellow, Department of Internal Medicine, Section on Infectious Diseases, Wake Forest School of Medicine, Winston-Salem, North Carolina

LATOYA A. FORRESTER, MPH, CIC
Hospital Epidemiology Service, National Institutes of Health Clinical Center, Bethesda, Maryland

JOLIE GALLAGHER, PharmD, BCCCP
Clinical Pharmacy Specialist, Department of Pharmacy, Emory University Hospital, Atlanta, Georgia

WENDY RICKETTS GREENE, MD, FACS, FCCM
Professor of Surgery, Emory University, Director of Acute and Critical Care Surgery, Emory University Hospital, Chair, Emory School of Medicine African American Women's Collaborative, Atlanta, Georgia; American College of Surgeons Board of Governors, Chicago, Illinois; Chair, Southeastern Surgical Congress ESC DEI Committee, Kansas City, Kansas; Co-Chair, ECCC IDEA Committee; Board member, Surgical Section of the National Medical Association and Surgical Leaders Foundation, Silverspring, Maryland

DAVID K. HENDERSON, MD
Hospital Epidemiology Service, National Institutes of Health Clinical Center, Bethesda, Maryland

ANGELA HEWLETT, MD, MS
Professor, Division of Infectious Diseases, Department of Internal Medicine, University of Nebraska Medical Center, Omaha, Nebraska

SAMEER S. KADRI, MD, MS, FIDSA
Tenure Track Investigator and Head, Clinical Epidemiology Section, Critical Care Medicine Department, National Institutes of Health Clinical Center, Bethesda, Maryland

ANDRE C. KALIL, MD, MPH
Professor, Division of Infectious Diseases, Department of Internal Medicine, University of Nebraska Medical Center, Omaha, Nebraska

MICHAEL KLOMPAS, MD, MPH
Department of Population Medicine, Harvard Medical School/Harvard Pilgrim Health Care Institute, Division of Infectious Diseases, Brigham and Women's Hospital, Boston, Massachusetts

ATUL MALHOTRA, MD
Professor, Division of Pulmonary, Critical Care, Sleep Medicine and Physiology, Department of Medicine, University of California, San Diego, La Jolla, California

RYAN C. MAVES, MD
Professor of Medicine and Anesthesiology, Department of Internal Medicine, Section on Infectious Diseases, Department of Anesthesiology, Section on Critical Care Medicine, Wake Forest School of Medicine, Winston-Salem, North Carolina

LENA M. NAPOLITANO, MD, FACS, FCCP, MCCM
Massey Foundation Professor of Surgery, Founding Division Chief, Acute Care Surgery, Director, Surgical Critical Care, Department of Surgery, University of Michigan Health System, Ann Arbor, Michigan

MINH HONG NGUYEN, MD
Professor, Department of Medicine, University of Pittsburgh, Pittsburgh, Pennsylvania

NAOMI P. O'GRADY, MD
Chief, Internal Medicine Services, Senior Research Physician, National Institutes of Health Clinical Center, Bethesda, Maryland

THEODORE R. PAK, MD, PhD
Division of Infectious Diseases, Massachusetts General Hospital, Department of Population Medicine, Harvard Medical School/Harvard Pilgrim Health Care Institute, Boston, Massachusetts

CHANU RHEE, MD, MPH
Department of Population Medicine, Harvard Medical School/Harvard Pilgrim Health Care Institute, Division of Infectious Diseases, Brigham and Women's Hospital, Boston, Massachusetts

RAMZY HUSAM RIMAWI, MD
Department of Medicine, Division of Pulmonary, Sleep, Allergy, and Critical Care Medicine, Assistant Professor of Medicine, Emory University School of Medicine, Atlanta, Georgia

DANIEL A. SWEENEY, MD
Associate Professor, Division of Pulmonary, Critical Care, Sleep Medicine and Physiology, Department of Medicine, University of California, San Diego, La Jolla, California

Contents

Sepsis guidelines and mandates encourage increasingly aggressive time-to-antibiotic targets for broad-spectrum antimicrobials for suspected sepsis and septic shock. This has caused considerable controversy due to weaknesses in the underlying evidence and fear that overly strict antibiotic deadlines may harm patients by perpetuating or escalating overtreatment. Indeed, a third or more of patients currently treated for sepsis and septic shock have noninfectious or nonbacterial conditions. These patients risk all the potential harms of antibiotics without their possible benefits. Updated Surviving Sepsis Campaign guidelines now emphasize the importance of tailoring antibiotics to each patient's likelihood of infection, risk for drug-resistant pathogens, and severity-of-illness.

Both cytokine release syndrome (CRS) and sepsis are clinical syndromes rather than distinct diseases and share considerable overlap. It can often be challenging to distinguish between the two, but it is important given the availability of targeted treatment options. In addition, several other clinical syndromes overlap with CRS and sepsis, further making it difficult to differentiate them. This has particularly been highlighted in the recent coronavirus disease-2019 pandemic. As we start to understand the differences in the inflammatory markers and presentations in these syndromes, hopefully we will be able to enhance treatment and improve outcomes.

Future pandemics will certainly arise and continue to have a profound impact on health care, including management within the intensive care unit. Robust preparedness plans require specific attention to detail as it pertains to incident management, surge capacity, infection control practices, and the health care workforce. The COVID-19 pandemic highlighted many gaps in prior preparedness efforts, and those lessons learned must be integrated into updated preparedness work. Additionally, ensuring health care workforce wellness, decreasing health care disparities, strengthening networks for rapid research and response, and active roles in dispelling misinformation within the media should be integrated into pandemic preparedness plans.

Following the reduction in mortality demonstrated by dexamethasone treatment in severe COVID-19, many targeted immunotherapies have been investigated. Thus far, inhibition of IL-6 and JAK pathways have the most robust data and have been granted Emergency Use Authorization for treatment of severe disease. However, it must be noted that critically ill patients comprised a relatively small proportion of most of the trials of COVID-19 therapeutics, despite bearing a disproportionate burden of morbidity and mortality. Furthermore, the rapidity and fluidity with which clinical trials have been conducted in the pandemic setting have contributed to difficulty in extrapolating available trial data to critically ill patients. The exclusion of many patients requiring invasive mechanical ventilation, preponderance of ordinal scale based endpoints, and frequent lack of blinding are particular challenges. More data is needed to identify beneficial treatments in the complex milieu of critical illness from COVID-19 infection.

Specific therapies for the treatment of coronavirus disease 2019 (COVID-19) have limited efficacy in the event a patient worsens clinically and requires admission to the intensive care unit (ICU). Thus, providing quality supportive care is essential to the overall management of patients with critical COVID-19. Patients with respiratory failure not requiring intubation should be supported with noninvasive positive pressure ventilation, continuous positive airway pressure, or high flow oxygenation. Use of these respiratory modalities may prevent patients from subsequently requiring intubation. Basic components of supportive care for the critically ill should be applied equally to patients with COVID-19 in the ICU.

Antimicrobial-resistant bacterial infections, particularly those caused by Gram-negative bacteria, are major public health threats globally. Since 2015, several antibiotics with activity against highly antimicrobial-resistant Gram-negative bacteria have been approved, which offer alternatives to previous frontline agents such as polymyxins and aminoglycosides. Despite data that new drugs are more effective and better tolerated than older agents against at least some highly antimicrobial-resistant Gram-negative bacterial infections, clinicians remain uncertain about how best to incorporate them into clinical practice. In this article, we discuss the management of highly resistant Gram-negative bacterial infections in the era of new antibiotics, with particular attention to those caused by AmpC- and extended-spectrum β-lactamase-producing

Clostridioides difficile remains a major cause of morbidity and mortality in the intensive care unit, and therefore, C difficile guidelines are frequently being updated. Currently, fidaxomicin is the suggested treatment of initial and recurrent infection. Oral vancomycin is an acceptable alternative, followed by rifaximin and fecal microbiota transplantation. Bezlotoxumab is suggested in recurrent cases within 6 months. If patients fail to improve within 3 to 5 days of therapy, especially in patients who have had nasogastric tubes or emergent surgery, fulminant colitis is possible and surgical consultation should be considered for total colectomy.

Procalcitonin is a commonly used biomarker for infection and severity in the intensive care unit. Although relatively specific for bacterial, as opposed to viral, infections, serum procalcitonin levels also correlate with disease severity and thus cannot reliably distinguish between bacterial and nonbacterial infections in the setting of critical illness, particularly in cases of severe influenza and coronavirus disease-2019. Baseline procalcitonin levels are insufficiently discriminative to permit the withholding of antibiotics in patients with critical illness and suspected sepsis. Trends in procalcitonin levels over time, however, give us the opportunity to individualize the duration of antibiotics without negative impacts on mortality.

INFECTIOUS DISEASE CLINICS
OF NORTH AMERICA

nfections in the Critically
Il during the COVID-19 Pandemic:
nfectious Diseases on Steroids

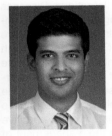 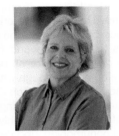

Sameer S. Kadri, MD, MS   Naomi P. O'Grady, MD

Editors

The first issue of "Complex Infectious Diseases Issues in the Intensive Care Unit" in *Infectious Disease Clinics of North America* highlighted the overwhelming presence of infection in the intensive care unit (ICU) and the unique intersection of infectious disease and critical care medicine. Now, 5 years later, the COVID-19 pandemic has highlighted the intersection of these two subspecialties in an obvious way and has made abundantly clear that the partnership should be strengthened. The second issue of "Update on Complex Infectious Diseases Issues in the Intensive Care Unit" is a compilation of articles that combines current evidence with the opinions of experts to highlight important nuances in caring for patients in the ICU in this new era of COVID-19.

The pandemic has raised the world's guard around infectious diseases in general. It has undoubtedly heightened interest in the infections that tend to make us very sick, the ones that challenge the paradigms in medicine, the ones that keep clinicians up worrying at night. It has made health care leaders and society reflect on the multiple mishaps that occurred during the pandemic due to lack of planning, and to work on bolstering resilience so we are better prepared for the next one, as there surely will be. It is also why 5 years ago, before the pandemic, we put together the original issue of this *Infectious Disease Clinics of North America* collection, "Complex Infectious Diseases Issues in the Intensive Care Unit."

Now well into the third year of the pandemic, as we write this Preface, we can't help it but marvel at one remarkable accomplishment of our time when basic scientists, clinicians, industry, funding, and regulatory agencies joined forces to develop and test effective vaccines in record time. This certainly should set a standard for a model going forward. We also note how the practice of medicine has changed, and how the demeanor of our colleagues has been impacted: despair at the thought of millions losing their lives needlessly to an avoidable tragedy; respect for our colleagues on the frontline, whose dedication, sacrifice, hours, and in some cases their own health,

Infect Dis Clin N Am 36 (2022) xiii–xiv
https://doi.org/10.1016/j.idc.2022.09.001
0891-5520/22/© 2022 Published by Elsevier Inc.

id.theclinics.com

have been at risk while they maintained the patient as their top priority; acceptance of the fact that the doctor—patient relationship will be adversely affected by the need for personal protective equipment for the foreseeable future. As we, as a profession, grapple with these changes, this issue of "Update on Complex Infectious Diseases Issues in the Intensive Care Unit" will leverage these changes in medical practice into an opportunity to better equip our fellow clinicians to follow the evidence, learn from the opinions of world experts, and save more lives.

This issue disentangles ongoing and additional "Complex Infectious Diseases Issues in the Intensive Care Unit" continues to disentangle ongoing and additional clinical controversies and provides evidence-based updates on cutting-edge critical care management of patients with serious infections beyond just COVID-19. Although COVID-19 has impacted the way we deliver care for all patients in the ICU, there are still some areas of ICU care that are complex enough without COVID-19 and warrant a discussion of a detailed evidence-based approach. These topics include the timing and spectrum of antibiotic therapy in sepsis, distinguishing cytokine release syndrome from sepsis, management of infections with highly resistant gram-negative bacteria, management of some unique pneumonias, updates on the management of severe streptococcal infections, and an updated discussion of the management of *Clostridioides difficile* infections. Of course, this issue would not be complete if we did not address topics that are COVID-19 related, such as preparing an ICU for a lethal respiratory virus pandemic, management of serious COVID-19 infections with immunotherapies, and addressing supportive ICU care in patients with COVID-19.

Crises, wars, and major disasters have historically been coupled with significant advances and opportunities. COVID-19 was no exception; we should in turn take it, learn from the last several years, and prepare for the next pandemic.

Sameer S. Kadri, MD, MS
Clinical Epidemiology Section
Critical Care Medicine Department
National Institutes of Health Clinical Center
10 Center Drive, Room 2C145
Bethesda, MD 20892-1662, USA

Naomi P. O'Grady, MD
Internal Medicine Services
National Institutes of Health Clinical Center
10 Center Drive, Room 2-2731
Bethesda, MD 20892-1662, USA

E-mail addresses:
sameer.kadri@nih.gov (S.S. Kadri)
nogrady@cc.nih.gov (N.P. O'Grady)

Timing and Spectrum of Antibiotic Treatment for Suspected Sepsis and Septic Shock

Why so Controversial?

Theodore R. Pak, MD, PhD[a,b], Chanu Rhee, MD, MPH[b,c], Michael Klompas, MD, MPH[b,c],*

KEYWORDS

- Sepsis • Evidence-based medicine • Retrospective studies • time-to-antibiotics
- antibiotic stewardship • quality improvement

KEY POINTS

- A third or more of patients treated for possible sepsis or septic shock have noninfectious conditions or nonbacterial infections.
- The literature on the association between time-to-antibiotics and mortality is almost exclusively observational and at high risk of bias. Sources of bias include failure to differentiate between sepsis and septic shock, insufficient adjustment for potential confounders, and blending together the high increases in mortality associated with very long delays until antibiotics with the small or absent effects associated with short delays until antibiotics, thus generating a misleading impression that every hour until antibiotics increases mortality and does so equally.
- Choosing appropriate empiric antibiotics for patients with possible sepsis or septic shock is a balancing act: both failure to cover the active pathogen and treating with unnecessarily broad regimens are associated with increased mortality.
- Clinicians are advised to tailor the timing and breadth of antibiotics for each patient with possible sepsis and septic shock to each individual's likelihood of infection, risk factors for resistant pathogens, and severity of illness.

[a] Division of Infectious Diseases, Massachusetts General Hospital, 55 Fruit Street, Cox Building, Suite #515, Boston, MA 02114, USA; [b] Department of Population Medicine, Harvard Medical School/Harvard Pilgrim Health Care Institute, 401 Park Drive, Suite 401 East, Boston, MA 02215, USA; [c] Division of Infectious Diseases, Brigham and Women's Hospital, 75 Francis Street, Boston, MA 02115, USA
* Corresponding author. 401 Park Drive, Suite 401 East, Boston, MA 02215.
E-mail address: mklompas@bwh.harvard.edu

Infect Dis Clin N Am 36 (2022) 719–733
https://doi.org/10.1016/j.idc.2022.08.001
0891-5520/22/© 2022 Elsevier Inc. All rights reserved.

id.theclinics.com

BACKGROUND

Sepsis, defined as a dysregulated host response to infection leading to acute organ dysfunction, affects millions of patients per year. It is associated with 850,000 visits to US emergency departments (EDs) annually[1] and one-third of US hospitalizations that end in death or discharge to hospice.[2] Guidelines on sepsis management have long emphasized that early recognition and treatment are key to lowering mortality. Many observational studies have attempted to quantify the association between delays in antibiotics and mortality risk. One of the earliest studies analyzed 2,731 cases of septic shock and estimated that mortality increased by 7.6% for every hour until effective antimicrobials were administered after the onset of recurrent or persistent hypotension.[3] Subsequent studies have not replicated as dramatic a result,[4] but associations of about 1% absolute increase in mortality risk per hour have been reported by several large studies that included tens of thousands of patients.[5-7]

Based in part upon these data, the Surviving Sepsis Campaign (SSC), the Centers for Medicaid and Medicare Services (CMS), the New York State Department of Health, and other state regulators have promoted 1-h or 3-h bundles of care for sepsis that include requirements to give empiric broad-spectrum antibiotics within brief time windows.[8-11] In 2016, SSC guidelines reaffirmed a target of less than 1 h to deliver antibiotics for all patients with sepsis (per Sepsis-3 definitions) or septic shock.[10,12,13] The Severe Sepsis and Septic Shock Management (SEP-1) bundle by CMS was implemented in 2015 and modeled on SSC guidelines.[14] It requires lactate measurements, blood cultures, and broad-spectrum antibiotics within 3 h of meeting specific physiologic criteria for severe sepsis with or without shock (per Sepsis-2 definitions).

These recommendations stirred considerable controversy. The Infectious Diseases Society of America (IDSA), for example, withheld their endorsement from the 2016 SSC guidelines.[15] One of their primary concerns was the SSC guidelines' failure to acknowledge the high levels of uncertainty inherent to the diagnosis of sepsis. Up to 40% of patients treated with antibacterials for possible sepsis turn out to have noninfectious conditions or nonbacterial infections.[16,17] These patients risk suffering the potential harms of antibacterial treatments without their potential benefits. These potential harms are not insignificant; a growing body of literature associates unnecessary antibiotics and unnecessarily broad antibiotics with higher rates of *Clostridioides difficile* infections, acute kidney injury, selection for resistant pathogens, and in some studies higher mortality rates.[18-20] IDSA feared that 1-h or even 3-h time-to-treatment requirements would perpetuate or exacerbate the problem of overtreatment given the difficulty of establishing a clear diagnosis within this timeframe, and thus inadvertently cause more harm than benefit to patients.

Moreover, IDSA noted substantial weaknesses in the data being used to support sepsis management bundles and their strict time-to-antibiotic deadlines, finding that nearly all studies on the association between time-to-antibiotics and mortality were at substantial risk of bias.[4,15] As such, the premise driving strict time-to-treatment mandates was potentially flawed. Finally, the 2016 SSC guidelines equated patients with *suspected sepsis* and *suspected septic shock* for the purposes of recommending the 1 h time-to-treatment, even though these groups have very different associations between time-to-antibiotics and mortality.[7,9] Studies published after the 2016 guidelines were released have reported that the association between time-to-antibiotics and mortality for sepsis without shock is much weaker than that for septic shock, and when present, the signal suggesting increased mortality in sepsis without shock only becomes apparent after delays of three to 5 h, not 1 h.[21,22]

Challenges in Interpreting Evidence on Antibiotic Delays and Associated Outcomes

How has the evidence regarding timing of antibiotics for sepsis patients led to such a wide range of conclusions? First, most of the evidence available for this question is from retrospective observational studies, given the difficulty of performing prospective trials that randomize patients to different antibiotic strategies during emergency care. We are only aware of two randomized controlled trials (RCTs) specifically examining the impact of faster time-to-antibiotics for sepsis on patient outcomes. One was a randomized trial of antibiotics in the prehospital setting versus the ED for patients with suspected sepsis.[23] Despite a 96-min difference in median time to antibiotics between groups there were no significant differences in mortality. The second study was a randomized trial comparing a multifaceted set of interventions focusing on reducing time-to-antibiotics versus conventional continuous medical education.[24] Unfortunately, this study did not achieve a significant difference in time-to-antibiotics between groups and thus was uninformative on this specific question. All the other evidence for the existence of an association between time-to-antibiotics and increased mortality is from observational studies, which carry inherent risks of confounding and are more difficult to interpret as causal evidence.

Second, most early observational studies (particularly those cited by SSC in 2016) were limited to intensive care unit (ICU) populations and thus enriched with a high proportion of patients with septic shock, potentially introducing unintended bias when formulating guidelines for all sepsis patients, including those without shock. Most of these studies did not perform subgroup analyses comparing sepsis with and without shock, and the few studies that included subgroup analyses found smaller associations or no significant association for sepsis without shock.[21] For example, in 35,000 presentations of sepsis to California EDs, there was an absolute increase in mortality of 1.8% (95% confidence interval [CI], 0.8%–3.0%; adjusted odds ratio [aOR], 1.14; aOR 95% CI, 1.06 to 1.23) associated with each hour of delay in antibiotics for patients with septic shock, whereas for severe sepsis patients without shock, this association shrank to 0.4% (95% CI, 0.1%–0.8%; aOR, 1.07; aOR 95% CI, 1.01–1.24).[7] Similarly, a study of 49,331 patients triggering sepsis protocols in New York EDs found a significant association between in-hospital death and hourly delays in completing a bundle that included antibiotics among patients that required vasopressors (aOR, 1.07; 95% CI, 1.05–1.09), but the association was not significant for patients not requiring vasopressors (aOR, 1.01; 95% CI, 0.99–1.04).[9] So too, in a study of 10,811 adult ED patients in Utah with sepsis predominantly without shock (92% did *not* have septic shock) there was no impact on 30-day mortality until $\geq$5 h had elapsed from ED triage until antibiotics were given.[5] And in a study of 74,114 adult ED patients with suspected infection without shock, there was an association between time-to-antibiotics and progression to shock (aOR 1.03 per hour, 95% CI 1.02–1.04) but no association between time-to-antibiotics and hospital mortality (aOR 1.02, 95% CI 0.99–1.04).[25] Most recently, a *prospective* non-randomized study of 178 Japanese ICU patients with sepsis found an association between decreased in-hospital mortality and completion of a 1-h bundle including antibiotics (aOR, 1.28; 95% CI, 1.04–1.57).[26] But once more, in risk-adjusted subgroup analyses comparing patients with and without shock, the association between in-hospital mortality and hourly bundle delays was only significant for the 55% of patients with septic shock (aOR, 1.25; 95% CI, 1.03–1.52), there was no significant association for the 45% of patients without shock (aOR, 1.17; 95% CI, 0.73–1.87).[26]

Third, most studies have linearized the relationship between time-to-antibiotics and mortality and reported a single blended estimate of the effect of each hour interval until antibiotics. This is highly problematic because inspection of the data underlying these studies shows clear nonlinear relationships.[21] Generally, very long intervals until antibiotics (typically >5 or 6 h) are associated with increased mortality but shorter intervals are not. Blending the effects of long intervals with the effects of shorter intervals gives the misimpression that each hour until treatment is associated with a clear and consistent increase in mortality. A very recent analysis of the impact of time-to-antibiotics in 4,792 patients with sepsis, for example, found that each additional hour until time-to-antibiotics was associated with a statistically significant 0.42% increase in 28-day mortality when combining data from all patients with time-to-antibiotic intervals ranging from <1 h to 48 h.[27] When the investigators compared intervals of 1 to 3 h versus <1 h and intervals of 3 to 6 h versus <1 h, however, there was no significant difference in 28-day mortality rates; only intervals of >6 h were associated with significantly higher mortality rates.[27]

Fourth, the timing of antibiotic administration in real-world practice is not random. Sicker patients with more obvious presentations of sepsis tend to be treated sooner. Confounders must be carefully controlled to disentangle the effects of time-to-antibiotics from patients' underlying mortality risk attributable to their preexisting comorbidities, presenting signs and symptoms, and severity of illness, all of which may influence the timing of antibiotics. Clinicians tend to order antibiotics more immediately for more ill-appearing patients and for those with higher baseline mortality risk, whether because of their demographics, medical history, or other data available at presentation, and for patients with more obvious clinical signs of infection (eg, fever).[28,29] Consequently, even in the largest observational studies, results change drastically when including different confounders in the model, going so far as to shift negative associations (earlier antibiotics paradoxically associated with greater mortality) to positive associations (earlier antibiotics associated with lower mortality).[7] Despite the clear importance of rigorously adjusting for potential confounders, studies vary widely in the number, breadth and granularity of the variables they use for this process; some do not even include age or comorbid diseases.[21] When medical history is included as a confounder, it is via simplifying rubrics such as Charlson or Elixhauser indices,[30,31] which conflate conditions with vastly different severities (eg, "mild intermittent asthma, uncomplicated" and "chronic obstructive pulmonary disease" incur equivalent risk in the Elixhauser Comborbidity Index).[32] Furthermore, these indices are not comprehensive; they omit key comorbidities (such as cystic fibrosis and some congenital immunodeficiencies) that may be uncommon but nonetheless clearly increase the risk of sepsis and death.[33] Few of the studies incorporate patients' prior infection-related data (culture results, recent antibiotic exposures, and recent infections) as confounders, even though these are often important determinants of clinicians' prescribing behavior and likely correlate with patients' likelihood of true sepsis and risk of death.

2016 to 2020: Conflicting Guidelines on a Time-To-Antibiotics Target

The net effect of these weaknesses and inconsistencies in source evidence as well as the controversy stirred by various sepsis guidelines and mandates is that guidelines on expected antibiotic timing for sepsis have changed frequently in the last 6 years, with contradictory recommendations between different professional societies. As described above, IDSA did not endorse the SSC 2016 guidelines, citing concerns regarding the promotion or perpetuation of antibiotic overuse, overdiagnosis of sepsis, weaknesses of the data supporting time-to-antibiotic goals, conflation of suspected sepsis and septic shock, and disagreement on specific recommendations regarding antimicrobial selection, blood cultures, procalcitonin, and treatment duration.[15] The concurrent release of the Third International Consensus definitions for sepsis ("Sepsis-3") sowed further confusion, partly because of terminology changes (redefining severe sepsis as sepsis)[34] and partly because different groups variably adopted the new definitions. SSC 2016 did adopt Sepsis-3 terminology but cited data using the old definitions to support their recommendations. Meanwhile, CMS continues to use the old definitions for their SEP-1 reporting requirement.

In 2018, the SSC released a "bundle update" combining its 3 h and 6 h bundles into a single 1 h bundle, which included lactate levels, blood cultures, volume resuscitation, vasopressors if fluid-refractory, and broad-spectrum antibiotics, all within 1 h of ED triage.[35] As more than 80% of sepsis is diagnosed on admission and initially managed in the ED,[1,2] concerns over the lack of evidence to support such a significant change to emergency medicine workflow were quickly raised.[36–38] In response to these concerns, the Society of Critical Care Medicine (SCCM) and American College of Emergency Physicians (ACEP) published a joint statement saying: "We recommend that hospitals not implement the Hour-1 Bundle in its present form in the United States at this time," whereas the authors of the SSC bundle update acknowledged that it was intended as a facilitative tool and not as a potential quality indicator.[39] "Time-zero" for bundle initiation was also revised from ED triage to time of sepsis recognition. Collectively, the net result was substantial confusion and/or disagreement among frontline providers, hospitals, and regulators on which components of the 2016 guidelines and the 2018 bundle update were in fact appropriate for implementation. Finally, in 2020, IDSA recommended revisions to the SEP-1 bundle created by CMS, again citing the lack of evidence supporting early antimicrobials for suspected sepsis without shock, concerns over the potential to drive antibiotic overuse, and the high complexity of SEP-1's "time-zero" definition.[22]

The Optimal Breadth of Broad-Spectrum Antibiotics

A parallel controversy has been determining the appropriate spectrum of empiric antibiotic coverage for sepsis, given similar mismatches between evolving guidelines and the level of evidence supporting them. In practice, just as important as *when* antibiotics are needed for sepsis is the corollary question of *which* antibiotics must be given. Antibiotic coverage is ideally tailored to causative pathogens and their susceptibility profiles, but these data are rarely available when antibiotics are started.

In 2016, SSC specified a number of overlapping terms for antimicrobial selection in sepsis ("empiric", "targeted/definitive", "broad-spectrum", "multidrug", and "combination").[10] IDSA felt that these terms were confusing, because differences between most of them would not be obvious even to experts in the field, and the terms were ultimately used inconsistently within the guidelines.[15] For example, SSC 2016 recommended "combination" therapy for septic shock—which they defined as the use of two or more antibiotics active against the patient's causative pathogen—"for several days." This recommendation was controversial for two reasons. First, many clinicians use "combination therapy" to refer to the empiric use of two agents active against gram-negative bacteria in order to increase the probability that the patient receives at least one agent active against their causative pathogen(s), that is, to broaden coverage. On the contrary, SSC defined it as two agents active against the same pathogen "to accelerate pathogen clearance rather than broaden antimicrobial coverage."[15] Second, the evidence supporting sustained use of two active agents for septic shock is very weak. Two large and rigorous randomized trials fail to support this approach, one focused on patients with sepsis in general[40] and one focused on patients with VAP.[41] Similarly, a meta-analysis of 13 randomized trials found no difference between empiric mono-versus combination antibiotic therapy on length-of-stay, mortality, or any other objective outcome among patients with sepsis.[42]

There is increasing evidence that the use of overly broad empiric antibiotics is not only unnecessary but may in fact cause harm.[43] A retrospective, propensity-weighted study of methicillin-resistant Staphylococcus aureus (MRSA) coverage in 88,605 Veterans' Affairs (VA) patients treated for community-acquired pneumonia (CAP) showed that the addition of anti-MRSA therapy was associated with increased adjusted risk of 30-day mortality and secondary infections including Clostridioides difficile, vancomycin-resistant Enterococcus (VRE), and gram-negative bacilli.[44] Counterintuitively, even when restricting to patients with MRSA found on cultures, there was no mortality benefit to adding anti-MRSA therapy, belying the complexity of diagnosing certain infections (did these patients have true pneumonias or mimicking conditions?) and the inconsistent relationships between antibiotic utilization and outcomes. Similar retrospective studies of 2,198 CAP patients in four US EDs, and a second VA cohort of 15,071 nonsevere pneumonia patients, showed increased mortality associated with broad-spectrum antibiotics.[45,46] A prospective cohort study of 303 ICU patients at risk for multidrug-resistant (MDR) pneumonia noted that guideline-directed (broader) therapy was associated with increased mortality.[47]

Regarding infections other than pneumonia, a 2-year quasi-experimental before-and-after observational cohort study of surgical ICU admissions at one hospital found that implementation of a conservative strategy for antimicrobial treatment, where antibiotics were started only after cultures or gram stain supported an infection, was associated with reduced mortality when compared with an aggressive strategy where broad empiric antimicrobials were started upon clinical suspicion and then stopped if cultures and gram stains were negative.[48] A retrospective study of 17,430 patients admitted to 104 US hospitals with sepsis and positive cultures (primarily blood, urine, or respiratory) found that unnecessarily broad empiric antibiotics, defined as including coverage of MRSA, VRE, Pseudomonas, or other MDR organisms when none of these were ultimately isolated on cultures, were independently associated with increased in-hospital mortality after adjusting for baseline characteristics and illness severity.[18] Identifying causes of these increases in mortality was outside the scope of these studies, but antibiotics have many known risks, including acute kidney injury, liver toxicity, cytopenias, selection for drug-resistant flora, mitochondrial toxicity, and disruption of the gut microbiome (an important modulator of the immune system).

On the contrary, empiric treatment of sepsis with a regimen that fails to cover the causative pathogen is also independently associated with increased mortality. Studies on this are limited to those with positive cultures so that antibiotic appropriateness can be determined, and therefore may not be representative of all suspected sepsis, for which a substantial fraction have negative cultures. Acknowledging this limitation, the aforementioned study of 17,430 patients with positive cultures did also show an association between inadequate empiric coverage and higher in-hospital mortality.[18] Similarly, a retrospective study of 21,608 patients from 131 US hospitals with bloodstream infections (about 20% of all sepsis cases)[2] found that among the 19% that received an inadequate initial regimen (failure to cover the bloodstream isolate), there was an independent association with increased mortality that was not affected by the presence or absence of drug resistance, sepsis, or septic shock.[49]

Therefore, the optimal "breadth" of broad-spectrum antibiotics for sepsis faces a Goldilocks problem[50]: evidence supports harms of both overly broad and overly narrow therapy, so in the face of diagnostic uncertainty, practical compromises have to be struck. As with time-to-antibiotics, the high rate of overdiagnosis of sepsis needs to be taken into account, as well as the variability in the signal between time-to-appropriate-antibiotics and mortality depending on patients' clinical syndrome and severity-of-illness. For conditions such as septic shock with less room for error, it is appropriate to use broader antibiotics up front, whereas ideally a stable patient with lower probability of infection should receive narrower or no antibiotics until a causative pathogen is confirmed.

2021 and Beyond: Toward Consensus in Sepsis Antimicrobial Guidelines

In July 2021, ACEP released its own set of guidelines on early sepsis care in the ED, which were endorsed by IDSA, SCCM, and 10 other professional societies. Taking a different tone from SSC 2016, ACEP's guidelines acknowledged the "inherent difficulty in establishing the early diagnosis of sepsis" in the ED.[51] Although prompt antibiotic administration is encouraged once sepsis is diagnosed, the authors concluded "there are insufficient data to recommend a specific time threshold for administration of antibiotics."[51] Regarding antibiotic spectrum, the guidelines avoided endorsing two-agent or "combination" therapy, instead recommending "initiation of broad-spectrum antibiotics with activity against gram-negative and gram-positive bacteria according to local susceptibility patterns."[51]

In November 2021, SSC published a new version of their guidelines that responded to much of the feedback from IDSA, ACEP, and other professional societies on antimicrobial management recommendations.[52] This update was endorsed by IDSA, signaling a shift back toward consensus. Although the general outline of antimicrobial-related recommendations remained similar, the evidence for many recommendations was downgraded from "moderate" quality evidence to "low" or "very low", and several crucial changes were made.

First, the new guidelines emphasize "the challenge of diagnostic uncertainty early in a patient's presentation," and now advise clinicians to "stratify antimicrobial timing recommendations based on the likelihood of sepsis and presence of shock."[53] Specifically, the cohort targeted for antimicrobials within 1 h has been narrowed from all patients with suspected sepsis or septic shock to just those patients with septic shock and possible sepsis "where likelihood of infection is high." For patients with an intermediate likelihood of infection, the guidelines now suggest a time-limited course of rapid investigation to determine a diagnosis, concluding with the administration of antimicrobials within 3 h only if concern for infection persists; the guidelines categorize evidence for this timeframe as weak instead of strong. Finally, the 2021 guidelines define an entirely new group of patients, "adults with low likelihood of infection and without shock," who explicitly do not need antimicrobials unless and until they are proven to have an infection. This recommendation will hopefully reinforce that many patients initially suspected of sepsis do not have a bacterial infection, and therefore it can be appropriate to do a diagnostic workup before starting antibiotics.

Second, a subtle but important change was added to the language of the SSC 2021 guidelines regarding time to antibiotics. The 2016 guidelines used durations of "within X hours" with the starting point left unnamed, leaving open an implication that this referred to the onset of sepsis. As the time of sepsis onset is not known for many patients entering the hospital, and could have occurred hours to days before admission, this is difficult to incorporate into metrics for hospital performance or observational studies, setting aside the minority case of hospital-onset sepsis.[2] Therefore, when creating bundles and cohort definitions, SSC, CMS, and sepsis researchers have all chosen different "time-zero" definitions—ranging from ED triage time in SSC's 2018 bundle update,[35] a combination of documentation and physiologic data within a sliding 6 h window in SEP-1,[8] and variations on these themes among the time-to-antibiotics studies.[21] By contrast, the SSC 2021 guidelines now explicitly refer to the clock on antibiotics starting "from the time when sepsis was first recognized," acknowledging the reality of a clinician needing time to evaluate the patient and consider other diagnoses before management can begin. Some time-to-antibiotics studies have also tried to use clinical recognition as their time-zero, although it is a labor-intensive and subjective concept to abstract from charts. Even time-zero definitions based on vital signs and laboratory measures are subject to high interobserver variability. Manual abstractors of SEP-1's time-zero, for example, disagree over half of the time on when time-zero occurred.[54] Nevertheless, by including a conceptual time-zero (sepsis recognition) for the first time, the 2021 guidelines helped narrow down potential interpretations of time-to-antibiotics and may encourage future researchers to build consensus on an operational definition.

Finally, the SSC 2021 guidelines made significant changes to recommendations on spectrum of coverage. The artificial terminology of "empiric", "targeted/definitive," "combination," "multidrug," etc., was eliminated. Instead, the new guidelines frame spectrum of coverage around specific categories of pathogens that should be considered when starting antimicrobials. For instance, there is a new best practice statement on including empiric MRSA coverage for sepsis only when the patient is judged to have "high risk of MRSA infection," and a similar "weak" suggestion for antifungal coverage only if the patient is at "high risk for fungal infection." There still is a "weak" suggestion for using two antimicrobial agents (previously called "combination therapy") to cover gram-negative bacteria, but instead of applying to all patients with suspected sepsis, it is aimed at patients specifically with high risk for MDR organisms. There is a parallel recommendation to narrow this regimen to a single agent once the causative pathogen(s) and susceptibilities are known, and the evidence categorization for these suggestions has been downgraded to "very low quality." Overall, although evidence ratings for the new antimicrobial spectrum recommendations are modest, by framing them around categories with specific microbiologic correlates such as "MRSA coverage," they have increased clarity and adaptability to local data, such as the use of community prevalence of MRSA and MDR organisms to help determine the appropriateness of broader empiric coverage.

DISCUSSION

Overall, the 2021 SSC and ACEP guidelines have made significant progress in building consensus recommendations for antimicrobial timing and breadth, balancing the importance of rapid treatment for potentially septic patients with bona fide infections against the potential harms associated with antibiotics for those who are not infected. By casting a more critical light upon the limitations of existing evidence, they also forecast several areas where higher quality evidence is needed. For instance, although the 2021 SSC guidelines now emphasize concepts intrinsic to the early clinical evaluation and management of sepsis, including "sepsis where the likelihood of infection is high," "the time when sepsis was first recognized," "high risk for MDRs," and "high risk for fungal infection," the onus is on researchers to characterize these probabilities and timepoints more concretely so that clinicians may leverage them for decision-making.

The fundamental challenge in sepsis management remains: how might we better identify which patients along the spectra of sepsis risk and severity benefit most from earlier antibiotics, and which merit broader versus narrower coverage? One approach might be to raise the standard for large observational studies on time-to-antibiotics, which are increasingly robust in terms of sample size but have been less rigorous about the methods used to control for confounders. Future studies can and should expand their input variables to incorporate more of the richness and breadth of the data available in electronic medical records (EMRs). For example, studies rarely use data from prior encounters to formulate confounders and the likelihood for a patient's subsequent presentation of suspected sepsis. Incorporating more detailed measures of current and prior clinical markers of organ dysfunction as well as their trajectories could improve differentiation and quantification of acute changes catalyzed by infection vs chronic underlying conditions—something that clinicians do routinely when evaluating patients, but has been left out of cohort definitions and adjustment models underlying nearly all time-to-antibiotics studies. In addition, machine-learning techniques may disentangle the vast heterogeneity in EMR data from sepsis populations by identifying distinct sub-phenotypes of sepsis using clustering and similar techniques.[55–59] Future work could integrate machine-learning sub-phenotyping with data on antibiotic timing, breadth, and outcomes to generate predictive models of the sub-phenotypes that most likely benefit from earlier antibiotics or broader-spectrum coverage.

Translational research on rapid diagnostics for sepsis may also permit a more tailored approach. After decades of research, likely due to the biological heterogeneity of the syndrome,[60] there still are no gold-standard diagnostic tests or biomarkers for sepsis, which remains a clinical diagnosis based on the same kinds of data that were first used to describe the "systemic inflammatory response syndrome" in 1992.[61] Nonetheless, earlier accurate identification of sepsis caused by bacteria and their susceptibility profiles could both accelerate the time-to-antibiotics and mitigate antibiotic overuse. Over 200 biomarkers for sepsis have been investigated,[62] with C-reactive protein and procalcitonin among the most popular, but as these two markers are both upregulated in noninfectious inflammation, neither is sensitive nor specific enough to reliably guide initial sepsis treatment. Procalcitonin has shown more promise as a longitudinal marker of antibiotic response in serious infections, permitting shortened antibiotic courses that are associated with lower in-hospital mortality in meta-analyses.[63,64] Of the other biomarkers, only 26 have been investigated in samples of at least 300 patients, and it seems increasingly unlikely that any single host biomarker will "break through" and significantly alter early sepsis diagnosis or management.[62]

Other researchers have focused on molecular diagnostics targeting bacterial nucleic acids, such as polymerase chain reaction (PCR) of 16S ribosomal RNA and microarrays. In principle, these may yield equally accurate and slightly faster results compared with blood cultures,[65,66] but their utility is less clear for non-bloodstream infections. Similarly, mass spectrometry is increasingly integrated into culturing workflows, providing the greatest speed benefit when identifying slow growing and less common organisms.[67] Recent methods have attempted to decrease turnaround time for mass spectrometry on blood culture isolates by replacing subculturing with centrifugation and protein extraction, although this still requires waiting for growth in the initial blood culture bottle.[68,69] Whole-genome sequencing of pathogens provides high-resolution data useful for genotyping and molecular epidemiology, but is unlikely to usurp culturing and mass spectrometry on turnaround time for species identification, except for pathogens that are difficult to culture.[70] Researchers have also directed omics assays toward the host immune response, finding potential sepsis sub-phenotypes in meta-analysis of microarray data from 600 patients,[71] and more recently, a unique CD14$^+$ monocyte state distinguishing 29 sepsis patients from 36 controls using single-cell RNA sequencing.[72] New diagnostics leveraging these insights are still undergoing development and validation for potential clinical applications.

SUMMARY

From 2016 to 2020, sepsis guidelines and regulatory mandates encouraged increasingly brief targets—as short as 1 h—for initiating broad-spectrum antimicrobials for patients with suspected sepsis or septic shock. This sparked considerable controversy due to weaknesses in the underlying evidence and concern that strict antibiotic deadlines cause inadvertent harm by perpetuating or accelerating overtreatment at the expense of diagnostic inquiry. A third or more of patients treated for sepsis and septic shock have noninfectious or nonbacterial conditions. These patients risk harm from unnecessary antibiotics. New guidelines from both ACEP and SSC in 2021 now emphasize the importance of tailoring treatment to each patient's likelihood of infection, risk for drug-resistant pathogens, and severity of illness. These guidelines will benefit from future research that raises the standards for evidence derived from observational studies of time-to-antibiotics and associated outcomes. New diagnostics that rapidly quantify the likelihood of infection by bacteria, MDR organisms, fungi, and other pathogen groups relevant to antimicrobial selection could also have a major clinical impact, given the emphasis on these concepts in the latest guidelines.

CLINICS CARE POINTS

- A third or more of patients treated for sepsis turn out to have noninfectious conditions or nonbacterial infections.

- When evaluating a patient for possible sepsis, tailor the urgency of antibiotics to the patient's likelihood of infection and severity of illness.

- In patients with possible septic shock, administer antibiotics immediately. In patients with less severe illness, undertake a rapid course of diagnostics (eg, lab studies, imaging, microbiological assays, etc.) and treat for noninfectious possibilities if present (eg, fluids, diuretics, bronchodilators, heart rate control, etc.). Continually reevaluate the likelihood of infection based on the results of diagnostic studies and response to treatments for noninfectious conditions. If high concern for infection persists at 3 h from when sepsis was first suspected, then administer antimicrobials.

- Choose the spectrum of antibiotics according to severity of illness (as critically ill patients have less margin for error) and the local distribution of organisms and their resistance patterns as well as each patient's individual risk factors for antibiotic-resistant organisms.

DISCLOSURE

T.R. Pak, author, reports grant funding from the National Institute of Allergy and Infectious Diseases (5T32AI007061). C. Rhee and M. Klompas report grant funding from the Centers for Disease Control and Prevention and Agency for Healthcare Research and Quality to conduct research related to sepsis. C. Rhee reports royalties from UpToDate, Inc. for chapters related to procalcitonin use. MK reports royalties from UpToDate, Inc. for chapters related to hospital-acquired pneumonia.

REFERENCES

1. Wang HE, Jones AR, Donnelly JP. Revised National Estimates of Emergency Department Visits for Sepsis in the United States. Crit Care Med 2017;45(9): 1443–9.

2. Rhee C, Dantes R, Epstein L, et al. Incidence and trends of sepsis in US hospitals using clinical vs claims data, 2009-2014. JAMA 2017;318(13):1241-9.

3. Kumar A, Roberts D, Wood KE, et al. Duration of hypotension before initiation of effective antimicrobial therapy is the critical determinant of survival in human septic shock. Crit Care Med 2006;34(6):1589-96.

4. Sterling SA, Miller WR, Pryor J, et al. The Impact of Timing of Antibiotics on Outcomes in Severe Sepsis and Septic Shock: A Systematic Review and Meta-Analysis. Crit Care Med 2015;43(9):1907-15.

5. Door-to-Antibiotic Time and Long-term Mortality in Sepsis. In: Peltan ID, Brown SM, Bledsoe JR, et al, editors. Chest 2019;155(5):938-46.

6. Ferrer R, Martin-Loeches I, Phillips G, et al. Empiric antibiotic treatment reduces mortality in severe sepsis and septic shock from the first hour: Results from a guideline-based performance improvement program. Crit Care Med 2014; 42(8):1749-55.

7. Liu VX, Fielding-Singh V, Greene JD, et al. The Timing of Early Antibiotics and Hospital Mortality in Sepsis. Am J Respir Crit Care Med 2017;196(7):856-63.

8. Centers for Medicare & Medicaid Services. Hospital Inpatient Specifications Manuals. 2020. Available at: https://qualitynet.cms.gov/inpatient/specifications-manuals. Accessed February 8, 2022.

9. Seymour CW, Gesten F, Prescott HC, et al. Time to Treatment and Mortality during Mandated Emergency Care for Sepsis. N Engl J Med 2017;376(23):2235-44.

10. Rhodes A, Evans LE, Alhazzani W, et al. Surviving Sepsis Campaign: International Guidelines for Management of Sepsis and Septic Shock: 2016. Crit Care Med 2017;45(3):486-552.

11. Dwyer J. One boy's death moves state to action to prevent others. The New York Times; 2012. Available at: https://www.nytimes.com/2012/12/21/nyregion/one-boys-death-moves-state-to-action-to-prevent-others.html. Accessed February 13, 2022.

12. Seymour CW, Liu VX, Iwashyna TJ, et al. Assessment of Clinical Criteria for Sepsis: For the Third International Consensus Definitions for Sepsis and Septic Shock (Sepsis-3). JAMA 2016;315(8):762-74.

13. Dellinger RP, Levy MM, Rhodes A, et al. Surviving sepsis campaign: International guidelines for management of severe sepsis and septic shock, 2012. Intensive Care Med 2013;39(2):165-228.

14. Pepper DJ, Jaswal D, Sun J, et al. Evidence underpinning the centers for medicare & medicaid services' severe sepsis and septic shock management bundle (SEP-1) a systematic review. Ann Intern Med 2018;168(8):1-11.

15. IDSA Sepsis Task Force, Kalil AC, Gilbert DN, Winslow DL, et al. Infectious Diseases Society of America (IDSA) POSITION STATEMENT: Why IDSA Did Not Endorse the Surviving Sepsis Campaign Guidelines. Clin Infect Dis 2018; 66(10):1631-5.

16. Klein Klouwenberg PMC, Cremer OL, van Vught LA, et al. Likelihood of infection in patients with presumed sepsis at the time of intensive care unit admission: A cohort study. Crit Care 2015;19(1):1-8.

17. Shappell CN, Klompas M, Ochoa A, et al. Likelihood of Bacterial Infection in Patients Treated With Broad-Spectrum IV Antibiotics in the Emergency Department. Crit Care Med 2021;49(11):e1144-50.

18. Rhee C, Kadri SS, Dekker JP, et al. Prevalence of Antibiotic-Resistant Pathogens in Culture-Proven Sepsis and Outcomes Associated With Inadequate and Broad-Spectrum Empiric Antibiotic Use. JAMA Netw Open 2020;3(4):e202899.

19. Tamma PD, Avdic E, Li DX, et al. Association of Adverse Events With Antibiotic Use in Hospitalized Patients. JAMA Intern Med 2017;177(9):1308–15.

20. Ong DSY, Frencken JF, Klein Klouwenberg PMC, et al. Short-Course Adjunctive Gentamicin as Empirical Therapy in Patients With Severe Sepsis and Septic Shock: A Prospective Observational Cohort Study. Clin Infect Dis 2017;64(12): 1731–6.

21. Weinberger J, Rhee C, Klompas M. A critical analysis of the literature on time-to-antibiotics in suspected sepsis. J Infect Dis 2021;222:S110–8.

22. Rhee C, Chiotos K, Cosgrove SE, et al. Infectious Diseases Society of America Position Paper: Recommended Revisions to the National Severe Sepsis and Septic Shock Early Management Bundle (SEP-1) Sepsis Quality Measure. Clin Infect Dis 2021;72(4):541–52.

23. Alam N, Oskam E, Stassen PM, et al. Prehospital antibiotics in the ambulance for sepsis: a multicentre, open label, randomised trial. Lancet Respir Med 2018;6(1): 40–50.

24. Bloos F, Rüddel H, Thomas-Rüddel D, et al. Effect of a multifaceted educational intervention for anti-infectious measures on sepsis mortality: a cluster randomized trial. Intensive Care Med 2017;43(11):1602–12.

25. Bisarya R, Song X, Salle J, et al. Antibiotic Timing and Progression to Septic Shock Among Patients in the ED With Suspected Infection. Chest 2022;161(1): 112–20.

26. Umemura Y, Abe T, Ogura H, et al. Hour-1 bundle adherence was associated with reduction of in-hospital mortality among patients with sepsis in Japan. PLoS One 2022;17(2):1–12.

27. Rüddel H, Thomas-Rüddel DO, Reinhart K, et al. Adverse effects of delayed antimicrobial treatment and surgical source control in adults with sepsis: results of a planned secondary analysis of a cluster-randomized controlled trial. Crit Care 2022;26(1):51.

28. Filbin MR, Lynch J, Gillingham TD, et al. Presenting symptoms independently predict mortality in septic shock: Importance of a previously unmeasured confounder. Crit Care Med 2018;46(10):1592–9.

29. Henning DJ, Carey JR, Oedorf K, et al. The absence of fever is associated with higher mortality and decreased antibiotic and IV fluid administration in emergency department patients with suspected septic shock. Crit Care Med 2017; 45(6):e575–82.

30. Van Walraven C, Austin PC, Jennings A, et al. A modification of the elixhauser comorbidity measures into a point system for hospital death using administrative data. Med Care 2009;47(6):626–33.

31. Charlson ME, Pompei P, Ales KL, et al. A new method of classifying prognostic comorbidity in longitudinal studies: development and validation. J Chronic Dis 1987;40(5):373–83.

32. Agency for Healthcare Research and Quality. Elixhauser comorbidity software refined for ICD-10-CM reference file, v2022.1. Available at: https://www.hcup-us.ahrq.gov/toolssoftware/comorbidityicd10/CMR-Reference-File-v2022-1.xlsx. Accessed March 13, 2022.

33. Alrawashdeh M, Klompas M, Simpson SQQ, et al. Prevalence and Outcomes of Previously Healthy Adults Among Patients Hospitalized With Community-Onset Sepsis. Chest 2022;1–10. https://doi.org/10.1016/j.chest.2022.01.016.

34. Singer M, Deutschman CS, Seymour CW, et al. The Third International Consensus Definitions for Sepsis and Septic Shock (Sepsis-3). JAMA 2016;315(8):801–10.

35. Levy MM, Evans LE, Rhodes A. The Surviving Sepsis Campaign Bundle: 2018 update. Intensive Care Med 2018;44(6):925–8.
36. Marik PE, Farkas JD, Spiegel R, et al. POINT: Should the Surviving Sepsis Campaign Guidelines Be Retired? Yes *Chest* 2019;155(1):12–4.
37. Kalantari A, Rezaie SR. Challenging the one-hour sepsis bundle. West J Emerg Med 2019;20(2):185–90.
38. Talan DA, Yealy DM. Challenging the One-Hour Bundle Goal for Sepsis Antibiotics. Ann Emerg Med 2019;73(4):359–62.
39. Levy MM, Rhodes A, Evans LE. Steering and Executive Committee of the Surviving Sepsis Campaign. COUNTERPOINT: Should the Surviving Sepsis Campaign Guidelines Be Retired? No. Chest 2019;155(1):14–7.
40. Brunkhorst FM, Oppert M, Marx G, et al. Effect of empirical treatment with moxifloxacin and meropenem vs meropenem on sepsis-related organ dysfunction in patients with severe sepsis: A randomized trial. JAMA 2012;307(22):2390–9.
41. Heyland DK, Dodek P, Muscedere J, et al. Randomized trial of combination versus monotherapy for the empiric treatment of suspected ventilator-associated pneumonia. Crit Care Med 2008;36(3):737–44.
42. Sjövall F, Perner A, Hylander Møller M. Empirical mono- versus combination antibiotic therapy in adult intensive care patients with severe sepsis – A systematic review with meta-analysis and trial sequential analysis. J Infect 2017;74(4):331–44.
43. Arulkumaran N, Routledge M, Schlebusch S, et al. Antimicrobial-associated harm in critical care: a narrative review. Intensive Care Med 2020;46(2):225–35.
44. Jones BE, Ying J, Stevens V, et al. Empirical Anti-MRSA vs Standard Antibiotic Therapy and Risk of 30-Day Mortality in Patients Hospitalized for Pneumonia. JAMA Intern Med 2020;180(4):552–60.
45. Webb BJ, Sorensen J, Jephson A, et al. Broad-spectrum antibiotic use and poor outcomes in community-onset pneumonia: A cohort study. Eur Respir J 2019;54(1):1–9.
46. Attridge RT, Frei CR, Restrepo MI, et al. Guideline-concordant therapy and outcomes in healthcare-associated pneumonia. Eur Respir J 2011;38(4):878–87.
47. Kett DH, Cano E, Quartin AA, et al. Implementation of guidelines for management of possible multidrug-resistant pneumonia in intensive care: An observational, multicentre cohort study. Lancet Infect Dis 2011;11(3):181–9.
48. Hranjec T, Rosenberger LH, Swenson B, et al. Aggressive versus conservative initiation of antimicrobial treatment in critically ill surgical patients with suspected intensive-care-unit-acquired infection: A quasi-experimental, before and after observational cohort study. Lancet Infect Dis 2012;12(10):774–80.
49. Kadri SS, Lai YL, Warner S, et al. Inappropriate empirical antibiotic therapy for bloodstream infections based on discordant in-vitro susceptibilities: a retrospective cohort analysis of prevalence, predictors, and mortality risk in US hospitals. Lancet Infect Dis 2021;21(2):241–51.
50. Leisman DE. The Goldilocks Effect in the ICU—When the Data Speak, but Not the Truth. Crit Care Med 2020;48(12):1887–9.
51. Yealy DM, Mohr NM, Shapiro NI, et al. Early Care of Adults With Suspected Sepsis in the Emergency Department and Out-of-Hospital Environment: A Consensus-Based Task Force Report. Ann Emerg Med 2021;78(1):1–19.
52. Evans L, Rhodes A, Alhazzani W, et al. Surviving Sepsis Campaign: International Guidelines for Management of Sepsis and Septic Shock 2021. Crit Care Med 2021;49(11):e1063–143.

53. Evans L, Rhodes A, Alhazzani W, et al. Executive Summary: Surviving Sepsis Campaign: International Guidelines for the Management of Sepsis and Septic Shock 2021. Crit Care Med 2021;49(11):1974–82.

54. Rhee C, Brown SR, Jones TM, et al. Variability in determining sepsis time zero and bundle compliance rates for the centers for medicare and medicaid services SEP-1 measure. Infect Control Hosp Epidemiol 2018;39(8):994–6.

55. Zhang Z, Zhang G, Goyal H, et al. Identification of subclasses of sepsis that showed different clinical outcomes and responses to amount of fluid resuscitation: a latent profile analysis. Crit Care 2018;22(1):347.

56. Gårdlund B, Dmitrieva NO, Pieper CF, et al. Six subphenotypes in septic shock: Latent class analysis of the PROWESS Shock study. J Crit Care 2018;47:70–9.

57. Han X, Spicer A, Carey KA, et al. Identifying High-Risk Subphenotypes and Associated Harms From Delayed Antibiotic Orders and Delivery. Crit Care Med 2021; 49(10):1694–705.

58. Seymour CW, Kennedy JN, Wang S, et al. Derivation, Validation, and Potential Treatment Implications of Novel Clinical Phenotypes for Sepsis. JAMA 2019; 321(20):2003–17.

59. Ibrahim ZM, Wu H, Hamoud A, et al. On classifying sepsis heterogeneity in the ICU: Insight using machine learning. J Am Med Inform Assoc 2020;27(3):437–43.

60. Stanski NL, Wong HR. Prognostic and predictive enrichment in sepsis. Nat Rev Nephrol 2020;16(1):20–31.

61. Bone RC, Balk RA, Cerra FB, et al. Definitions for sepsis and organ failure and guidelines for the use of innovative therapies in sepsis. Chest 1992;101(6): 1644–55.

62. Pierrakos C, Velissaris D, Bisdorff M, et al. Biomarkers of sepsis: Time for a reappraisal. Crit Care 2020;24(1):1–15.

63. Pepper DJ, Sun J, Rhee C, et al. Procalcitonin-Guided Antibiotic Discontinuation and Mortality in Critically Ill Adults: A Systematic Review and Meta-analysis. Chest 2019;155(6):1109–18.

64. Elnajdy D, El-Dahiyat F. Antibiotics duration guided by biomarkers in hospitalized adult patients; a systematic review and meta-analysis. Infect Dis (Auckl) 2022; 0(0):1–16.

65. Järvinen AKK, Laakso S, Piiparinen P, et al. Rapid identification of bacterial pathogens using a PCR- and microarray-based assay. BMC Microbiol 2009;9. https://doi.org/10.1186/1471-2180-9-161.

66. Shang S, Chen G, Wu Y, et al. Rapid diagnosis of bacterial sepsis with PCR amplification and microarray hybridization in 16S rRNA gene. Pediatr Res 2005;58(1):143–8.

67. Altun O, Botero-Kleiven S, Carlsson S, et al. Rapid identification of bacteria from positive blood culture bottles by MALDI-TOF MS following short-term incubation on solid media. J Med Microbiol 2015;64(11):1346–52.

68. Watanabe N, Koyama S, Taji Y, et al. Direct microorganism species identification and antimicrobial susceptibility tests from positive blood culture bottles using rapid Sepsityper Kit. J Infect Chemother 2022;2021(2). https://doi.org/10.1016/j.jiac.2021.12.030.

69. Lin JFF, Ge MCC, Liu TPP, et al. A simple method for rapid microbial identification from positive monomicrobial blood culture bottles through matrix-assisted laser desorption ionization time-of-flight mass spectrometry. J Microbiol Immunol Infect 2018;51(5):659–65.

70. Pak TR, Kasarskis A. How Next-Generation Sequencing and Multiscale Data Analysis Will Transform Infectious Disease Management. Clin Infect Dis 2015; 61(11):1695–702.
71. Sweeney TE, Azad TD, Donato M, et al. Unsupervised analysis of transcriptomics in bacterial sepsis across multiple datasets reveals three robust clusters. Crit Care Med 2018;46(6):915–25.
72. Reyes M, Filbin MR, Bhattacharyya RP, et al. An immune-cell signature of bacterial sepsis. Nat Med 2020;26(3):333–40.

Cytokine Release Syndrome and Sepsis

Analogous Clinical Syndromes with Distinct Causes and Challenges in Management

Janhavi Athale, MD[a], Lindsay M. Busch, MD[b],
Naomi P. O'Grady, MD[c],*

KEYWORDS

- Cytokine release syndtome • Sepsis • Inflammatory clinical syndromes • COVID-19
- Tocilizumab

KEY POINTS

- Differentiate between sepsis and cytokine release syndrome (CRS).
- Identify CRS triggers.
- Discuss syndromes with clinical overlap between sepsis and CRS.

INTRODUCTION

Cytokine release syndrome (CRS) and sepsis are clinical syndromes with considerable overlap and heterogeneous clinical presentations. The goal of this review is to define a spectrum of diseases that are associated with CRS and sepsis, including other closely related immunopathologic syndromes such as hemophagocytic lymphohistiocytosis (HLH), to describe several well-recognized CRS triggers (including chimeric antigen receptor [CAR] T-cell therapy, allogeneic transplants, novel drugs, and coronavirus disease-2019 [COVID-19]), and to provide a framework for delivering therapy that covers both clinical syndromes when the etiology is not yet known.

CRS was first described to define the body's hyperinflammatory immune response to a stimulus, including infection or sterile inflammatory processes.[1] One of the first reported descriptions of CRS in the literature was in a patient who developed acute graft-versus-host disease (GVHD) during hematopoietic stem cell transplantation (HSCT) in the early 1990s.[2] CRS has been used to describe the clinical syndrome of

[a] Department of Critical Care Medicine, Division of Hematology and Oncology, Mayo Clinic Arizona, 5777 East Mayo Boulevard, Phoenix, AZ 85054, USA; [b] Department of Medicine, Emory University Hospital, 550 Peachtree Street Northeast, Atlanta, GA 30308, USA; [c] Internal Medicine Services, National Institutes of Health, Room 2-2734, Bethesda, MD 20892-1662, USA
* Corresponding author.
E-mail address: nogrady@mail.cc.nih.gov

Infect Dis Clin N Am 36 (2022) 735–748
https://doi.org/10.1016/j.idc.2022.07.001
0891-5520/22/Published by Elsevier Inc.

id.theclinics.com

elevated cytokines with exaggerated inflammation and organ dysfunction.[1] This definition bears similarity to the Society of Critical Care Medicine/European Society of Intensive Care Medicine guidelines most recent definition of sepsis as "life-threatening organ dysfunction caused by a dysregulated host response to infection."[3] Neither the definition of CRS nor sepsis have complete consensus, and there is significant overlap in the clinical presentations of both. Furthermore, the two entities may be linked, as many of the underlying disorders and treatments that predispose to CRS are states of profound immunosuppression, which carry an increased risk of infection and sepsis. However, as management strategies for both syndromes have become more targeted in recent years, accurate diagnosis is essential to facilitate the early initiation of appropriate therapies.

CYTOKINE RELEASE SYNDROME TRIGGERS
Chimeric Antigen Receptor T-Cell Therapies

Over the past decade, CRS has been used more specifically to describe the syndrome of elevated cytokines with associated fevers, hypotension, hypoxia, and multiorgan dysfunction that can result after CAR-T.[4] CRS associated with CAR-T cells has been well studied with now agreed upon standardized classification[5] (**Table 1**). In addition to fever (defined as temp $\geq$ 38°C), the extent of hypotension and hypoxia are used to classify the grade of CRS, with grade 5 signifying death due to CRS. Furthermore, central nervous system-associated toxicities, often referred to as immune effector cell-associated neurotoxicity syndrome (ICANS) or less commonly cytokine release encephalopathy syndrome (CRES), are classified separately given their distinct treatments and outcomes.[5,6] However, as discussed previously, CRS is not unique to CAR-T cell therapies and can be seen in several novel therapies, including the now widely used checkpoint inhibitors (CPIs).

Checkpoint Inhibitor Therapy-Associated Cytokine Release Syndrome, and the Overlap with Sepsis

There are three widely used categories of CPIs: cytotoxic T-lymphocyte-associated protein 4 (CTLA-4) inhibitor (ipilimumab), programmed cell death protein 1 (PD-1) inhibitors (cemiplimab, nivolumab, and pembrolizumab), and programmed death ligand 1 (PD-L1) inhibitors (atezolizumab, avelumab, and durvalumab), with several new targets (LAG-3, TIM-2, B7-H3, and others) in ongoing clinical trials.[7] CPIs have revolutionized outcomes in oncology. The mechanism of CRS associated with CPIs is not well known, but presumably arises from the priming of T cells/cancer cells with resultant cellular destruction and subsequent inflammation.[8] A recent World Health

Table 1
Cytokine release syndrome clinical grading criteria as agreed upon by the American Society for Transplantation and Cellular Therapy

CRS Grade	Hypotension	Hypoxia
1	None	None
2	Not requiring a vasopressor	Requiring NC or blow-by oxygen
3	Requiring a single vasopressor (with or without vasopressin)	HFNC, facemask, NRB, or Venturi
4	Requiring multiple vasopressors	Requiring invasive or noninvasive positive pressure ventilation

All CRS grades must have a temperature $\geq$ 38°C.
Abbreviations: HFNC, high-flow nasal cannula; NC, nasal cannula; NRB, non-rebreather.

Organization (WHO) global database survey noted 58 cases of worldwide CRS in over 130 member countries surveyed, with the highest total cases in North America (United States and Canada with $n = 37$), and with the highest incidence in Australia (0.14%).[9] The malignancies most associated with CPI-related CRS included melanoma ($n = 17$) and hematologic malignancies ($n = 16$). Six of the cases ($\sim 10\%$) had concurrent infections, thereby suggesting some overlap between sepsis and CRS.[9] Another study evaluated 25 patients with CRS after CPI therapy in two tertiary hospitals and classified these patients using the CRS grading scale detailed in **Table 1**.[10] In this study, three patients suffered from Grade 5 (fatal) CRS, and Grade 3 to 4 CRS was seen in another five patients.[10] This study raises concerns that the overall incidence of CRS after CPI is underreported when compared with numbers in the WHO global database.

Underreporting could also be due to the overlap in immune-related adverse events (IRAEs) associated with CPI use.[11] IRAEs affect multiple organ systems and are used to describe organ-specific toxicities that result after CPI use. Most commonly, dermatitis, pneumonitis, and gastroenteritis can be seen.[12] The IRAEs can result in disruption of the epithelial barrier and predispose to secondary infections, including sepsis. In addition, IRAEs are treated with immunosuppression which can result in additional infectious risks. When IRAEs are associated with hypotension due to secondary infection or hypophysitis with multi-organ involvement, there can be overlap with CRS, and even sepsis. Thus, the exact classification of the syndrome impacting these patients can be challenging. Would the patient benefit from additional immunosuppression versus antimicrobial therapy versus immunomodulation of cytokines? These questions remain challenging for the bedside clinician.

CPIs are now being considered for use in sepsis with ongoing clinical trials.[13] Septic patients have been noted to have marked immunosuppression and defects in adaptive immune cell responses to infection, thus placing them at an increased risk of infection.[14,15] This phenomenon of immune exhaustion during sepsis is similar to the immune exhaustion seen in patients with cancer.[16] Hence, it is not surprising that immunotherapy is now being considered for the potential treatment of sepsis in non-cancer patients. CPIs have shown remarkable responses in certain infections, such as JC virus-associated progressive multifocal leukoencephalopathy, but it is notable that even in that small study one patient (of eight studied) was identified as having an inflammatory syndrome classified as immune reconstitution inflammatory syndrome (IRIS).[17] Thus, as the indications for CPIs broaden, in addition to CRS, overlap with infectious diseases/sepsis, and additional inflammatory syndromes (IRAEs or IRIS) will likely become more common.[18]

Cytokine Release Syndrome Associated with Antibody Therapy

Apart from the CPIs, almost all monoclonal antibodies could be associated with CRS.[19,20] The incidence of CRS after the use of muromonab-CD3 (OKT3) was among the first published cases of CRS in the literature.[20] Antibody-mediated reactions may result in the production of excessive cytokines resulting in a hyperinflammatory syndrome that could be classified as CRS.[21] Specifically, the novel CD19/CD3 bispecific T-cell receptor-engaging (BiTE) antibody, blinatumomab, has been associated with CRS along with neurologic toxicities. The CRS and neurologic toxicities associated with blinatumomab are treated with steroids and CRS-specific anti-cytokine antibody treatment.[22] Several other BiTEs are now in clinical trials with their unique side-effect CRS profiles. In addition to CRS, certain antibody therapies are associated with very specific side effects. For example, the novel agent tagraxofusp-erzs is a CD123 targeting IL-3 antibody fused with diphtheria toxin that has revolutionized responses to blastic plasmacytoid dendritic-cell neoplasm (BPDCN) but is associated with capillary leak syndrome, which will be discussed later in this article.[23]

Cytokine Release Syndrome Associated with Hematopoietic Stem Cell Transplantation

With the availability of haploidentical (or half-matched donors), the ability to provide allogeneic HSCT has greatly increased.[24] The infusion of hematopoietic stem cells, particularly from a haploidentical donor, has been associated with an increased incidence of CRS akin to what is seen after CAR-T cell therapy.[25] Several risk factors, perhaps most predominantly the use of peripheral blood stem cells, have been associated with an increased incidence of CRS with higher grades of CRS corresponding to increased mortality and worse overall outcomes.[25–28] Haploidentical HSCT-associated CRS generally abates with the administration of cyclophosphamide on day three and four post-transplant, but in high CRS grades with multiorgan dysfunction, the elevated interleukin (IL)-6 levels in particular are highly responsive to steroids and tocilizumab, an IL-6 receptor antibody.[29–31]

This patient population is generally neutropenic following conditioning chemotherapy treatment in anticipation of a new hematopoietic stem cell population, and thus is also at an increased risk of sepsis, and particularly neutropenic sepsis necessitating early intervention with supportive care and appropriate antimicrobial therapy. In addition to the overlap with sepsis, several other peri-transplant syndromes, including acute GVHD and engraftment syndrome may also be present in this patient population, further complicating the diagnosis.[32]

Cytokine Release Syndrome after Engineered Virus-Specific T Cells

In addition to CAR-T cells, other engineered cellular products may also contribute to CRS. With the advent of new virus-specific T cells (VST), case reports have noted associated CRS.[33,34] With VST therapy, T cells are obtained either from a viral-experienced allogeneic donor or more recently virus-naïve umbilical cord blood or adult donors, stimulated and expanded ex-vivo against a single or multivalent viral target, and infused into the recipient to confer immediate antiviral immunity.[35] Although this method provides a potentially powerful tool against difficult-to-treat viruses, the direct infusion of a large number of primed T cells into a host with a significant antigen burden poses a risk for acute release of inflammatory cytokines resulting in CRS and subsequent infiltrative tissue damage. Several groups have reported success with VST in Phase 1 and 2 studies and case series, showing microbiologic and clinical cures with limited adverse events.[34,36,37] In total, CRS is felt to be rare post-VST, complicating less than 2% of recipients in one study.[38] However, it must be noted that these patients are largely clinically stable at the time of infusion and although they may have evidence of tissue-invasive disease (ie, cytomegalovirus pneumonitis or retinitis, BK virus-associated hemorrhagic cystitis), they are not generally critically ill with evidence of multisystem organ dysfunction. There are limited data to guide whether VST may be of potential clinical benefit or harm in patients who are systemically ill with concurrent organ dysfunction, and thus remains an important clinical question about the optimal timing of treatment. Clinically significant and potentially fatal CRS has been reported following VST.[33] The authors show an acute rise in serum ferritin and IL-6 levels and concurrent fall in C-reactive protein (CRP) and interferon (IFN) γ, immediately following anti-BK VSTs in a patient with severe BK virus hemorrhagic cystitis. The patient received tocilizumab but developed progressive multiorgan failure secondary to sinusoidal obstructive syndrome (SOS)/veno-occlusive disease (VOD) and acute hypoxic respiratory failure and subsequent death on day 63 posttransplant. Postmortem sampling showed hepatic SOS/VOD with hemorrhagic necrosis, acute renal tubular injury, and early pulmonary exudative phase diffuse alveolar damage without any evidence of polyomavirus on SV40 staining, supporting the hypothesis that the fatal organ injury was likely driven by overwhelming inflammatory cytokines and cellular damage rather than direct microbial-mediated damage. Thus, although VST is an important weapon in a limited arsenal of therapy against challenging viral infections, it is not without risk. Vigilance for signs of CRS is essential, and further data are needed to evaluate for safety in the setting of systemic illness.

Inflammatory syndromes resembling cytokine release syndrome

Hemophagocytic lymphohistiocytosis. HLH clinically presents similarly to sepsis and CRS but has well-established criteria for the diagnosis. A vast majority of the HLH in adult patients arises because of ongoing stimulation from either an infection, malignancy, or autoimmune disease. This type of HLH is referred to as a secondary HLH, rather than genetic or primary HLH which is more common in pediatric patients.[39] The diagnosis of secondary HLH requires five of the following eight criteria: (1) fever, (2) cytopenias in at least two cell lines, (3) hypertriglyceridemia or hypofibrinogenemia, (4) splenomegaly, (5) elevated soluble IL-2 receptor α (CD25), (6) decreased or absent NK cell activity, (7) ferritin elevation, and (8) hemophagocytosis in tissue.[40] Once this diagnosis is established, the primary objective is to treat the underlying trigger. In general, over a third of secondary HLH is due to malignancy, under a third due to infection, over 10% due to autoimmune disease (referred to as macrophage activation syndrome),[41] and about 10% remain idiopathic.[42] Thus, as expected there is a significant overlap between HLH, CRS, and sepsis. In one of the largest retrospective intensive care unit (ICU) studies of HLH (40 patients with HLH of 2643 total ICU patients), the authors found that a higher ferritin cut-off value (9083 μg/L; AUC 0.963, 95% CI, 0.949–0.978) correlated with HLH when compared with patients with sepsis.[43] Given that 1/3 of HLH is triggered by infection, distinguishing sepsis from HLH can be difficult.

In patients that develop refractory CRS after CAR-T cell therapy, there is a concern that their clinical disease may start to resemble HLH. Based on the HLH diagnostic criteria, several patients with CRS would meet the criteria for HLH at baseline (or merely Grade 1–2 CRS toxicity), and thus deciding whether therapy targeting the HLH is merited can be challenging. Several institutions have adapted treatment guidelines to further distinguish refractory CRS and HLH. For instance, most centers recommend first treating for CRS, and then monitoring for improvement at 48 h, before initiating chemotherapy (generally etoposide).[44] Regardless, these patients are often covered for sepsis as well with broad-spectrum antibiotics given for their immunosuppressed state.

Immune reconstitution inflammatory syndrome and human immunodeficiency virus malignancies. IRIS is generally used to describe the phenomenon of immune recovery, and specifically T-cell recovery, in patients with human immunodeficiency virus (HIV) after initiation of antiretroviral therapy.[45] Although IRIS can be applied to a variety of immune reconstitution phenomenon, it is characterized by elevated cytokines and diffuse organ involvement with vasodilation, and thus can have overlap with CRS and sepsis syndromes. In addition, several HIV and human herpes virus-8 associated malignancies, including Kaposi sarcoma, primary effusion lymphoma, and multicentric Castleman's disease are characterized by elevated cytokines, and a "cytokine storm" like phenomenon akin to CRS, and even sepsis.[46,47] Smaller studies have shown the role of tocilizumab (commonly used in CAR-T-associated CRS) in these patients.[48,49]

Capillary leak syndrome. Capillary leak syndrome is another clinical syndrome with a significant overlap between CRS and sepsis. It is characterized by increasing capillary permeability with loss of oncotic pressure, and resultant leakage of fluid into the interstitium and hypotension.[50] It can be idiopathic, secondary to sepsis, secondary to the treatment of sepsis, or it can be seen with acute respiratory distress syndrome (ARDS). It can also be associated with the use of certain targeted therapies employing toxins. For instance, Tagraxofusp-erzs is a novel CD123-directed cytotoxin of IL-3 fused to truncated diphtheria toxin that is used for the treatment of blastic plasmacytoid dendritic cell neoplasm and is sometimes complicated by capillary leak syndrome.[23] In this disease with poor outcomes, Tagraxofusp-erzs showed a 90% overall response rate. However, two of the 47 patients enrolled died from capillary leak syndrome. The package insert for the drug recommends aggressive management of capillary leak syndrome in these patients. As newer antibody and cytokine-mediated therapies develop, we are likely to see more patients with CRS and associated syndromes.[51–53]

Distinguishing between cytokine release syndrome and sepsis to target clinical management

Both CRS and sepsis can be associated with fever, hypotension, vasodilatory shock, and multiorgan failure. Making the distinction between CRS and sepsis can be challenging but important such that targeted therapy can be initiated promptly. When one is unable to distinguish between CRS and sepsis it is imperative to treat both, focusing on maintaining end-organ perfusion, maintaining oxygenation, supporting hemodynamics, and monitoring inflammatory markers frequently. Supportive treatment of coagulopathies and symptom relief are also important parts of clinical management. Understanding the timing of CRS may also help distinguish this from sepsis and allow for targeted therapies. In general, the timing of CRS after infusion of CAR-T depends on the CAR-T cellular construct, but on an average is seen 7 days after infusion.[54] Although delayed complications can be seen in a subset of population.[55]

Anti-interleukin-6 therapy and steroids. CAR-T cell therapy revolutionized outcomes in refractory diseases, but initially there was a concern for an unacceptably high mortality associated with CRS. This was mitigated using tocilizumab, an anti-IL-6 receptor antibody.[56–58] Tocilizumab is being explored for sepsis in clinical trials, and the results of these studies are still pending.[59] In higher grade CRS, or ICANS, rapid initiation of steroids is recommended for their cytolytic and anti-inflammatory activity on CAR-T cells, along with their ability to cross the blood–brain barrier.[60] However, this infusion of steroids and resultant cytolysis of the CAR-T cells could be deleterious. A recent single-center study evaluated 60 CAR-T recipients (of 100 total) who had received steroids.[61] The study found that higher doses of steroids and earlier use of steroids after infusion of CAR-T cells were both associated with overall shorter survival. The role of steroids in septic shock remains contentious though large studies have shown a trend toward accelerated recovery and possible improved mortality.[62,63] Most guidelines recommend steroids in patients with refractory septic shock.[64]

Fluid resuscitation strategy. Recent studies have highlighted challenges with guideline-mandated volume resuscitation in sepsis, along with choices of fluid (balanced crystalloid vs normal saline).[65] Unlike sepsis, in CRS, cautious and judicious use of fluids is recommended given a tendency for patients to develop pulmonary edema.[58,66] Most institutional guidelines recommend early use of vasopressors after a modest fluid challenge to minimize expected third-spacing of fluid.[60]

Antimicrobial therapy. In septic shock, early antibiotic administration has been shown to improve mortality.[67] Patients with CRS after CAR-T therapy have a high risk of concomitant infection, and most guidelines recommend early administration of antibiotics with first fever.[51,68] In fact, several patients with CRS have concomitant neutropenia after conditioning therapy requiring immediate initiation of broad-spectrum antibacterial agents. The European Society for Blood and Marrow Transplantation has also recommended the initiation of antiviral prophylaxis (along with Cytomegalovirus monitoring), with delayed initiation of pneumocystis pneumonia prophylaxis, along with conditional mold prophylaxis and immunoglobulin replacement.[69] Centers in the United States tend to follow a similar paradigm, with more institution-specific guidelines.[70,71]

Coronavirus disease-2019 complicated with cytokine release syndrome and sepsis

The interplay between CRS and sepsis has further been highlighted with the recent COVID-19 pandemic. Early in the pandemic, clinicians noticed a hyperinflammatory subtype in some of the patients with COVID-19 which mimicked a secondary HLH.[72] This response represented the exaggerated host immune response to the viral infection, and the need to mitigate this response became the focus of several trials. RECOVERY remains among the first studies in COVID-19 to show a mortality benefit in hypoxic patients that were treated with steroids.[73] The role of steroids in CRS and sepsis has been discussed above.

On the heels of the RECOVERY trial, several studies assessed the roles additional anti-inflammatory agents may play in COVID-19. The recommended treatments for COVID-19 include anti-IL-6 agents, specifically tocilizumab and sarilumab (anti-IL-6 receptor antibodies). These agents have been shown to prevent the need for mechanical ventilation and death.[74–76] In addition, inhibition of the janus tyrosine kinase (JAK) and signal transducers and activators of transcription (STAT) pathway with agents such as baricitinib and ruxolitinib has been shown to help in recovery from COVID-19.[77,78] Interestingly, these agents have also been used in HLH with some success.[79]

A particularly inflammatory endotype of patients with hyperinflammation and COVID-19 has been classified as multisystem inflammatory syndrome (MIS) in adults (A) and children (C). The clinical criteria for MIS-C are slightly variable among the WHO, Centers for Disease Control and Prevention (CDC), and the Royal College of Pediatrics and Child Health.[80] For the purposes of this review, we have focused on the CDC definitions.[81] **Table 2** details the clinical criteria for the definition of MIS-A. Patients must present with fevers and elevated inflammatory markers in the presence of confirmation of infection with SARS-CoV-2, followed by the inclusion of at least three clinical criteria, with one being a primary clinical criterion. MIS-C, by CDC definition, is used to describe patients less than 21 years with COVID-19 who are hospitalized with elevated inflammatory markers and evidence of two or more organ system dysfunction without other plausible explanations.

In the largest case series of MIS-C published in the United States, 186 patients with a median age of 8.5 years were included with almost 80% requiring ICU care and four deaths (though almost a third of the patients remained hospitalized at the time of study publication).[81] This hyperinflammatory state has been treated with immunomodulators including intravenous immunoglobulins, steroids, IL-6 antagonists, and anakinra (IL-1 receptor inhibitor).

Beyond the inflammatory subtype of COVID-19, there has also been a concern for secondary infections, particularly pneumonia, in damaged lungs of patients with COVID-19 resulting in increased mortality and septic shock.[82] Yet, larger group

Table 2
Classification of multisystem inflammatory syndrome in adults

Age	$\geq$ 21 y
Duration	Hospitalized for $\geq$ 24 h, or with illness resulting in death
Fever	($\geq$38.0 C) for $\geq$ 24 h before hospitalization, or fevers within 3 days of hospitalization

Primary (must include at least one of the following)	1. Severe cardiac dysfunction (cardiac arrest alone does not qualify)
	   • Myocarditis
	   • Pericarditis
	   • Coronary artery dilation or aneurysm
	   • New left ventricular or right ventricular dysfunction
	   • Second/third degree A–V block
	   • Ventricular tachycardia
	2. Rash and non-purulent conjunctivitis

Secondary (must have at least one primary, and two additional secondary to meet criteria)	1. Neurologic dysfunction:
	   • Encephalopathy
	   • Seizures
	   • Meningismus
	   • Peripheral neuropathy
	   • Acute inflammatory demyelinating polyneuropathy (Guillain–Barré syndrome)
	2. Shock or hypotension
	3. Gastrointestinal symptoms: abdominal pain, vomiting, or diarrhea
	4. Thrombocytopenia (platelet count <150,000/mL)

Laboratory markers	1. Elevated levels of at least two of the following: C-reactive protein, ferritin, interleukin-6, erythrocyte sedimentation rate, and procalcitonin 2. A positive SARS-CoV-2 test for current or recent infection by RT-PCR, serology, or antigen detection

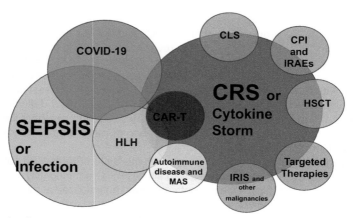

Fig. 1. Overlap between CRS and sepsis with the inclusion of other diseases and clinical syndromes. CAR-T, chimeric antigen receptor T cell; CLS, capillary leak syndrome; CPI, checkpoint inhibitor; HLH, hemophagocytic lymphohistiocytosis; HSCT, hematopoietic stem cell transplant; IRAE, immune-related adverse events; IRIS, immune reconstitution inflammatory syndrome; MAS, macrophage activation syndrome.

studies have recommended judicious use of antibiotics given the lower incidence of concomitant bacterial or fungal infection.[83] There may be some utility in using infectious markers, such as CRP and procalcitonin, in making decisions regarding antimicrobial stewardship.[84] Overall, infection with COVID-19 serves to highlight the overlap between sepsis and CRS, and the challenges in distinguishing between the two.

SUMMARY

This review provides a broad framework for understanding CRS and other closely related syndromes. We have discussed several triggers of CRS, along with clinical syndromes that share significant overlap with both CRS and sepsis. **Fig. 1** details CRS-associated conditions and shows the overlap between CRS and sepsis, along with the interplay of HLH and the COVID-19 pandemic. Given that both CRS and sepsis are clinical syndromes rather than distinct diseases, identifying and classifying patients at the bedside as having one or the other, or both, will remain challenging. The backbone for treatment of both CRS and sepsis remains excellent supportive care to maintain oxygenation and end-organ perfusion, with a focus on making the distinction quickly such that targeted therapies can be used.

CLINICS CARE POINTS

- Sepsis and CRS are both clinical syndromes with significant overlap that can make distinction between the two challenging.
- In addition, there are several other clinical syndromes and diseases which also share features of both sepsis and CRS.
- Learning to recognize the features of both sepsis and CRS will allow for more targeted therapies, and hopefully overtime improved outcomes.

DISCLOSURE

Dr. O'Grady: This article has been partially funded by the Intramural Program at the National Institutes of Health.

REFERENCES

1. Fajgenbaum DC, June CH. Cytokine Storm. N Engl J Med 2020;383(23):2255–73.
2. Ferrara JL, Abhyankar S, Gilliland DG. Cytokine storm of graft-versus-host disease: a critical effector role for interleukin-1. Transplant Proc 1993;25(1 Pt 2): 1216–7.
3. Singer M, Deutschman CS, Seymour CW, et al. The Third International Consensus Definitions for Sepsis and Septic Shock (Sepsis-3). JAMA 2016;315(8):801–10.
4. Morgan RA, Yang JC, Kitano M, et al. Case report of a serious adverse event following the administration of T cells transduced with a chimeric antigen receptor recognizing ERBB2. Mol Ther 2010;18(4):843–51.
5. Lee DW, Santomasso BD, Locke FL, et al. ASTCT Consensus Grading for Cytokine Release Syndrome and Neurologic Toxicity Associated with Immune Effector Cells. Biol Blood Marrow Transplant 2019;25(4):625–38.
6. Neelapu SS. Managing the toxicities of CAR T-cell therapy. Hematol Oncol 2019; 37(Suppl 1):48–52.

7. Marin-Acevedo JA, Kimbrough EO, Lou Y. Next generation of immune checkpoint inhibitors and beyond. J Hematol Oncol 2021;14(1):45.

8. Ciner AT, Hochster HS, August DA, et al. Delayed cytokine release syndrome after neoadjuvant nivolumab: a case report and literature review. Immunotherapy 2021;13(13):1071–8.

9. Ceschi A, Noseda R, Palin K, et al. Immune Checkpoint Inhibitor-Related Cytokine Release Syndrome: Analysis of WHO Global Pharmacovigilance Database. Front Pharmacol 2020;11:557.

10. Tay SH, Toh MMX, Thian YL, et al. Cytokine Release Syndrome in Cancer Patients Receiving Immune Checkpoint Inhibitors: A Case Series of 25 Patients and Review of the Literature. Front Immunol 2022;13:807050.

11. Thompson JA, Schneider BJ, Brahmer J, et al. NCCN Guidelines Insights: Management of Immunotherapy-Related Toxicities, Version 1.2020. J Natl Compr Canc Netw 2020;18(3):230–41.

12. Postow MA, Sidlow R, Hellmann MD. Immune-Related Adverse Events Associated with Immune Checkpoint Blockade. N Engl J Med 2018;378(2):158–68.

13. Hotchkiss RS, Colston E, Yende S, et al. Immune Checkpoint Inhibition in Sepsis: A Phase 1b Randomized, Placebo-Controlled, Single Ascending Dose Study of Antiprogrammed Cell Death-Ligand 1 Antibody (BMS-936559). Crit Care Med 2019;47(5):632–42.

14. Otto GP, Sossdorf M, Claus RA, et al. The late phase of sepsis is characterized by an increased microbiological burden and death rate. Crit Care 2011;15(4):R183.

15. Boomer JS, To K, Chang KC, et al. Immunosuppression in patients who die of sepsis and multiple organ failure. JAMA 2011;306(23):2594–605.

16. Dyck L, Mills KHG. Immune checkpoints and their inhibition in cancer and infectious diseases. Eur J Immunol 2017;47(5):765–79.

17. Cortese I, Muranski P, Enose-Akahata Y, et al. Pembrolizumab Treatment for Progressive Multifocal Leukoencephalopathy. N Engl J Med 2019;380(17):1597–605.

18. Brahmer JR, Lacchetti C, Schneider BJ, et al. Management of Immune-Related Adverse Events in Patients Treated With Immune Checkpoint Inhibitor Therapy: American Society of Clinical Oncology Clinical Practice Guideline. J Clin Oncol 2018;36(17):1714–68.

19. Winkler U, Jensen M, Manzke O, et al. Cytokine-release syndrome in patients with B-cell chronic lymphocytic leukemia and high lymphocyte counts after treatment with an anti-CD20 monoclonal antibody (rituximab, IDEC-C2B8). Blood 1999;94(7):2217–24.

20. Chatenoud L, Ferran C, Bach JF. The anti-CD3-induced syndrome: a consequence of massive in vivo cell activation. Curr Top Microbiol Immunol 1991;174:121–34.

21. Bugelski PJ, Achuthanandam R, Capocasale RJ, et al. Monoclonal antibody-induced cytokine-release syndrome. Expert Rev Clin Immunol 2009;5(5):499–521.

22. Teachey DT, Rheingold SR, Maude SL, et al. Cytokine release syndrome after blinatumomab treatment related to abnormal macrophage activation and ameliorated with cytokine-directed therapy. Blood 2013;121(26):5154–7.

23. Pemmaraju N, Lane AA, Sweet KL, et al. Tagraxofusp in Blastic Plasmacytoid Dendritic-Cell Neoplasm. N Engl J Med 2019;380(17):1628–37.

24. Luznik L, O'Donnell PV, Symons HJ, et al. HLA-haploidentical bone marrow transplantation for hematologic malignancies using nonmyeloablative conditioning

and high-dose, posttransplantation cyclophosphamide. Biol Blood Marrow Transplant 2008;14(6):641–50.

25. Abboud R, Wan F, Mariotti J, et al. Cytokine release syndrome after haploidentical hematopoietic cell transplantation: an international multicenter analysis. Bone Marrow Transplant 2021;56(11):2763–70.

26. Modi D, Albanyan O, Kim S, et al. Grade 3-4 cytokine release syndrome is associated with poor survival in haploidentical peripheral blood stem cell transplantation. Leuk Lymphoma 2021;62(8):1982–9.

27. Otoukesh S, Elmariah H, Yang D, et al. Cytokine Release Syndrome Following Peripheral Blood Stem Cell Haploidentical Hematopoietic Cell Transplantation with Post-Transplantation Cyclophosphamide. Transplant Cell Ther 2022;28(2): 111.e1-8.

28. Imus PH, Blackford AL, Bettinotti M, et al. Severe Cytokine Release Syndrome after Haploidentical Peripheral Blood Stem Cell Transplantation. Biol Blood Marrow Transplant 2019;25(12):2431–7.

29. Farias MG, de Mello Vicente B, Habigzang M, et al. High plasma IL-6 levels following haploidentical allogeneic hematopoietic stem cell transplantation post-transplant cyclophosphamide as predictor of early death and worse outcome. Transpl Immunol 2022;71:101543.

30. Nishimoto M, Hirose A, Koh H, et al. Clinical Impacts of Using Serum IL-6 Level as an Indicator of Cytokine Release Syndrome after HLA-Haploidentical Transplantation with Post-Transplantation Cyclophosphamide. Biol Blood Marrow Transplant 2019;25(10):2061–9.

31. Abboud R, Keller J, Slade M, et al. Severe Cytokine-Release Syndrome after T Cell-Replete Peripheral Blood Haploidentical Donor Transplantation Is Associated with Poor Survival and Anti-IL-6 Therapy Is Safe and Well Tolerated. Biol Blood Marrow Transplant 2016;22(10):1851–60.

32. Fornwalt RA, Brigham EP, Scott Stephens R. Critical Care of Hematopoietic Stem Cell Transplant Patients. Crit Care Clin 2021;37(1):29–46.

33. Holland EM, Gonzalez C, Levy E, et al. Case Report: Fatal Complications of BK Virus-Hemorrhagic Cystitis and Severe Cytokine Release Syndrome Following BK Virus-Specific T-Cells. Front Immunol 2021;12:801281.

34. Tzannou I, Papadopoulou A, Naik S, et al. Off-the-Shelf Virus-Specific T Cells to Treat BK Virus, Human Herpesvirus 6, Cytomegalovirus, Epstein-Barr Virus, and Adenovirus Infections After Allogeneic Hematopoietic Stem-Cell Transplantation. J Clin Oncol 2017;35(31):3547–57.

35. Sutrave G, Blyth E, Gottlieb DJ. Cellular therapy for multiple pathogen infections after hematopoietic stem cell transplant. Cytotherapy 2017;19(11):1284–301.

36. Papadopoulou A, Gerdemann U, Katari UL, et al. Activity of broad-spectrum T cells as treatment for AdV, EBV, CMV, BKV, and HHV6 infections after HSCT. Sci Transl Med 2014;6(242):242ra283.

37. Koehne G, Hasan A, Doubrovina E, et al. Immunotherapy with Donor T Cells Sensitized with Overlapping Pentadecapeptides for Treatment of Persistent Cytomegalovirus Infection or Viremia. Biol Blood Marrow Transplant 2015;21(9): 1663–78.

38. Keller MD, Bollard CM. Virus-specific T-cell therapies for patients with primary immune deficiency. Blood 2020;135(9):620–8.

39. George MR. Hemophagocytic lymphohistiocytosis: review of etiologies and management. J Blood Med 2014;5:69–86.

40. Henter JI, Horne A, Aricó M, et al. HLH-2004: Diagnostic and therapeutic guidelines for hemophagocytic lymphohistiocytosis. Pediatr Blood Cancer 2007;48(2): 124–31.
41. Crayne CB, Albeituni S, Nichols KE, et al. The Immunology of Macrophage Activation Syndrome. Front Immunol 2019;10:119.
42. Merrill SA, Naik R, Streiff MB, et al. A prospective quality improvement initiative in adult hemophagocytic lymphohistiocytosis to improve testing and a framework to facilitate trigger identification and mitigate hemorrhage from retrospective analysis. Medicine (Baltimore) 2018;97(31):e11579.
43. Lachmann G, Knaak C, Vorderwülbecke G, et al. Hyperferritinemia in Critically Ill Patients. Crit Care Med 2020;48(4):459–65.
44. Neelapu SS, Tummala S, Kebriaei P, et al. Chimeric antigen receptor T-cell therapy - assessment and management of toxicities. Nat Rev Clin Oncol 2018;15(1): 47–62.
45. Martin-Blondel G, Mars LT, Liblau RS. Pathogenesis of the immune reconstitution inflammatory syndrome in HIV-infected patients. Curr Opin Infect Dis 2012;25(3): 312–20.
46. Yarchoan R, Uldrick TS. HIV-Associated Cancers and Related Diseases. N Engl J Med 2018;378(11):1029–41.
47. Ramaswami R, Lurain K, Polizzotto MN, et al. Characteristics and outcomes of KSHV-associated multicentric Castleman disease with or without other KSHV diseases. Blood Adv 2021;5(6):1660–70.
48. Barlingay G, Findakly D, Hartmann C, et al. The Potential Clinical Benefit of Tocilizumab Therapy for Patients with HHV-8-infected AIDS-related Multicentric Castleman Disease: A Case Report and Literature Review. Cureus 2020;12(4):e7589.
49. Ramaswami R, Lurain K, Peer CJ, et al. Tocilizumab in patients with symptomatic Kaposi sarcoma herpesvirus-associated multicentric Castleman disease. Blood 2020;135(25):2316–9.
50. Siddall E, Khatri M, Radhakrishnan J. Capillary leak syndrome: etiologies, pathophysiology, and management. Kidney Int 2017;92(1):37–46.
51. Gutierrez C, McEvoy C, Munshi L, et al. Critical Care Management of Toxicities Associated With Targeted Agents and Immunotherapies for Cancer. Crit Care Med 2020;48(1):10–21.
52. Shimabukuro-Vornhagen A, Gödel P, Subklewe M, et al. Cytokine release syndrome. J Immunother Cancer 2018;6(1):56.
53. Kroschinsky F, Stölzel F, von Bonin S, et al. New drugs, new toxicities: severe side effects of modern targeted and immunotherapy of cancer and their management. Crit Care 2017;21(1):89.
54. Santomasso B, Bachier C, Westin J, et al. The Other Side of CAR T-Cell Therapy: Cytokine Release Syndrome, Neurologic Toxicity, and Financial Burden. Am Soc Clin Oncol Educ Book 2019;39:433–44.
55. Cordeiro A, Bezerra ED, Hirayama AV, et al. Late Events after Treatment with CD19-Targeted Chimeric Antigen Receptor Modified T Cells. Biol Blood Marrow Transplant 2020;26(1):26–33.
56. Le RQ, Li L, Yuan W, et al. FDA Approval Summary: Tocilizumab for Treatment of Chimeric Antigen Receptor T Cell-Induced Severe or Life-Threatening Cytokine Release Syndrome. Oncologist 2018;23(8):943–7.
57. Gutierrez C, Brown ART, May HP, et al. Critically Ill Patients Treated for Chimeric Antigen Receptor-Related Toxicity: A Multicenter Study. Crit Care Med 2022; 50(1):81–92.

58. Brudno JN, Kochenderfer JN. Recent advances in CAR T-cell toxicity: Mechanisms, manifestations and management. Blood Rev 2019;34:45–55.

59. Rizvi MS, Gallo De Moraes A. New Decade, Old Debate: Blocking the Cytokine Pathways in Infection-Induced Cytokine Cascade. Crit Care Explor 2021;3(3): e0364.

60. Gutierrez C, McEvoy C, Mead E, et al. Management of the Critically Ill Adult Chimeric Antigen Receptor-T Cell Therapy Patient: A Critical Care Perspective. Crit Care Med 2018;46(9):1402–10.

61. Strati P, Ahmed S, Furqan F, et al. Prognostic impact of corticosteroids on efficacy of chimeric antigen receptor T-cell therapy in large B-cell lymphoma. Blood 2021; 137(23):3272–6.

62. Annane D, Renault A, Brun-Buisson C, et al. Hydrocortisone plus Fludrocortisone for Adults with Septic Shock. N Engl J Med 2018;378(9):809–18.

63. Venkatesh B, Finfer S, Cohen J, et al. Adjunctive Glucocorticoid Therapy in Patients with Septic Shock. N Engl J Med 2018;378(9):797–808.

64. Dugar S, Choudhary C, Duggal A. Sepsis and septic shock: Guideline-based management. Cleve Clin J Med 2020;87(1):53–64.

65. Lat I, Coopersmith CM, De Backer D. The Surviving Sepsis Campaign: Fluid Resuscitation and Vasopressor Therapy Research Priorities in Adult Patients. Crit Care Med 2021;49(4):623–35.

66. Gutierrez C, Brown ART, Herr MM, et al. The chimeric antigen receptor-intensive care unit (CAR-ICU) initiative: Surveying intensive care unit practices in the management of CAR T-cell associated toxicities. J Crit Care 2020;58:58–64.

67. Seymour CW, Gesten F, Prescott HC, et al. Time to Treatment and Mortality during Mandated Emergency Care for Sepsis. N Engl J Med 2017;376(23):2235–44.

68. Hill JA, Li D, Hay KA, et al. Infectious complications of CD19-targeted chimeric antigen receptor-modified T-cell immunotherapy. Blood 2018;131(1):121–30.

69. Yakoub-Agha I, Chabannon C, Bader P, et al. Management of adults and children undergoing chimeric antigen receptor T-cell therapy: best practice recommendations of the European Society for Blood and Marrow Transplantation (EBMT) and the Joint Accreditation Committee of ISCT and EBMT (JACIE). Haematologica 2020;105(2):297–316.

70. Haidar G, Garner W, Hill JA. Infections after anti-CD19 chimeric antigen receptor T-cell therapy for hematologic malignancies: timeline, prevention, and uncertainties. Curr Opin Infect Dis 2020;33(6):449–57.

71. Hill JA, Seo SK. How I prevent infections in patients receiving CD19-targeted chimeric antigen receptor T cells for B-cell malignancies. Blood 2020;136(8): 925–35.

72. Mehta P, McAuley DF, Brown M, et al. COVID-19: consider cytokine storm syndromes and immunosuppression. Lancet 2020;395(10229):1033–4.

73. Horby P, Lim WS, Emberson JR, et al. Dexamethasone in Hospitalized Patients with Covid-19. N Engl J Med 2021;384(8):693–704.

74. Hermine O, Mariette X, Tharaux PL, et al. Effect of Tocilizumab vs Usual Care in Adults Hospitalized With COVID-19 and Moderate or Severe Pneumonia: A Randomized Clinical Trial. JAMA Intern Med 2021;181(1):32–40.

75. Salama C, Han J, Yau L, et al. Tocilizumab in Patients Hospitalized with Covid-19 Pneumonia. N Engl J Med 2021;384(1):20–30.

76. Gordon AC, Mouncey PR, Al-Beidh F, et al. Interleukin-6 Receptor Antagonists in Critically Ill Patients with Covid-19. N Engl J Med 2021;384(16):1491–502.

77. Kalil AC, Patterson TF, Mehta AK, et al. Baricitinib plus Remdesivir for Hospitalized Adults with Covid-19. N Engl J Med 2021;384(9):795–807.

78. Marconi VC, Ramanan AV, de Bono S, et al. Efficacy and safety of baricitinib for the treatment of hospitalised adults with COVID-19 (COV-BARRIER): a randomised, double-blind, parallel-group, placebo-controlled phase 3 trial. Lancet Respir Med 2021;9(12):1407–18.

79. Setiadi A, Zoref-Lorenz A, Lee CY, et al. Malignancy-associated haemophagocytic lymphohistiocytosis. Lancet Haematol 2022;9(3):e217–27.

80. Vogel TP, Top KA, Karatzios C, et al. Multisystem inflammatory syndrome in children and adults (MIS-C/A): Case definition & guidelines for data collection, analysis, and presentation of immunization safety data. Vaccine 2021;39(22): 3037–49.

81. Feldstein LR, Rose EB, Horwitz SM, et al. Multisystem Inflammatory Syndrome in U.S. Children and Adolescents. N Engl J Med 2020;383(4):334–46.

82. Ripa M, Galli L, Poli A, et al. Secondary infections in patients hospitalized with COVID-19: incidence and predictive factors. Clin Microbiol Infect 2021;27(3): 451–7.

83. Rawson TM, Moore LSP, Zhu N, et al. Bacterial and Fungal Coinfection in Individuals With Coronavirus: A Rapid Review To Support COVID-19 Antimicrobial Prescribing. Clin Infect Dis 2020;71(9):2459–68.

84. Pink I, Raupach D, Fuge J, et al. C-reactive protein and procalcitonin for antimicrobial stewardship in COVID-19. Infection 2021;49(5):935–43.

Preparing the Intensive Care Unit for a Lethal Viral Respiratory Pandemic

Kelly Cawcutt, MD, MS*, Andre C. Kalil, MD, MPH,
Angela Hewlett, MD, MS

KEYWORDS

• Pandemic • Preparedness • Critical care • Virus

KEY POINTS

- Prior pandemics have provided key lessons to aid in the development and execution of preparedness plans.
- COVID-19 highlighted many gaps in preparedness plans, including supply chain, surge capacity, risks within the health care workforce, and the impact of misinformation in the media.
- Robust preparedness plans should include the assessment and integration of the four S's, the phases of incident management, the hierarchy of controls, with added aspects of implementation of medical research, identifying and decreasing health care disparities, and ensuring the wellness of the health care, and ICU, workforce.

Those who fail to learn from history are doomed to repeat it.
— *Winston Churchill*

INTRODUCTION

Recent years have demonstrated the impact epidemics and pandemics can have on health care systems, from SARS to H1N1 to Ebola, and now, the unprecedented and devastating impact of the COVID-19 pandemic in health care systems around the world. Historically, many organizations had previously developed pandemic preparedness plans, with a focus on contagious respiratory infections, such as influenza. Many of these plans were implemented and practiced in 2009 during the H1N1 influenza pandemic, a pandemic that heavily impacted intensive care units (ICUs). Hospital preparedness plans were then revised during the Ebola outbreak in 2014 to 2016, which primarily occurred in West Africa but resulted in a small number of patients being

Division of Infectious Diseases, Department of Internal Medicine, University of Nebraska Medical Center, Omaha, NE, USA
* Corresponding author. 985400 Nebraska Medical Center, Omaha, NE 68198.
E-mail address: Kelly.cawcutt@unmc.edu
Twitter: @KellyCawcuttMD (K.C.)

Infect Dis Clin N Am 36 (2022) 749–759
https://doi.org/10.1016/j.idc.2022.08.002
0891-5520/22/© 2022 Elsevier Inc. All rights reserved.

id.theclinics.com

medically evacuated for care at specialized biocontainment centers in the United States and Europe, and several patients who developed symptoms following travel from West Africa and presented to health care facilities.[1] The Ebola outbreak, the ongoing outbreak of Middle East respiratory syndrome (MERS-CoV) in the Arabian Peninsula, and subsequent imported cases to other parts of the world also stimulated preparedness efforts and the development of screening protocols for returning travelers.[2] However, these best laid plans were not sufficient to deter the rapid rise of the COVID-19 pandemic, highlighting the need for improved preparedness for future waves of COVID-19, but also for the likelihood of future pandemics from highly contagious, and lethal, respiratory viral infections.

Prior viral pandemics have been drivers of improved medical care, particularly in the realm of critical illness and the evolution of critical care medicine as a specialty.[3] The advent of artificial ventilation during the polio epidemic in the 1950s was touted to be the "treatment of choice" by Bjorn Ibsen, and from within the devastation of polio, the concept of critical care medicine and the first ICUs arose.[3] Since that time, critical care medicine and ICUs have evolved to robust, multidisciplinary teams with increasingly complex interventions to preserve life, although access to this level of care because of ICU bed capacity was a well-known limitation before the COVID-19 pandemic.[3] Additional epidemics and pandemics have continued to test health care systems, medical capacity, and resources for maintaining care, including experiences with H1N1 and Ebola. H1N1 brought an era of limited resources, such as the use of extracorporeal membrane oxygenation. The Ebola outbreak resulted in the need for development of capacity and capability to care for patients with highly hazardous communicable diseases, including the need for dedicated hospital space, well-practiced infection prevention procedures and protocols, and specialized multidisciplinary care teams with the ability to provide intensive care to patients in the biocontainment environment.

Following the Ebola outbreak in 2014 to 2016, the Centers for Disease Control and Prevention and Department of Health and Human Services (DHHS) developed a tiered system for the triage and clinical management of patients suspected or confirmed to have a highly hazardous communicable disease.[4,5] This system includes 10 designated Regional Ebola and Other Special Pathogen Treatment Centers (RESPTCs) in the United States (in each of the 10 DHHS regions).[6] The RESPTCs possess enhanced infection control, high-level isolation patient care capabilities, and highly trained teams, and these centers serve as leaders for other facilities within their DHHS region. Other health care facilities were designated as Ebola Treatment Centers, Ebola Assessment Hospitals, or Frontline facilities depending on their capabilities. Although these designations were initially made in response to Ebola, the intent was to elevate hospital preparedness, and efforts have been made to transition to general preparedness for highly hazardous communicable diseases, including viral respiratory infections.

Despite these experiences and improvements in preparedness, the COVID-19 pandemic demonstrated the gaps in knowledge, stockpiles, surge capacity, mitigation strategies, and the fragility of the health care workforce.

COVID-19 PANDEMIC: LESSONS LEARNED

The COVID-19 pandemic has provided enumerable lessons regarding gaps, failures, and risks in health care overall, and in the setting of a pandemic. Among early lessons learned were the lack of adequate supplies and established supply chains for multitudes of care items from masks to tests to hand sanitizer to gloves and gowns to durable medical equipment, such as ventilators. In addition, the supply of human resources was found to be finite, given attrition from the stress of working in an under-resourced setting, lack of adequate numbers of staff, absenteeism because of personal or family illness, and an inability to train medical personnel fast enough to replace staff. In fact, in early 2020, a survey of critical care health care workers noted widespread concern for inadequate preparedness within organization pandemic plans.[7]

In many areas, a diversion of resources was required, with some diversions being costly to the overall health care system. The diversion of infection control and antibiotic stewardship staff is one area in which these small pools of staff with this expertise, who also often overlap, were diverted to COVID-19-related efforts, at the costs of the inability to remain as focused on prevention and maintenance of health care–associated infections and horizontal measures, respectively.[8] This resulted in increased health care–associated infections in many areas, and the repercussions and long-term impact are still not fully understood.[9]

Additional lessons surrounded the impact of ethics as it pertains to treatments for COVID-19, vaccination, mask use, and in the most severe case, discussion of crisis standards of care. Many ethical questions surrounded the provision of care to those who declined vaccination and who declined evidence-based therapies, with many discussions regarding which patients would have access to the limited ICU level care, given the beds high occupancy, low availability of ventilators, and staffing shortage, especially during the highest surges. These scenarios highlighted the need for robust ethical plans to manage care in a pandemic; provide quality care to the highest number of patients possible; and the need for well-established crisis standards of care plans to rely on, and refine as needed. Ethical controversy clearly extended into the health care workforce also, particularly regarding mandatory vaccination to maintain employment.

Media has played a pivotal role in pandemics, in the past and now, particularly given the rapid sharing of digital information via social media. Accurate information on social media provides key opportunities to decrease fear, stress, and uncertainty.[10] However, not all information is accurate, and this was a major lesson learned during the COVID-19 pandemic. Misinformation, the sharing of inaccurate information without intent to cause harm, and disinformation, the sharing of inaccurate information with the intent to cause harm, have been well demonstrated. Prior studies have reported large variation in misinformation on social media, with 4.5% on Twitter related to H1N1 influenza, 23.8% on YouTube pertaining to Zika virus, and 55.5% on Twitter related to Ebola.[11] Early in the COVID-19 pandemic, research demonstrated up to nearly 30% of social media posts related to COVID-19 contained misinformation or disinformation.[11] Additionally, some studies indicated that such misinformation resulted in fear and panic.[11] Several strategies have been recommended to address misinformation and disinformation, and can include ensuring dissemination of trustworthy information, debunking of misinformation and disinformation, increasing the health literacy and training of social media users, increasing research, and considering more aggressive monitoring of social media, with implementation of additional regulations and policies to reduce misinformation and disinformation.[11,12] Given the prevalence of misinformation and disinformation, the importance of supporting the expertise of local, state, and national public health authorities in a pandemic cannot be overstated, and should be a tenet of preparedness for the next pandemic.

Not all of the lessons learned as a result of the COVID-19 pandemic were negative, because there is also an abundance of innovation and creative solutions that evolved during the pandemic. First, the rapid development of therapeutics and vaccines, and high-quality randomized double-blind controlled trials to assess these cannot be underscored. Medical research may never have moved as quickly and efficiently. Some potential innovations included the use of ultraviolet germicidal decontamination of N95s to extend use[13]; "intubation boxes"[14] to decrease risk for aerosolization, particularly with personal protective equipment (PPE) shortages; and creative use of existing supplies, such as transesophageal echocardiography probe covers[15] and the transition of intravenous pumps[16] to hallways.

THE FOUR S'S OF SURGE CAPACITY, AS PERTAINING TO THE INTENSIVE CARE UNIT

Surge capacity is perhaps the most critical aspect of preparedness that must be addressed in detail and encapsulates many of the lessons learned from the COVID-19 pandemic that can aid in preparing for future events. Surge capacity is the ability to provide medical care to a significantly higher number of patients that challenges, and frequently surpasses, standard operating capacity.[17] One suggested target is to be able to quickly expand baseline capacity in the ICU by at least 20%.[7,18] Key aspects of how to address this are noted in the "four S's of surge capacity": staffing, space, supplies, and systems (**Fig. 1**).[7] Each of these is particularly relevant to the ICU environment given the need to provide and maintain the ability of critical care services in a surge scenario.

Staffing

The importance of staffing within the health care system is a lesson learned as a result of the COVID-19 pandemic. The availability of physical space to care for patients with a highly transmissible respiratory disease is a small part of the patient care equation, because available space is useless without adequate staffing. This is especially important in the ICU environment, where critical care is provided to the sickest patients in a multidisciplinary manner. Unit leaders should be established, and leaders should actively participate in all aspects of planning and protocol development and being present in the unit frequently to support staff and assess the need for modifications or enhancements in protocols. Multidisciplinary care teams should participate and demonstrate competency in infection control practices, and it is of utmost importance to consider staff safety and patient safety when creating staffing models. The ICU staffing model should also take into account the time required for the donning and doffing of PPE and the time while in PPE, so shift times and staffing ratios may differ from those used for routine ICU care. Infection control personnel or others with specific training in PPE donning and doffing protocols can be deployed to the ICU to assist

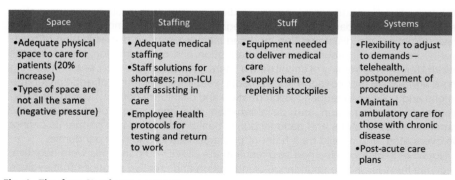

Space	Staffing	Stuff	Systems
•Adequate physical space to care for patients (20% increase) •Types of space are not all the same (negative pressure)	• Adequate medical staffing •Staff solutions for shortages; non-ICU staff assisting in care •Employee Health protocols for testing and return to work	•Equipment needed to deliver medical care •Supply chain to replenish stockpiles	•Flexibility to adjust to demands – telehealth, postponement of procedures •Maintain ambulatory care for those with chronic disease •Post-acute care plans

Fig. 1. The four S's of surge capacity.

and provide support to the care teams with these processes. Staff can also be cross-trained to perform appropriate tasks, even if it is outside of their usual job description, to aid in preserving staff as a resource. Cross-trained staff, including physicians and other health care workers, may be used in a tiered staffing model under an intensivist to further extend the patient care capacity within the ICU depending on capacity, and whether or not the organization is functioning within contingency or crisis models.[7,18] Certain tasks can also be delegated to special care teams to alleviate pressure on the nursing staff, such as the proning teams used at some centers during the COVID-19 pandemic, who were responsible for placing patients in the prone position to improve oxygenation.[19] The nursing staffing model must also take into account the need and availability of specialized services, such as extracorporeal membrane oxygenation, which requires well-trained nursing staff who are familiar with the process. Facilities should choose and maintain an effective physician team based on the potential needs of the patients. Critical care physicians typically serve as the primary physician team in most care models, but it is important to assess the need for procedures, consultants, and other specialized services and ensure the availability of appropriate physicians to perform these services. Determinations should be made regarding the involvement of all levels of trainees and students in direct patient care after a risk versus benefit assessment. The COVID-19 pandemic illustrated the need to ensure that ample back-up staffing plans are in place, because front-line health care workers may become ill and not be able to report to work. These may include redeploying health care workers with previous critical care expertise who are working in other areas, expediting the credentialing process for new staff, providing ample and ongoing training opportunities and just-in-time training, and restructuring ICU teams to use a tiered staffing model to allow experienced critical care staff to care for as many patients as possible.[20] Maintenance of preparedness activities should be ongoing, and can include continuous protocol revisions and updates as new data emerge, participation in multidisciplinary drills and exercises, and team engagement via teambuilding events. Given the psychological and emotional toll of caring for patients in a pandemic, facilities should maintain robust on-site or telemedicine behavioral health support for unit staff, and seeking support should be encouraged by unit leadership.

Space

The appropriate use of clinical care space should be determined based on multiple factors, including the availability and use of preexisting space, along with the potential use of alternate surge spaces if capacity exceeds routine space availability. In the case of a respiratory pathogen, the number and availability of current airborne infection isolation rooms and the potential for facility modifications to create temporary negative pressure isolation should be evaluated, and the facilities manager should be consulted to provide input.[21] The designation of an entire unit or units within the facility to provide ICU-level care to patients with a suspected or confirmed highly hazardous respiratory disease may be necessary depending on the case burden, but when this is not possible or case numbers are low, cohorting is considered. The use of shared spaces and multipatient rooms is not ideal, but may be necessary when surge capacity is overwhelming. Areas for donning/doffing PPE, as close to the patient care room as possible, should be predetermined and practiced.

Supplies

Assessment of the availability of necessary patient care equipment should occur before receiving patients, and inventory evaluation should be part of ongoing preparedness efforts. This includes everything from testing supplies to critical patient care equipment, such as ventilators, dialysis machines, and ultrasounds. Some of this equipment is prepositioned and stocked, whereas other equipment is brought to the unit in a just-in-time fashion. Equipment should be dedicated to the patient care unit if possible, to ensure availability and access. The availability of PPE has been a hallmark of the COVID-19 pandemic and is constantly in flux. Attention should be paid to the evaluation of the supply chain and available stockpile of PPE within and outside of health care facilities. Expert guidance on recommended PPE should be followed based on the specific pathogen. When PPE shortages occur, extended use and decontamination strategies are considered, and these processes were used for N95 respirators at some centers during the COVID-19 pandemic.[13,22,23] Appropriate personnel should monitor for equipment shortages and potential signals of disruptions in the supply chain, paying special attention to vulnerabilities. Notifications should occur immediately when a potential shortage is expected to allow time for the creation of alternative plans and protocols. Consideration should also be given to the designation of back-up vendors because supplies from a primary vendor may not be available. It may be appropriate to request supplies from the Strategic National Stockpile in certain scenarios.[24]

Systems

Systematic approaches to hospital and ICU preparedness help prevent gaps and should be used. There are several key aspects of such planning, starting with phases of incident management, for broad assessment of preparedness plans, how to execute plans, and including the key component of review and revising plans. Pandemic planning will continue to require frequent assessment and revision, through the continued phases of the COVID-19 pandemic, but also in preparing for future pandemics.

Phases of incident management include aspects of preparedness, mitigation, response, and recovery (**Fig. 2**).[17,25] In essence, preparedness is heavily focused on planning and training to be prepared for future events. Mitigation requires concentration on how to identify and reduce risks within an incident, including plans to ensure adequate supplies and resources are present, and to provide communication regarding the situation. Of note, the important of communication must not be underestimated. Pandemic communications that are internal and external facing is critical and must start early, be easily accessible, and occur frequently via various delivery methods.[17] Response relates to the actual execution of the plans and procedures in a real-life situation, and requires an after-action assessment for where improvements

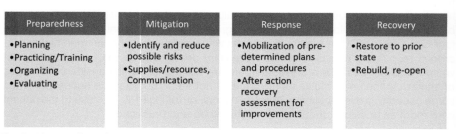

Preparedness	Mitigation	Response	Recovery
•Planning •Practicing/Training •Organizing •Evaluating	•Identify and reduce possible risks •Supplies/resources, Communication	•Mobilization of pre-determined plans and procedures •After action recovery assessment for improvements	•Restore to prior state •Rebuild, re-open

Fig. 2. Phases of incident management.

could be made based on lessons learned during the response. Finally, recovery focuses on restoring systems to prior states and reopening at preincident levels. It should be noted that innovation and quality of care concerns identified within the response component should be carried forward, not blindly reestablishing the prior state if there are valuable changes that should be maintained.

Policies and procedures regarding the ability to provide and maintain safe and effective ICU care during a pandemic should be created before the event and modified, as necessary. The COVID-19 pandemic highlighted the importance of providing telemedicine services for expert consultation, particularly in hospitals with limited ICU resources. Prevention of transmission of viruses through infection control measures, including considerations within the hierarchy of controls (**Fig. 3**) to protect patients and health care workers, must also be combined with provisions for readily available, quick, and efficient testing of symptomatic staff through employee health and clear return-to-work protocols for ill employees should be established to preserve the critical ICU workforce.[17] In prior outbreaks, health care workers have had higher rates of infection often caused by gaps within infection control practices and caring for patients not known to have an active infection.[17] An appropriate ICU visitor policy should be established in coordination with hospital leadership, ICU leadership, and with infection control, and methods of support for patient families, such as facilitation of communication through telephone calls and teleconferencing, should be readily available.

Routine systems and practices may need to be modified during a patient surge. Some examples of this that occurred at some health care facilities during the COVID-19 pandemic are the cancellation of elective procedures[7] and reevaluation of where patient care equipment is placed to facilitate clinical care while minimizing exposure risk. Facilities placed medication pumps outside of the immediate patient care room, so medications could be adjusted quickly and without entering the room to decrease the potential for health care worker exposure and preserve PPE.[16] Special attention should be given to protocols for respiratory specimen collection, specimen transport, and processing, and this may differ depending on the specific pathogen.[16] Some pathogens also require confirmatory testing in specialized laboratories, so hospital systems should ensure availability and access to these resources.

Systems-based infection control practices should be established and modified if necessary to fit special scenarios in the ICU setting. It is of utmost importance to

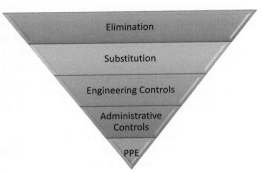

Fig. 3. Hierarchy of infection controls and components. (*Adapted from* Hierarchy of controls. Centers for Disease Control and Prevention. Available at https://www.cdc.gov/niosh/topics/hierarchy/default.html. Published January 13, 2015.)

provide 24/7 support from infection control, and that an infection preventionist with expertise in the ICU sets rounds in the units frequently, discusses process improvements with leadership and staff, and is available for questions. Processes for transporting patients to alternate locations, such as radiology, cardiac catheterization laboratory, operating room, and through all areas of the hospital, should be assessed and modified to ensure that safe and efficient transport of patients can occur. Interhospital transfers also need to be assessed regarding whether surge capacity allows acceptance of patients from other organizations,[7] and additionally, strategies for safe transfers must be developed. Waste management protocols should be discussed because some pathogens may require specific processes for the safe handling and disposal of medical waste. Expert consultation on clinical management, including testing, the provision of therapeutics, and discontinuation of isolation, can also be provided by infectious diseases specialists to support the primary ICU teams, and this was done in many centers during the COVID-19 pandemic. Systems also must consider post-ICU and acute care needs for patients in a pandemic, because many patients from the ICU have prolonged recoveries and require additional medical resources, along with possible placement at skilled nursing facilities.[7] If there are a paucity of beds, or staffing, available in postacute care, discharges may be delayed, further compounding the surge capacity limitations.

On a national scale, the Assistant Secretary for Preparedness and Response and the National Emerging Special Pathogens Training and Education Center, in cooperation with other agencies, developed the concept of the National Special Pathogen System of Care to further address preparedness gaps in the United States. The National Special Pathogen System of Care further defines and delineates a tiered network of health care facilities based on capacity and capability.[26] Health care facilities should fully use these resources to seek expert advice and consultation, including identifying the appropriate Regional Emerging Special Pathogens Treatment Center (NETEC.org) in their DHHS region.[6] Facilities should also maintain relationships with city, county, state, and regional partners, including health departments, emergency medical services, and the state public health laboratory.

ADDITIONAL CONSIDERATIONS

Media engagement and participation to fight misinformation and disinformation will remain crucial in future pandemics. Understanding organizational media policies before engaging should be pursued, with additional development of organizational media liaisons and public relations contacts to ensure accurate information is shared on various platforms to increase audience reach. Ensuring a diverse presence of health care expertise in media is also critical. This should include diversity of profession, but also diversity in age, gender identity, race/ethnic identity, and geographic and socioeconomic status. Principles from the Centers for Disease Control and Prevention within their Crisis and Emergency Risk Communication tool, include the need to "be first, be right, express empathy, promote action, and show respect."[17] These principles need to be used consistently in the breadth of different communication tools used.

The need for pandemic preparedness based on the four S's, the hierarchy of controls, and phases of incident management provide a broad framework to assess plans and consider revisions. In specific concern for staffing, future efforts toward ensuring an adequate health care workforce will require additional efforts surrounding ensuring health care workforce wellness including addressing burnout, moral injury, psychological safety, and management of acute stress.[17]

Rigorous research is essential to improve the preparedness for future viral pandemics. Pathways for rapid response institution review board assessments and approvals because of critical needs are required. Optimal methods for recruitment and enrollment of patients into clinical studies require greater understanding. These pieces are critical to support the necessity of investigational therapeutics, vaccines, determination of optimal supportive cares and mitigation measures, and communication strategies targeted at internal and external audiences. Engagement of broader, multidisciplinary teams for research, with experience to deploy such teams on short notice, for additional research that is qualitative and quantitative would further increase the speed to greater understanding, knowledge, and optimal outcomes in future pandemics.

Finally, inequities within health care have been increasingly recognized during this pandemic. This includes disproportionate rates of infection, hospitalization (including ICU stays), and death among multiple minority groups as defined by race.[27] These inequities are not the same among all groups, with recent data demonstrating increased in-hospital mortality among American Indian and Alaska Native populations, despite these two groups having lower comorbidity scores.[28] Disparities and inequities that exist in communities extend into hospitals and ICUs. Continued research and efforts to decrease these are critical to current health, but rapid research, assessment of, and action toward any disparities in future pandemics is of paramount importance.

SUMMARY

With understanding the preparedness that evolved from prior pandemics, and the lessons learned from the COVID-19 pandemic, it is prudent to consider how to address preparedness in health systems overall, but also with particular concern for ICU-level preparedness. With respiratory transmission being a common route of transmission in pandemics, being prepared for surges of future lethal respiratory viruses, or other pathogens, is critically necessary.

If history has taught us anything, it is that future pandemics are inevitable. COVID-19 highlighted the critical infrastructure failures in preparedness for a large-scale lethal respiratory viral pandemic and those failures must be the lessons on which future pandemic preparedness strategies are built. This must be a multidisciplinary, broad reaching strategy, and perhaps there are no areas more critical to ensure preparedness than within ICUs.

DISCLOSURE

K. Cawcutt has no disclosures relevant to this article. A. Hewlett has no disclosures relevant to this article. A.C. Kalil has no disclosures relevant to this article.

REFERENCES

1. Uyeki TM, Mehta AK, Davey RT Jr, et al. Clinical management of Ebola virus disease in the United States and Europe. N Engl J Med 2016;374(7):636–46.
2. Schwedhelm MM, Herstein JJ, Watson SM, et al. Can you catch it? Lessons learned and modification of ED triage symptom-and travel-screening strategy. J Emerg Nurs 2020;46(6):932–40.
3. Kelly FE, Fong K, Hirsch N, et al. Intensive care medicine is 60 years old: the history and future of the intensive care unit. Clin Med 2014;14(4):376.
4. Centers for Disease Control and Prevention. Preparing U.S. Hospitals for Ebola. Available at: https://www.cdc.gov/vhf/ebola/pdf/preparing-hospitals-ebola-P.pdf. Accessed March 25, 2022.

5. Centers for Disease Control and Prevention. Interim Guidance for U.S. Hospital Preparedness for Patients Under Investigation (PUIs) or with Confirmed Ebola Virus Disease (EVD): A Framework for a Tiered Approach. Available at: https://www.cdc.gov/vhf/ebola/healthcare-us/preparing/hospitals.html. Accessed March 25, 2022.

6. Available at: https://netec.org/about-netec/partners-regional-contacts/. Accessed March 25, 2022.

7. Harris G, Adalja A. ICU preparedness in pandemics: lessons learned from the coronavirus disease-2019 outbreak. Curr Opin Pulm Med 2021;27(2):73.

8. Stevens MP, Doll M, Pryor R, et al. Impact of COVID-19 on traditional healthcare-associated infection prevention efforts. Infect Control Hosp Epidemiol 2020;41(8):946–7.

9. Weiner-Lastinger LM, Pattabiraman V, Konnor RY, et al. The impact of coronavirus disease 2019 (COVID-19) on healthcare-associated infections in 2020: a summary of data reported to the National Healthcare Safety Network. Infect Control Hosp Epidemiol 2022;43(1):12–25.

10. Abbas J, Wang D, Su Z, et al. The role of social media in the advent of COVID-19 pandemic: crisis management, mental health challenges and implications. Risk Manag Healthc Pol 2021;14:1917.

11. Gabarron E, Oyeyemi SO, Wynn R. COVID-19-related misinformation on social media: a systematic review. Bull World Health Organ 2021;99(6):455.

12. Arora VM, Bloomgarden E, Jain S. Supporting health care workers to address misinformation on social media. N Engl J Med 2022. https://doi.org/10.1056/NEJMp2117180.

13. Lowe J, Paladino K, Farke J, et al. N95 filtering facepiece respirator ultraviolet germicidal irradiation (UVGI) process for decontamination and reuse. Nebraska Medicine; 2020.

14. Canelli R, Connor CW, Gonzalez M, et al. Barrier enclosure during endotracheal intubation. N Engl J Med 2020;382(20):1957–8.

15. Markin NW, Cawcutt KA, Sayyed SH, et al. Transesophageal echocardiography probe sheath to decrease provider and environment contamination. Anesthesiology 2020;133(2):475–7.

16. Blake JW, Giuliano KK, Butterfield RD, et al. Extending tubing to place intravenous smart pumps outside of patient rooms during COVID-19: an innovation that increases medication dead volume and risk to patients. BMJ Innov 2021;7(2).

17. Godshall CE, Banach DB. Pandemic preparedness. Infect Dis Clin 2021;35(4):1077–89.

18. Harris GH, Baldisseri MR, Reynolds BR, et al. Design for implementation of a system-level ICU pandemic surge staffing plan. Crit Care Explorations 2020;2(6).

19. Miguel K, Snydeman C, Capasso V, et al. Development of a prone team and exploration of staff perceptions during COVID-19. AACN Adv Crit Care 2021;32(2):159–68.

20. Aziz S, Arabi YM, Alhazzani W, et al. Managing ICU surge during the COVID-19 crisis: rapid guidelines. Intensive Care Med 2020;46(7):1303–25.

21. Jeanna Anderson AG, Streifel A. Airborne Infectious Disease Management Methods for Temporary Negative Pressure Isolation 2007. Available at: https://www.health.state.mn.us/communities/ep/surge/infectious/airbornenegative.pdf. Accessed March 25, 2022.

22. O'Hearn K, Gertsman S, Sampson M, et al. Decontaminating N95 and SN95 masks with ultraviolet germicidal irradiation does not impair mask efficacy and safety. J Hosp Infect 2020;106(1):163–75.

23. Ontiveros C, Sweeney CL, Smith C, et al. Assessing the impact of multiple ultra-violet disinfection cycles on N95 filtering facepiece respirator integrity. Scientific Rep 2021;11(1):1–9.
24. Available at: https://www.phe.gov/about/sns/Pages/about.aspx. Accessed March 25, 2022.
25. Lindsay BR. Federal Emergency Management: A Brief Introduction. Available at: https://training.fema.gov/hiedu/highref/federal%20em-a%20brief%20introduction-r42845%20-%20lindsay.pdf. Accessed March 25, 2022.
26. Committee NNSPSoCS. National Special Pathogen System of Care (NSPS) Strategy Summary. 2021. Available at: https://netec.org/wp-content/uploads/2021/12/NETEC_NSPS-Strategy-Summary-1.pdf. Accessed March 25, 2022.
27. Acosta AM, Garg S, Pham H, et al. Racial and ethnic disparities in rates of COVID-19–associated hospitalization, intensive care unit admission, and in-hospital death in the United States from March 2020 to February 2021. JAMA Netw Open 2021;4(10):e2130479.
28. Musshafen LA, El-Sadek L, Lirette ST, et al. In-hospital mortality disparities among American Indian and Alaska Native, Black, and White patients with COVID-19. JAMA Netw Open 2022;5(3):e224822.

Management of Severe and Critical COVID-19 Infection with Immunotherapies

Janhavi Athale, MD[a], Jolie Gallagher, PharmD, BCCCP[b],
Lindsay M. Busch, MD[c,d,*]

KEYWORDS

- Severe COVID-19 infection • Critical COVID-19 infection • Immunotherapy

KEY POINTS

- The only immunomodulators granted FDA Emergency Use Authorization for severe COVID-19 infection are tocilizumab and baricitinib, though their benefit in critical illness is less clear.
- Additional targets for immunomodulators under investigation for COVID-19 include, but are not limited to: IL-1, GM-CSF, Bruton's tyrosine kinase.
- Monoclonal antibody therapy is not recommended in severe or critical COVID-19 disease, though data are lacking regarding the potential for benefit in patients unable to mount an endogenous antibody response.
- Severe COVID-19 infection comprises a wide spectrum of disease, and clinicians should interpret new clinical trial data thoughtfully with particular attention to baseline characteristics of disease severity, blinding procedures, concurrent use of other immunomodulatory agents, and clinical endpoint selection.

INTRODUCTION

Early in the COVID-19 pandemic, clinicians and researchers sought to rapidly repurpose available candidate therapies for SARS-CoV-2 infection pending the development of directed antivirals and novel vaccines. Slowly, anecdotal case series and single-arm observational trials gave way to randomized control trials (RCTs) as the global research community mobilized to design, implement, and analyze studies in the midst of unprecedented pressure on health care systems. Despite the early

[a] Critical Care Medicine Department, Mayo Clinic, Phoenix, AZ, USA; [b] Department of Pharmacy, Emory University Hospital, Atlanta, GA, USA; [c] Division of Infectious Diseases, Emory University School of Medicine, 101 Woodruff Memorial Building, Suite 2101, Atlanta, GA 30322, USA; [d] Emory Critical Care Center, Atlanta, GA, USA
* Corresponding author. Division of Infectious Diseases, Emory University School of Medicine, 101 Woodruff Memorial Building, Suite 2101, Atlanta, GA 30322.
E-mail address: lindsay.margoles.busch@emory.edu

Infect Dis Clin N Am 36 (2022) 761–775
https://doi.org/10.1016/j.idc.2022.07.002
0891-5520/22/© 2022 Elsevier Inc. All rights reserved.
id.theclinics.com

controversy surrounding the Emergency Use Authorization (EUA) and politicization of hydroxychloroquine therapy, progress soon followed in the form of remdesivir and dexamethasone, which became the standard of care following EUA by the Food and Drug Administration (FDA) in May 2020[1] and release of the RECOVERY trial results in June 2020.[2] Propelled by the dramatic impact on mortality conferred by the nonspecific immunosuppression of steroids, earnest investigation into directed immunomodulation soon followed, with modest mortality benefit demonstrated with these agents and an on-going need for larger studies.

A full discussion of steroid therapy in COVID-19 is beyond the scope of this article, but the initial practice-changing studies bear mention given their impact on the standard of care and interpretation of subsequent immunotherapy trials. RECOVERY was the first therapeutic trial to improve mortality in COVID-19. Dexamethasone treatment was associated with a 27% reduction in mortality (risk ratio (RR): 0.83, 95% confidence interval (CI): [0.75, 0.93]) from severe COVID-19 disease, quickly changing the standard of care for hospitalized patients globally.[2] Notably, however, subsequent studies have not demonstrated such dramatic mortality benefit, and clinical practice has evolved to include a variety of different steroid regimens despite comparatively smaller trial sizes and modest outcomes. There were 3 trials evaluating corticosteroid use in critically ill patients with COVID-19 which had to stop enrollment following the release of RECOVERY data: REMAP-CAP, CoDEX, and CAPE COVID. The results from REMAP-CAP (n = 403; endpoint: number of days alive and free of organ support on Day 21) suggested that hydrocortisone therapy had a high probability of benefit, though due to early stoppage they were unable to confirm this nor define an optimal regimen.[3] CoDEX reported an increase in the number of ventilator-free days on Day 28 with dexamethasone vs control (6.6 vs 4.0 d, p = 0.04), though no benefit in mortality (56.3% vs 61.5%, p = 0.83).[4] CAPE COVID reported no difference in their endpoint of treatment failure (composite death or ongoing respiratory support mechanical ventilation [MV] or high flow nasal cannula [HFNC]) on Day 21 (42.1% vs 50.7%, p = 0.29) in patients randomized to hydrocortisone vs placebo.[5] A concurrently published prospective meta-analysis from the World Health Organization (WHO) of 7 RCTs examining corticosteroid administration in 1703 critically ill patients reported results favoring steroids for improved mortality, with a summary odds ratio (OR): 0.66 (95% CI: [0.53, 0.82]).[6] A 2021 Cochrane systematic review included 11 available RCTs testing steroid use in hospitalized patients with COVID-19 with summary findings of probable reduction in all-cause mortality (9 RCTs, 7930 subjects; RR: 0.89, 95% CI: 0.8, 1.0). Unfortunately, due to the inability to adjust for the impact of early deaths and wide intertrial heterogeneity, they were unable to provide further analysis regarding new initiation of mechanical ventilation, serious adverse events, or comparison of different steroid regimens.[7] With the loss of equipoise for placebo-controlled steroid trials in the wake of RECOVERY, the clinical focus shifted to the type of steroid and dosing regimen. Many providers and institutions protocolized the RECOVERY dexamethasone regimen, while others looked to the broader ARDS literature, such as the DEXA ARDS trial,[8] for alternative dosing regimens. While the landscape of steroid treatment in severe COVID-19 infection continues to evolve, investigation into targeted immunomodulatory therapies has grown rapidly. The agents with the most data and clinical experience to date are baricitinib and tocilizumab. We will focus on available data for the treatment of severe COVID-19 infection, with specific attention to critical illness. This population represents a particular challenge with regard to directed therapeutics for many reasons: the high rate of mortality, dependence on life support measures, increased risk of secondary infections, complications of critical illness (e.g., gastrointestinal bleeding, limb ischemia, neuromuscular weakness), unique pharmacokinetic considerations, and high incidence of concurrent organ dysfunctions (e.g., renal failure, liver injury, coagulopathy, cardiac dysfunction). Furthermore, prolonged critical illness is itself associated with dysregulation and suppression of the immune system,[9–11] and understanding how potential immunomodulatory therapies perform in this complex milieu is essential to maximize medical therapies in this vulnerable population, without predisposing to undo risk of infectious complications.

IMMUNOMODULATION FOR COVID-19

The goal of immunotherapy for infectious diseases is to facilitate the functions of immune cells that are essential for microbial clearance while curbing potentially damaging aspects of host inflammation which can exacerbate organ injury. Infection with SARS-CoV-2 begins with the binding of the viral spike glycoprotein to the angiotensin-conversing enzyme-2 (ACE2) receptor on the respiratory epithelial cells, entry into which is facilitated by the host transmembrane protease serine 2 (TMPRSS2). Recognition by immune cell pattern-recognition receptors spurs the host response, largely governed by interleukin (IL)-1 and IL-6 signaling.[12] Infections result in a wide spectrum of disease, from asymptomatic to mild influenza-like illness to severe pneumonia with acute respiratory distress syndrome (ARDS), multisystem organ failure, and death. The T cell response in severe COVID-19 infection shows some similarities to the immune dysregulation observed in bacterial sepsis including circulating monocyte downregulation of HLA-DR expression and CD4+ and CD8+ T cell lymphopenia. Interestingly, while T cell production of type II interferons is reduced, the cells retain the capacity to produce other inflammatory cytokines—one target for potential therapeutics. Several case series have sought to describe T cell phenotypic and functional changes associated with COVID-19 infection,[13–15] although it should be noted that the landmark RCTs and adaptive trials published to date have included few or no immunologic endpoints, so we lack data directly linking immunophenotypes with therapeutic responses. Later in discussion, we will discuss several classes of immunomodulatory agents currently in use or under investigation for severe COVID-19 disease, with specific attention to the applicability of these data to critical illness.

ANTICYTOKINE THERAPY
IL-6 Inhibition

The aggressive hyperinflammatory response known as cytokine storm (CS) is a well-described feature of severe COVID-19 disease. IL-6 plays an important role in viral immunity and is a key cytokine associated with CS.[16] Initial reports of elevated IL-6 levels associated with adverse outcomes coupled with the finding that critically ill patients with COVID-19 had significantly higher levels of IL-6 compared to patients with moderate disease spawned early investigations targeting this pathway to mitigate adverse effects.[17–19] There are 2 classes of anti-IL-6 agents that are currently approved by the FDA, the IL-6 receptor monoclonal antibodies (IL-6ra) tocilizumab and sarilumab, and the IL-6 monoclonal antibody, siltuximab. The IL-6ra agents have the most robust data for the treatment of COVID-19 disease, while no data are available for siltuximab at the time of this review. Data from 3 large studies (RECOVERY, REMAP-CAP, and COVACTA) were published in early 2021 with conflicting results regarding efficacy, and with notable differences in study design and adjunct therapies.[20–22] Both RECOVERY and REMAP-CAP demonstrated improved clinical outcomes associated with tocilizumab, while COVACTA found no difference in 28-day mortality when compared to placebo. The RECOVERY study enrolled all hospitalized patients with COVID-19 disease and elevated CRP, regardless of severity, with almost half (~45%) of patients requiring either no or low-flow supplemental oxygen. Investigators reported that tocilizumab compared to usual care alone significantly improved 28-day mortality, 31% vs 35% (RR: 0.85, 95% CI: 0.76–0.94, p = 0.0028). Tocilizumab was also associated with a greater probability of hospital discharge on Day 28 and a lower risk of new initiation of mechanical ventilation or death.[20] The REMAP-CAP study specifically enrolled critically ill patients with COVID-19 disease receiving either respiratory support (e.g., HFNC, noninvasive positive pressure ventilation [NIPPV], or MV) or cardiovascular support. Rather than mortality, however, the primary outcome of this study was the number of respiratory or cardiovascular organ support-free days on day 21. At the time of publication of the anti-IL-6 data in 2021, of the 2,274 patients enrolled in the Immunomodulatory Domain, 353 were assigned to the tocilizumab group, 48 to sarilumab, and 402 to the standard of care (control). Patients in the tocilizumab and sarilumab arms had a greater median number of organ support-free days, 10 (IQR -1 to 15) and 11 (IQR 0 to 16), respectively, compared to 0 days in the control arm (IQR -1 to 15). Tocilizumab and sarilumab were also both associated with a significantly lower in-hospital mortality, 28% and 22%, respectively, compared to the control arm (36%).[21] These data are supported in the preprint edition of the complete REMAP-CAP Immunotherapy Domain RCT, which is pending peer review at the time of this article preparation.[23] Lastly, the COVACTA study enrolled hospitalized patients with severe COVID-19 disease with approximately two-thirds admitted to the ICU with high oxygen requirements (HFNC or greater). However, it is notable that the mortality in both groups was fairly low at 19%, despite the apparent high acuity of the population. This study found no difference in their primary outcome of clinical status improvement as measured by seven-point ordinal scale (OS) or secondary endpoint of mortality. One major difference between the RECOVERY and REMAP-CAP studies compared to COVACTA was the use of steroids in addition to IL-6ra or usual care.[22] Fewer than 30% of patients in either arm of the COVACTA study received corticosteroids—just 19.4% in the tocilizumab arm vs 28.5% in the control arm. In contrast, greater than 80% of patients in RECOVERY and 90% of patients in REMAP-CAP received steroids. Furthermore, a meta-analysis that included all 3 studies found a signal toward improved survival in patients receiving steroids in addition to IL-6ras in a subgroup analysis.[24] Thus, the current NIH treatment guidelines state that IL-6ras should only be given in combination with steroid treatment.[25]

While the current literature suggests a benefit with the use of IL-6ras in patients with COVID-19 disease when used with steroids, it is important to note that most studies included patients with moderate–severe disease, and several studies excluded patients who were mechanically ventilated at baseline. REMAP-CAP is the only study to have investigated IL-6ra therapy specifically in critically ill patients with COVID-19 and even then only 30% of patients in the tocilizumab arm, 17% in the sarilumab arm, and 30% in the control arm required mechanical ventilation at baseline.[21] Consequently, the highest acuity patients with COVID-19 remain underrepresented, and it is difficult to draw firm conclusions regarding the benefit of IL-6ras in this subgroup of critically ill patients.

IL-1 Inhibition

Although the IL-1 antagonist anakinra and canakinumab hold FDA approval for moderate-to-severe rheumatoid arthritis, they are often used in other acute conditions identified clinically by cytokine storm or capillary leaks such as CAR-T cell-associated cytokine release syndrome (CRS) and macrophage activation syndrome (MAS). These agents have not been submitted to the FDA for EUA in COVID-19 disease at the time of this writing, nor are they recommended by the NIH Treatment Guidelines Panel due to limited demonstrable efficacy in several trials. A brief summary of the data from the REMAP-CAP,[23] SAVE-MORE,[26] CORIMUNO-ANA-1,[27] and CAN-COVID[28] is included later in discussion.

Of the 2,274 participants in REMAP-CAP randomized into the Immunomodulatory Domain, 365 were assigned to receive anakinra and 406 were assigned to the control arm. Of the available trials, this is the only one to specifically enroll critically ill subjects. Thirty-seven percent of the patients assigned to anakinra were receiving invasive MV at baseline, compared with 32% for the other arms. The median number of organ support-free days was similar between the groups (0 days [IQR 1 to 15 days] vs 1 day [IQR -1 to 15 days]); aOR: 0.99 (95% CrI 0.74,1.35, 46.6% posterior probability of superiority to control). Mortality was also similar at 60% vs 63% (43.6% posterior probability of superiority to control). The SAVE-MORE trial randomized 594 patients hospitalized with moderate or severe COVID-19 pneumonia, using a plasma soluble urokinase plasminogen receptor (suPAR) level greater than or equal to 6 ng/mL as an inclusion criterion to identify patients most likely to benefit from therapy (as determined by the preceding phase 2 SAVE study[29]). Unfortunately, patients receiving noninvasive or invasive mechanical ventilation were excluded from the study. Subjects in the anakinra group demonstrated a lower odds of progression of disease based on the WHO-Clinical Progression Scale (CPS), as well as favorable secondary endpoints including an absolute decrease in sequential organ failure assessment (SOFA) score from baseline to Day 7, median time to hospital discharge, median duration of ICU stay, and lower 28-day mortality (3.2% vs 6.9%; hazard ratio (HR): 0.45 [95% CI: 0.21, 0.98,] p = 0.045). Unfortunately, the suPAR assay is not widely available, limiting incorporation and further evaluation of these findings.

The CORIMUNO-ANA-1 randomized 116 subjects with severe COVID-19 requiring greater than three liters per minute of supplemental oxygen to either anakinra or standard of care. Of note, patients requiring HFNC oxygen, MV, or ICU admission were excluded. There was no difference between the groups in the 2 coprimary endpoints of the proportion of patients who died or required noninvasive or invasive mechanical ventilation on Day 4 and proportion of patients who survived without the use of noninvasive or invasive MV (including HFNC) on Day 14. Of note, there were more serious adverse events in the treatment group (46% vs 38%), including an increased incidence of fungal infections in the anakinra group (18.6% vs 7.3%). CAN-COVID randomized 454 patients with severe COVID-19 that were hypoxemic but not requiring mechanical ventilation to receive either canakinumab or placebo. There was no difference in the primary endpoint of the proportion of patients who survived without MV from Days 3–29 (88.8% vs 85.7%, p = 0.29). Of note, mortality was low in both groups (4.9% vs 7.7%, OR: 0.67 [95% CI: 0.30, 1.50]). The results are confounded by an imbalance in the administration of both steroids and tocilizumab between the treatment and placebo groups (41% vs 32%, and 2.2% vs 8.8%, respectively).

Some smaller series and cohort studies have examined critically ill patients,[30–32] providing some potential insights for further consideration by clinicians, but the results are significantly limited by small numbers and variable methodologies.

JAK INHIBITION

As discussed above, the rationale for immunomodulation in COVID-19 relies on the inhibition of cytokines that result in inflammatory organ injury.[33] Thus, it is not surprising that rather than targeting individual cytokines, the attention turned to blocking the Janus Tyrosine Kinase (JAK) and Signal Transducers and Activators of Transcription (STAT) pathway.[34] The JAK-STAT pathway is a pivotal cell signaling pathway that leads to downstream activation of several cytokines and subsequent immune proliferation and adaptation. Several drugs target the JAK-STAT pathway, and most of the studies on COVID-19 have focused on baricitinib (JAK 1/2 inhibitor) and ruxolitinib (JAK 1/2 inhibitor). The main difference between the 2 being that baricitinib is not metabolized via cytochrome P450 and is renally cleared.[35] A third JAK3 inhibitor, tofacitinib, has also been assessed in smaller studies, along with additional JAK-STAT inhibitors.

The largest among the JAK inhibitor studies, the Adaptive COVID-19 Treatment Trial 2 (ACTT-2), assessed the role of baricitinib and remdesivir when compared to remdesivir alone.[36] The trial was a multicenter international randomized double-blind placebo-controlled trial of 1033 hospitalized patients with a primary outcome of time to recovery on an eight-point OS. The study included about 30% of patients in each group who were receiving either NIPPV, HFNC, MV, or extracorporeal membrane oxygenation (ECMO) support. Across the board, the study demonstrated a benefit of the combination treatment when compared to remdesivir alone. Importantly, while the rates of glucocorticoid and dexamethasone use after enrollment were not significantly different between the 2 groups, they were relatively low in both groups—as per the intent of the study. This is particularly noteworthy for dexamethasone, which was used in just 6% and 7% of the investigational and control groups, respectively. This is vastly different than the subsequent adopted practice in which dexamethasone treatment became standard of care and baricitinib was often added after further review and assessment. The ACTT authors acknowledge that there is no head-to-head trial of steroids vs baricitinib, but do not postulate about the effect of real-world application of the concurrent use of steroids and baricitinib. Interestingly, the study did find that the patients who had received steroids had a higher incidence of infections (25.1% vs. 5.5% in patients not receiving steroids).[37]

Following ACTT-2, the COV-BARRIER trial studied patients receiving steroids (79.3% of the total patients) with the addition of baricitinib. The trial included a lower acuity population (only a quarter of patients in each group at the time of enrollment were on HFNC or NIPPV) and found no significant reduction in disease progression (primary outcome) but noted overall reduced mortality in hospitalized patients.[38] Regarding tofacitinib, a smaller study in Brazil randomized 289 inpatients (less than 20% in the ICU) to receive tofacitinib (89.3% of the patients were also on steroids) and noted a decrease in the incidence of their primary outcome of respiratory failure or death (RR: 0.63; 95% CI: 0.41 to 0.97; p = 0.04).[39]

A couple of smaller meta-analyses have assessed the role of JAK-STAT inhibitors and COVID-19. In one of the larger analyses (6 cohort studies and 5 clinical trials, for a total of 2367 patients), ruxolitinib and baricitinib led to a decreased use of mechanical ventilation, and possible trend toward decreased ICU admission and ARDS. The overall relative risk of death was 0.42 [95% CI: 0.30, 0.59]; p < 0.001.[40] Based on these studies, the NIH guidelines recommend steroids and a JAK-STAT inhibitor in hospitalized patients with COVID-19 requiring oxygen. There has always been concern about the combined immunosuppressive effects resulting in infectious complications, but few studies have systematically examined this complication.

OTHER AGENTS UNDER INVESTIGATION
Granulocyte Macrophage Colony Stimulating Factor Inhibition

The OSCAR[41] and LIVE-AIR[42] trials have reported results for the investigation of anti-granulocyte macrophage colony stimulating factor (GM-CSF) therapy with otilimab and lenzilumab, respectively, for severe COVID-19 infection. OSCAR was a large phase II trial (n = 793) of hospitalized patients with new onset severe COVID-19 infection requiring HFNC, NIPPV, or invasive MV. It should be noted that patients with additional organ support needs including high dose vasopressor, dialysis, or ECMO were excluded. The primary endpoint was proportion of subjects alive and free of respiratory failure on Day 28, while secondary endpoints included all-cause mortality on Day 60. 52% of subjects were in the ICU without invasive MV and 22% required MV. 71% of subjects in the otilimab arm vs 67% of controls met the primary endpoint on Day 28, adjusted mean difference 5.3% (95% CI: -0.8, 11.4, p = 0.09). There was no difference in mortality between the groups. However, in a preplanned analysis, benefit of otilimab was observed for subjects >70 years old (n = 180): 65% vs 46% for primary endpoint (adjusted mean difference 19.1% [95% CI: 5.2, 33.3], p = 0.009), 27% vs 41% mortality (adjusted mean difference 14.4% [95% CI: 0.9, 27.9], p = 0.04). Despite the potential benefit for this vulnerable subgroup, GlaxoSmithKline ended the program for further development for this indication.[43] LIVE-AIR, a phase III RCT, randomized 479 hospitalized patients with COVID-19 not requiring MV to receive either lenzilumab or placebo in addition to standard of care. The primary endpoint was survival without MV on Day 28, with secondary endpoints including survival, proportion of MV, ECMO or death, and time to recovery. The population was of fairly high acuity, with 40% requiring HFNC or NIPPV. Lenzilumab improved ventilator-free survival, although there was no significant mortality difference of 9.6% vs 13.9% (HR: 1.38 [95% CI: 0.81, 2.37], p = 0.239).[42] Subsequently, the FDA declined the request for EUA for lenzilumab,[44] though this may be revisited pending the anticipated results of ACTIV-5/Big Effect Trial (BET-B) (NCT04583969). ACTIV-5/BET-B, evaluating the efficacy of remdesivir plus lenzilumab, is still pending at the time of preparation of this article. Primary outcomes for this study include: occurrence of MV or death through Day 29 in subjects with baseline OS 5 or 6; OS score 7 (hospitalized on MV or ECMO) or 8 (death) in subjections with baseline OS 5 or 6 and CRP <150 mg/L and age <85 years. Mortality is included as one of the many secondary endpoints in the study.

Tyrosine Kinase Inhibition

Imatinib, a Bruton's Tyrosine Kinase inhibitor, is proposed to provide benefit in the treatment of COVID-19 disease by direct viral inhibition, anti-inflammatory effect on cytokine and chemokine signaling, and mitigation of pulmonary capillary permeability.[45–48] The first reported trial of imatinib use in COVID-19 was the CounterCovid study, a randomized, double-blinded, placebo-controlled trial of hospitalized patients requiring oxygen supplementation.[49] The primary outcome of this trial was time to the discontinuation of mechanical ventilation and/or supplemental oxygen for more than 48 consecutive hours while alive on Day 28. The investigators did not find any difference in time to discontinuation between the imatinib and placebo groups (HR: 0.95 [95% CI: 0.76, 1.20], p = 0.69). The 28-day mortality was quite low at 8% in the imatinib group and 14% in placebo group and the unadjusted HR for mortality was significant, however, it became nonsignificant after adjusting for imbalances in baseline characteristics. The number of patients that were admitted to the ICU was low with only roughly 20% and 18% in the imatinib and placebo groups, respectively. The rate of mechanical ventilation was similarly low at 15% and 14%, respectively. At the time of preparation for this article, there are 4 trials investigating imatinib for the treatment of COVID-19 disease that is open and actively recruiting.

IMMUNE PRODUCTS FOR VIRAL ELIMINATION

While convalescent plasma and monoclonal antibodies directed against SARS-CoV-2 are not immunomodulators strictly speaking, a brief discussion is warranted. These immune therapies are designed to provide a ready-made humoral immune response without the time and cellular machinery required for an endogenous response to infection or vaccination. While this strategy may be beneficial in special populations, large-scale trials have not demonstrated efficacy in hospitalized patients with severe diseases.

Convalescent plasma failed to demonstrate improved 28-day mortality in a Cochrane review of 7 RCTs including over 12,000 subjects, nor did it reduce the new need for MV or promote liberation from ventilation.[50] Similarly, benefit was not demonstrated in either RECOVERY[51] or REMAP-CAP[52] trials. The initial EUA issued August 23, 2020 for COVID-19 convalescent plasma for the treatment of hospitalized patients was subsequently reissued on January 7, 2022 to limit the use of plasma with high titers of anti–SARS-CoV-2 antibodies for the treatment of disease in patients with immunosuppressive disease or receiving immunosuppressive treatment in the inpatient or outpatient settings. At the time of preparation of this article, the most recent update[53] states that data in this population remains limited and there remains a need for well-controlled randomized trials to determine demonstrable efficacy for this therapy. Access remains limited to administration under the EUA or investigational use (IND) pathways—both single patient and expanded access, and may be subject to further institutional protocols given the cost and availability of this product.[54]

Monoclonal antibodies (mAbs) engineered to interact with one or more predefined viral target with high neutralizing activity have enjoyed success in the outpatient treatment of high-risk patients, but have not been available for use in hospitalized patients with severe diseases. There have now been several products that have demonstrated efficacy in preventing progression to severe disease (eg, bamlanivumab,[55] casirivimab and imdevimab,[53] sotrovimab,[56] and tixagevimab plus cilgavimab[57]), but a notable drawback to these agents is that they are susceptible to immune escape mutations, potentially rendering them ineffective against subsequent SARS-CoV-2 variants.[58] Of note, the FDA EUA documents for all currently authorized mAbs state that benefit has not been observed in hospitalized patients and that monoclonals may be associated with worse clinical outcomes when administered to hospitalized patients requiring HFNC or mechanical ventilation. This recommendation stems from a safety signal observed in the ACTIV-3 trial, resulting in early stoppage of enrollment and unblinding of data safety monitoring board (DSMB) data for FDA review. On day 5, there was evidence of worsened clinical outcomes, most notable in the subjects requiring high flow nasal cannula at baseline (maximum support allowed per inclusion criteria). Further, there was increased incidence of grade 3 and 4 adverse events and death in one of the treatment groups. Ultimately, the DSMB review determined that there was no statistically significant difference in adverse events, deaths, or worsened pulmonary outcomes, but there was no evidence of benefit and bamlanivimab did not meet the criteria to advance in the platform trial and randomization did not resume.[59]

An important question remains: is there a role for monoclonal antibody therapy for patients with severe or critical illness, and without an endogenous antibody response? Patients with immunosuppressing conditions (e.g., those receiving anti-CD20 therapy, hematologic malignancies, or history of solid organ or hematopoietic stem cell transplantation) are at exceedingly high risk of poor outcomes. Given the limited efficacy of the available direct antiviral agents, exogenous antibody administration may be a useful tool to enhance viral clearance. Conducting trials in this immunosuppressed population is particularly challenging.

COVID-19 AND CRITICAL ILLNESS: FEW ANSWERS, MANY QUESTIONS

Despite the staggering number of deaths attributed to COVID-19 since the start of the pandemic, we remain limited in strong, evidence-based treatment recommendations for our most critically ill patients. Indeed, even in moderate and moderately severe diseases for which more evidence is available, demonstrable and durable efficacy has been elusive. In a recent publication evaluating the fragility index of available RCTs for COVID-19, Itaya and colleagues evaluated 36 treatment RCTs and found a fragility index (IQR) of just 2.5.[1–6,60] In the absence of robust data, clinicians must be prudent and realistic about their ability to extrapolate trial data to specific subgroups of patients, including those with severe and critical disease. Very few trials have been designed and powered specifically for the critically ill, a population that has been historically difficult to study.[61,62] Throughout the current pandemic, interpretation, and extrapolation of data in critical illness has been particularly challenging due to variability in trial design, rapidly evolving standards of care, and the impact of surging caseloads on depleted health care systems.

An interesting facet of this era of unprecedented investigation is the preponderance of phase III RCTs for COVID therapeutics utilizing OS-based clinical endpoints in lieu of more traditional "hard endpoints" such as mortality. For example, the OS developed by the NIH investigators early in the pandemic for the ACTT studies (NCT 04280705), influenced the design of many subsequent trials. When specifically considering the critical care population, however, the interpretation of OS measurements can be challenging. The NIH eight-point scale provides much more granularity on the lower end of the OS and assigns equal weight to clinical changes with vastly different implications. This is counterintuitive to our understanding of critically ill patients, in whom prognosis is dramatically impacted by sequential organ dysfunction.[63] That all mechanically ventilated and patients with ECMO receive the same score draws false equivalence between distinct phenotypes of patients, such as those with modest ventilator requirements, severe ARDS, need for renal replacement, liver failure, coagulopathy, or mechanical circulatory support. While the numeric distance for these patients to reach a recovery endpoint on the OS is the same, the clinical trajectory and risk of death are vastly different. Indeed, as one considers the myriad clinical challenges these subjects face and how relatively underrepresented they are in the majority of the landmark therapeutic trials, it becomes increasingly difficult to say with certainty what degree of benefit these patients may see from the same therapy as patients with moderate disease severity. Several publications have addressed the complexities of endpoint selection in this setting, including competing factors of the wide clinical spectrum of disease associated with SARS-CoV-2 infection, urgent need for rapid evaluation of therapies in the face of widespread morbidity and mortality, fluctuating standards of care over time, and impact of extrinsic factors such as surging caseloads on health care systems.[64–66] There are benefits to nonmortality endpoints in the setting of a global pandemic, and time-to-event endpoints such as used in ACTT attempt to overcome the risk of missing treatment effects due to the selection of an incorrect time point *a priori*. However, "time to recovery" may not capture the dynamic morbidity incurred or resources utilized over the course of a prolonged critical illness. Similarly, "time to recovery" is really time to first measured recovery endpoint and does not account for patients that developed subsequent complications, hospital readmission, or even death, all of which are frequent complications following critical illness.[67,68] Finally, the statistical handling of death in time to recovery analysis can also feel lacking when viewed from a clinical lens of a critical care provider, where mortality has been reported as high as 30–60%.[66] In ACTT, deaths are censored at the end of

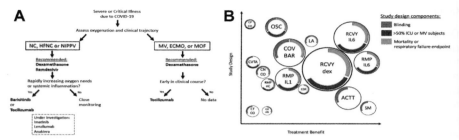

Fig. 1. Comparison of treatment recommendations for severe and critical COVID-19 infection and the relevance of clinical trial evidence to the ICU population. (*A*) Algorithm of currently recommended treatment guidelines for severe and critical COVID-19 infection. (*B*) Visual representation of the applicability and generalizability of the results of the cited trials to a critically ill population by comparing 3 aspects of study design with the magnitude of treatment effect observed in the trials. Treatment effect is a qualitative measure that includes comparison across multiple types of reported results including odds ratios, hazard ratios, survival analyses. The size of the circle corresponds to the size of the trial. ACTT, Adaptive COVID-19 Treatment Trial; CDX, CODEX; CO AN, CORIMMUNO-ANA-1; COV BAR, COVID BARRIER; CN CO, CAN-COVID; CP CO, CAPE COVID; CT CO, CounterCovid; CVTA, CO-VACTA; LA, LIVE AIR; OSC, OSCAR; RCVY dex, RECOVERY dexamethasone; RCVY IL6, RECOVERY tocilizumab; RMP IL1, REMAP CAP anakinra; RMP IL6, REMAP CAP tocilizumab/sarilumab; SM, SAVE MORE.

the study period and imputed as an "infinite time to recovery." While this may be a reasonable approach from a viewpoint of a statistician or trialist, there is clearly a huge clinical difference between a subject failing to meet a composite recovery endpoint and death. The statistical choices made by clinical trialists are understandably aligned with the public health objective to address the needs of the vast numbers of patients impacted by mild, moderate, and severe diseases with fairly modest and manageable clinical needs. Whether the results from these trials are meaningful and applicable to those with critical illness, however, is less clear. The accompanying **Fig. 1** provides a side-by-side comparison of the currently available treatment recommendations for severe and critical COVID-19[25,69,70] with a qualitative visual representation of the data discussed in this review, designed to reflect the applicability of the published immunotherapy trial results to a critically ill population. As depicted, only 2 studies possessed all 3 study design components examined, and these trials were relatively small and demonstrated minimal treatment benefit. Critically ill patients are physiologically distinct, have different pharmacokinetic and pharmacodynamic considerations, and, for those who do not die quickly, often require prolonged hospital courses with resultant increased risk of nosocomial complications. While extrapolation of data and therapeutics from a moderately ill population to the critically ill is not uncommon, it is fraught and likely to be inadequate. Unfortunately, for many of the reasons above, dedicated trials in the critically ill are challenging to perform and interpret. Thus, clinicians are often left to rely on subgroup analyses, Phase 1/2 data, small case series, and clinical experience to refine treatment protocols for the critically ill. Unfortunately, these data streams were also subjected to the constraints of the pandemic. Due to the immense clinical need, the rapidity with which investigations and regulatory review were occurring, and fluidity of trial designs during this period, immunologic endpoints and biomarker data were relatively devalued in regulatory review in lieu of clinical endpoints. While this was necessary, we likely lost granular immunologic data which may have allowed us to identify important physiologic differences between patients with moderate and severe disease in general, and those with critical illness specifically. Incorporating detailed immunophenotyping of patients across the wide spectrum of severe diseases alongside mortality and clinical outcome endpoints in large RCTs may allow us to discriminate between groups of patients and direct immunomodulator therapy to patients who may benefit most.

CLINICS CARE POINTS

- For patients with severe COVID-19 infection requiring oxygen supplementation by noninvasive measures, treatment is recommended with dexamethasone and remdesivir with consideration of tocilizumab or baricitinib for patients with rapidly progressive oxygen requirement or systemic inflammation.

- For patients with critical COVID-19 infection requiring invasive mechanical ventilation, extracorporeal membrane oxygenation, or multisystem organ failure, treatment recommendations are more limited, with guidelines endorsing dexamethasone alone and consideration of tocilizumab if early in the clinical course.

- Clinical trials linking immunophenotyping with response to therapeutics are in severe and critical COVID-19 infection.

REFERENCES

1. Administration UFaD. Pages. Accessed at US Food and Drug Administration at Available at: https://www.fda.gov/emergency-preparedness-and-response/mcm-legal-regulatory-and-policy-framework/emergency-use-authorization#coviddrugs. US FDA: accessed 2/1/2022.
2. Horby P, Lim WS, et al, Recovery Collaborative Group. Dexamethasone in hospitalized patients with Covid-19. N Engl J Med 2021;384(8):693–704.
3. Angus DC, Derde L, Al-Beidh F, et al. Effect of Hydrocortisone on mortality and organ support in patients with severe COVID-19: the REMAP-CAP COVID-19 corticosteroid domain randomized clinical trial. JAMA 2020;324(13):1317–29.
4. Tomazini BM, Maia IS, Cavalcanti AB, et al. Effect of dexamethasone on days alive and ventilator-free in patients with moderate or severe acute respiratory distress syndrome and COVID-19: the CoDEX randomized clinical trial. JAMA 2020;324(13):1307–16.
5. Dequin PF, Heming N, Meziani F, et al. Effect of hydrocortisone on 21-day mortality or respiratory support among critically ill patients with COVID-19: a randomized clinical trial. JAMA 2020;324(13):1298–306.
6. Group WHOREAfC-TW, Sterne JAC, Murthy S, et al. Association between administration of systemic corticosteroids and mortality among critically ill patients with COVID-19: a meta-analysis. JAMA 2020;324(13):1330–41.
7. Wagner C, Griesel M, Mikolajewska A, et al. Systemic corticosteroids for the treatment of COVID-19. Cochrane Database Syst Rev 2021;8:CD014963.
8. Villar J, Ferrando C, Martinez D, et al. Dexamethasone treatment for the acute respiratory distress syndrome: a multicentre, randomised controlled trial. Lancet Respir Med 2020;8(3):267–76.
9. Fenner BP, Darden DB, Kelly LS, et al. Immunological endotyping of chronic critical illness after severe sepsis. Front Med (Lausanne) 2020;7:616694.
10. Islam MN, Bradley BA, Ceredig R. Sterile post-traumatic immunosuppression. Clin Transl Immunol 2016;5(4):e77.

11. Zhao Q, Shen Y, Li R, et al. Cardiac arrest and resuscitation activates the hypothalamic-pituitary-adrenal axis and results in severe immunosuppression. J Cereb Blood Flow Metab 2021;41(5):1091–102.

12. van de Veerdonk FL, Giamarellos-Bourboulis E, Pickkers P, et al. A guide to immunotherapy for COVID-19. Nat Med 2022;28(1):39–50.

13. Ronit A, Berg RMG, Bay JT, et al. Compartmental immunophenotyping in COVID-19 ARDS: A case series. J Allergy Clin Immunol 2021;147(1):81–91.

14. Mathew D, Giles JR, Baxter AE, et al. Deep immune profiling of COVID-19 patients reveals distinct immunotypes with therapeutic implications. Science 2020;369(6508):eabc8511.

15. Laing AG, Lorenc A, Del Molino Del Barrio I, et al. A dynamic COVID-19 immune signature includes associations with poor prognosis. Nat Med 2020;26(10):1623–35.

16. Shekhawat J, Gauba K, Gupta S, et al. Interleukin-6 Perpetrator of the COVID-19 Cytokine Storm. Indian J Clin Biochem 2021;36(4):1–11.

17. Carvalho T, Krammer F, Iwasaki A. The first 12 months of COVID-19: a timeline of immunological insights. Nat Rev Immunol 2021;21(4):245–56.

18. Chen G, Wu D, Guo W, et al. Clinical and immunological features of severe and moderate coronavirus disease 2019. J Clin Invest 2020;130(5):2620–9.

19. Coomes EA, Haghbayan H. Interleukin-6 in Covid-19: a systematic review and meta-analysis. Rev Med Virol 2020;30(6):1–9.

20. Recovery Collaborative Group. Tocilizumab in patients admitted to hospital with COVID-19 (RECOVERY): a randomised, controlled, open-label, platform trial. Lancet 2021;397(10285):1637–45.

21. Gordon AC, Mouncey PR, et al, REMAP-CAP Investigators. Interleukin-6 receptor antagonists in critically ill patients with Covid-19. N Engl J Med 2021;384(16):1491–502.

22. Rosas IO, Brau N, Waters M, et al. Tocilizumab in hospitalized patients with severe Covid-19 pneumonia. N Engl J Med 2021;384(16):1503–16.

23. Derde LPG, et al, REMAP-CAP Investigators. Effectiveness of tocilizumab, sarilumab, and anakinra for critically ill patients with COVID-19 The REMAP-CAP COVID-19 immune modulation therapy domain randomized clinical trial. medRxiv 2021. 2021.06.18.21259133.

24. Belletti A, Campochiaro C, Marmiere M, et al. Efficacy and safety of IL-6 inhibitors in patients with COVID-19 pneumonia: a systematic review and meta-analysis of multicentre, randomized trials. Ann Intensive Care 2021;11(1):152.

25. Panel NC-TG. 2022. Pages. Available at: https://www.covid19treatmentguidelines.nih.gov/about-the-guidelines/table-of-contents/. NIH COVID-19 Treatment Guidelines: accessed 1/14/2022.

26. Kyriazopoulou E, Poulakou G, Milionis H, et al. Early treatment of COVID-19 with anakinra guided by soluble urokinase plasminogen receptor plasma levels: a double-blind, randomized controlled phase 3 trial. Nat Med 2021;27(10):1752–60.

27. CORIMMUNO-Collaborative Group. Effect of anakinra versus usual care in adults in hospital with COVID-19 and mild-to-moderate pneumonia (CORIMUNO-ANA-1): a randomised controlled trial. Lancet Respir Med 2021;9(3):295–304.

28. Caricchio R, Abbate A, Gordeev I, et al. Effect of canakinumab vs placebo on survival without invasive mechanical ventilation in patients hospitalized with severe COVID-19: a randomized clinical trial. JAMA 2021;326(3):230–9.

29. Rovina N, Akinosoglou K, Eugen-Olsen J, et al. Soluble urokinase plasminogen activator receptor (suPAR) as an early predictor of severe respiratory failure in patients with COVID-19 pneumonia. Crit Care 2020;24(1):187.

30. Kooistra EJ, Waalders NJB, Grondman I, et al. Anakinra treatment in critically ill COVID-19 patients: a prospective cohort study. Crit Care 2020;24(1):688.

31. Huet T, Beaussier H, Voisin O, et al. Anakinra for severe forms of COVID-19: a cohort study. Lancet Rheumatol 2020;2(7):e393–400.

32. Cavalli G, De Luca G, Campochiaro C, et al. Interleukin-1 blockade with high-dose anakinra in patients with COVID-19, acute respiratory distress syndrome, and hyperinflammation: a retrospective cohort study. Lancet Rheumatol 2020; 2(6):e325–31.

33. Mehta P, McAuley DF, Brown M, et al. COVID-19: consider cytokine storm syndromes and immunosuppression. Lancet 2020;395(10229):1033–4.

34. Bousoik E, Montazeri Aliabadi H. "Do We Know Jack" About JAK? A Closer Look at JAK/STAT Signaling Pathway. Front Oncol 2018;8:287.

35. Shi JG, Chen X, Lee F, et al. The pharmacokinetics, pharmacodynamics, and safety of baricitinib, an oral JAK 1/2 inhibitor, in healthy volunteers. J Clin Pharmacol 2014;54(12):1354–61.

36. Kalil AC, Patterson TF, Mehta AK, et al. Baricitinib plus Remdesivir for Hospitalized Adults with Covid-19. N Engl J Med 2021;384(9):795–807.

37. Kalil AC, Patterson TF, Mehta AK, et al. Baricitinib plus Remdesivir for Hospitalized Adults with Covid-19. N Engl J Med 2020;384(9):795–807.

38. Marconi VC, Ramanan AV, de Bono S, et al. Efficacy and safety of baricitinib for the treatment of hospitalised adults with COVID-19 (COV-BARRIER): a randomised, double-blind, parallel-group, placebo-controlled phase 3 trial. Lancet Respir Med 2021;9(12):1407–18.

39. Guimarães PO, Quirk D, Furtado RH, et al. Tofacitinib in Patients Hospitalized with Covid-19 Pneumonia. N Engl J Med 2021;385(5):406–15.

40. Chen CX, Wang JJ, Li H, et al. JAK-inhibitors for coronavirus disease-2019 (COVID-19): a meta-analysis. Leukemia 2021;35(9):2616–20.

41. Patel J, Beishuizen A, Ruiz XB, et al. A Randomized Trial of Otilimab in Severe COVID-19 Pneumonia (OSCAR). medRxiv 2021;2021. 04.14.21255475.

42. Temesgen Z, Burger CD, Baker J, et al. Lenzilumab in hospitalised patients with COVID-19 pneumonia (LIVE-AIR): a phase 3, randomised, placebo-controlled trial. Lancet Respir Med 2022;10(3):237–46.

43. GlaxoSmithKline. Press release: Third quarter 2021. gsk.com: GSK; 2021. https://www.gsk.com/media/7228/q3-2021-results-announcement.pdf. Accessed 2/1/2022

44. Humanigen. FDA has declined Humanigen's EUA request for Lenzilumab in hospitalized COVID-19 patients. Humanigen; 2021.

45. Coleman CM, Sisk JM, Mingo RM, et al. Abelson kinase inhibitors are potent inhibitors of severe acute respiratory syndrome coronavirus and middle east respiratory syndrome coronavirus fusion. J Virol 2016;90(19):8924–33.

46. Hui KP, Cheung MC, Lai KL, et al. Role of epithelial-endothelial cell interaction in the pathogenesis of severe acute respiratory syndrome coronavirus 2 (SARS-CoV-2) infection. Clin Infect Dis 2022;74(2):199–209.

47. Bernal-Bello D, Morales-Ortega A, Isabel Farfan-Sedano A, et al. Imatinib in COVID-19: hope and caution. Lancet Respir Med 2021;9(9):938–9.

48. Thompson BT, Chambers RC, Liu KD. Acute respiratory distress syndrome. N Engl J Med 2017;377(6):562–72.

49. Aman J, Duijvelaar E, Botros L, et al. Imatinib in patients with severe COVID-19: a randomised, double-blind, placebo-controlled, clinical trial. Lancet Respir Med 2021;9(9):957–68.

50. Piechotta V, Iannizzi C, Chai KL, et al. Convalescent plasma or hyperimmune immunoglobulin for people with COVID-19: a living systematic review. Cochrane Database Syst Rev 2021;5:CD013600.

51. Recovery Collaborative Group. Convalescent plasma in patients admitted to hospital with COVID-19 (RECOVERY): a randomised controlled, open-label, platform trial. Lancet 2021;397(10289):2049–59.

52. Estcourt LJ, Turgeon AF, et al, Writing Committee for the REMAP-CAP Investigators. Effect of convalescent plasma on organ support-free days in critically ill patients with COVID-19: a randomized clinical trial. JAMA 2021;326(17):1690–702.

53. Recovery Collaborative Group. Casirivimab and imdevimab in patients admitted to hospital with COVID-19 (RECOVERY): a randomised, controlled, open-label, platform trial. Lancet 2022;399(10325):665–76.

54. US FDA. Investigational COVID-19 Convalescent plasma: guidance for industry. In: Center for Biologics Evaluation and Research, editor. US FDA; 2022. Available at: https://www.fda.gov/media/136798/download. Accessed March 17, 2022.

55. Gottlieb RL, Nirula A, Chen P, et al. Effect of Bamlanivimab as monotherapy or in combination with etesevimab on viral load in patients with mild to moderate COVID-19: a randomized clinical trial. JAMA 2021;325(7):632–44.

56. Gupta A, Gonzalez-Rojas Y, Juarez E, et al. Early Treatment for Covid-19 with SARS-CoV-2 Neutralizing Antibody Sotrovimab. N Engl J Med 2021;385(21):1941–50.

57. Tixagevimab and Cilgavimab (Evusheld) for Pre-Exposure prophylaxis of COVID-19. JAMA 2022;327(4):384–5.

58. Jary A, Marot S, Faycal A, et al. Spike gene evolution and immune escape mutations in patients with mild or moderate forms of COVID-19 and treated with monoclonal antibodies therapies. Viruses 2022;14(2):226.

59. Pica N, et al, CDER. Emergency use authorization for bamlanivimab 700mg IV center for drug evaluation and research (CDER) review. In: Center for Biologics Evaluation and Research, editor. US FDA; 2020. Available at: https://www.fda.gov/media/144118/download. Accessed March 17, 2022.

60. Itaya T, Isobe Y, Suzuki S, et al. The Fragility of Statistically Significant Results in Randomized Clinical Trials for COVID-19. JAMA Netw Open 2022;5(3):e222973.

61. Granholm A, Alhazzani W, Derde LPG, et al. Randomised clinical trials in critical care: past, present and future. Intensive Care Med 2022;48(2):164–78.

62. Laffey JG, Kavanagh BP. Negative trials in critical care: why most research is probably wrong. Lancet Respir Med 2018;6(9):659–60.

63. Ferreira FL, Bota DP, Bross A, et al. Serial evaluation of the SOFA score to predict outcome in critically ill patients. JAMA 2001;286(14):1754–8.

64. Kadri SS, Sun J, Lawandi A, et al. Association between caseload surge and COVID-19 survival in 558 U.S. hospitals, march to august 2020. Ann Intern Med 2021;174(9):1240–51.

65. Dolin R, Hirsch MS. Remdesivir - an important first step. N Engl J Med 2020;383(19):1886–7.

66. Dodd LE, Follmann D, Wang J, et al. Endpoints for randomized controlled clinical trials for COVID-19 treatments. Clin Trials 2020;17(5):472–82.

67. Prescott HC, Osterholzer JJ, Langa KM, et al. Late mortality after sepsis: propensity matched cohort study. BMJ 2016;353:i2375.

68. Jones TK, Fuchs BD, Small DS, et al. Post-acute care use and hospital readmission after sepsis. Ann Am Thorac Soc 2015;12(6):904–13.
69. WHO 2022. Available at: Pageswww.who.int/publications/i/item/WHO-2019-nCoV-therapeutics-2022.2. Accessed 2/1/2022.
70. IDSA 2022. Available at: Pageswww.idsociety.org/practice-guideline/covid-19-guideline-treatment-and-management/#toc-1. Accessed Accessed 2/1/2022.

Supportive Care in Patients with Critical Coronavirus Disease 2019

Daniel A. Sweeney, MD*, Atul Malhotra, MD

KEYWORDS

- COVID-19 • Critical care • Supportive care • Prone ventilation
- Noninvasive positive pressure ventilation • High flow nasal cannula • Lung

KEY POINTS

- The COVID-19 pandemic has emphasized the importance of previously validated supportive care measures for critically ill patients, especially those with ARDS.
- For the patient with COVID-19 and ARDS, prone ventilation, low tidal volume ventilation, and ECMO consideration should be standard of care.
- Noninvasive positive pressure ventilation or high-flow nasal cannula may prevent the subsequent need for intubation.
- Prone ventilation in nonintubated patients has not been consistently shown to prevent the need for intubation.
- Providers should use well-established supportive care measures for critically ill patients with COVID-19, including chemical DVT prophylaxis, conservative fluid management, and strategies to minimize delirium.

INTRODUCTION

The mortality rate for patients with coronavirus disease 2019 (COVID-19) admitted to the intensive care unit (ICU) is approximately 30%.[1,2] Since the start of the pandemic therapeutic advances, including vaccines, monoclonal antibodies, antiviral agents, and immunomodulating therapies, have resulted in fewer patients with COVID-19 being hospitalized and requiring ICU admission. However, current therapeutics have not been consistently helpful once a patient with COVID-19 progresses to the point of requiring critical care support, with only baricitinib in a placebo-controlled trial and dexamethasone in an open-label trial demonstrating benefit in patients receiving mechanical ventilation.[3,4] Even vaccines, which have drastically reduced the burden of severe acute respiratory syndrome coronavirus 2 (SARS-CoV-2) infection worldwide,

Division of Pulmonary, Critical Care, Sleep Medicine and Physiology, Department of Medicine, University of California, San Diego, 9300 Campus Point Drive, La Jolla, CA 92037-7381, USA
* Corresponding author.
E-mail address: dasweeney@health.ucsd.edu

Infect Dis Clin N Am 36 (2022) 777–789
https://doi.org/10.1016/j.idc.2022.08.003
0891-5520/22/© 2022 Elsevier Inc. All rights reserved.

id.theclinics.com

do not measurably reduce either length of stay or mortality for fully vaccinated patients compared with unvaccinated patients who are admitted to the ICU.[5] In light of the dearth of therapeutic options for critically ill patients with COVID-19, optimization of supportive care is paramount. Although there has been great interest in expanding the application of prone ventilation to include nonintubated patients with COVID-19, current randomized trial data do not support its routine use. Rather, the pandemic experience has served to reinforce the importance of applying supportive critical care strategies that have been previously been proved to be beneficial in the management of patients with severe pneumonia and acute respiratory distress syndrome (ARDS). Accordingly, this article aims to highlight important aspects of supportive care for the critically ill patient with COVID-19, with an emphasis on a stepwise approach to the use of respiratory support for patients based on their severity of respiratory illness.

NONINVASIVE RESPIRATORY SUPPORT FOR CRITICALLY ILL PATIENTS WITH CORONAVIRUS DISEASE 2019

The need for additional respiratory support beyond low-flow oxygen therapy (<15 L/min [LPM]) is often the reason for admission to the ICU. For patients with COVID-19 who are hypoxemic (oxygen saturation <92%) despite receiving low-flow oxygen, but not requiring urgent intubation, the 3 advanced respiratory support options are continuous positive airway pressure (CPAP), noninvasive positive pressure ventilation (NIPPV, also known as noninvasive ventilation [NIV] or by its trade name, "BiPAP") or high-flow nasal cannula (HFNC). Although the data are limited, NIPPV and HFNC, both of which raised concerns for the potential to aerosolize viral particles, have not been shown to pose an increased risk of infection to health care workers who adhere to standards of personal protective equipment use.[6,7] Before discussing how to choose between CPAP, BiPAP, or HFNC for a particular patient, it is worth reviewing technical aspects of these respiratory support modalities.

Continuous Positive Airway Pressure

CPAP uses a tight-fitting nasal or face mask and delivers oxygen to a patient with a continuous positive pressure in the system during both patient inspiration and oxygenation. As such, CPAP is not a "ventilatory" mode because it does not provide additional pressure support during inspiration. Instead, the continuous airway pressure aids in oxygenation by preventing the collapse of alveoli during expiration. The clinician sets both the fraction of inspired oxygen (Fio_2) and the continuous pressure ranging from 4 to 20 cm H_2O.

Noninvasive Positive Pressure Ventilation

NIVPP delivers 2 levels of pressure: an expiratory pressure (EPAP, analogous to CPAP) and an inspiratory pressure (IPAP), additional pressure provided to the patient with each breath. In addition, the clinician sets a backup respiration rate (in the event the patient does not spontaneously breathe or to ensure a certain number of breaths per minute) and the Fio_2. An example of initial NIVPP settings include IPAP = 10 cm H_2O, EPAP = 5 cm H_2O, backup respiration rate = 10 breaths per minute, and Fio_2 = 100%. Patient oxygenation can be further improved by increasing the EPAP to prevent alveolar collapse. NIVPP is a ventilatory mode. Increasing the inspiratory pressure while maintaining the same expiratory pressure (IPAP – EPAP = "delta") will increase the patient's tidal volume. Although hypoxemia is a cardinal feature of pneumonia, increasing the delta will serve to improve ventilation and

CO_2 removal if hypercapnia requires correction, for example, in patients with concomitant asthma or chronic obstructive pulmonary disease (COPD).

High-Flow Nasal Cannula

HFNC systems deliver warmed and humidified oxygen (Fio_2 = 21%–100%) via nasal cannula at flow rates ranging from greater than or equal to 15 to 60 LPM. Typical HFNC settings are Fio_2 between 50% and 100% and a flow rate between 20 and 60 LPM. Both Fio_2 and flow rates are adjusted to improve a patient's oxygen saturation, because increasing the flow rate above the patient's intrinsic minute ventilation prevents entrainment of room air and thus ensures that the patient is receiving the set Fio_2; moreover, high flow rates provide a modest amount of end expiratory pressure that may further improve oxygenation by recruiting more alveoli. The flow rate can also be increased to relieve dyspnea and tachypnea, because HFNC serves to reduce anatomic dead space, thus reducing the work of breathing and aiding in CO_2 clearance.

Choosing Between Continuous Positive Airway, Noninvasive Positive Pressure Ventilation, and High-Flow Nasal Cannula Therapies for the Treatment of Patients with Coronavirus Disease 2019

Before the SARS-CoV-2 pandemic, the use of NIVPP and HFNC for the treatment of pneumonia was supported by limited clinical trial data.[8,9,10] In a study comparing the 2 modalities for the treatment of hypoxic respiratory failure (254 of 310 patients or 82% of trial participants with pneumonia), HFNC was associated with a greater number of ventilator-free days (P = .02) and a lower 90-day mortality rate (P = 0.006).[10]

For the treatment of patients with COVID-19, HFNC (vs low-flow oxygen therapy) has been shown in a retrospective study (n = 379) and in a randomized controlled trial (n = 220) to reduce the need for endotracheal intubation, but not impact mortality.[11,12] However, unlike the prepandemic experience, NIVPP may be superior to HFNC for the treatment of patients with COVID-19. In the Helmet Noninvasive Ventilation versus High-flow Oxygen Therapy in Acute Hypoxemic Respiratory Failure (HENIVOT) trial (n = 109), patients receiving NIPPV via a helmet device, compared with patients receiving HFNC therapy, were less likely to require mechanical ventilation (a secondary study outcome, 30% vs 51%, P = .03), although there was no difference in the number of days free of respiratory support (the primary study outcome).[13] Also, in the RECOVERY-RS trial (n = 1273), patients treated with CPAP compared with HFNC were less likely to reach the combined end point of endotracheal intubation or death within 30 days (36.3% vs 44.4%, P = .03), but this difference was due almost entirely to differences in intubation rates (33.4% vs 41.3%; odd ratio [OR], 0.71 [0.53–0.96]) and not mortality (16.7% vs 19.2%; OR, 0.84 [0.58–1.23]).[14] It should be noted that device intolerance (5.8% vs 0.7% of participants), adverse events (34.2% vs 20.6% of participants), and serious adverse events (1.8% vs 0% of participants), including pneumothoraces and vomiting requiring emergent intubation, were more common in patients receiving CPAP, compared with patients receiving HFNC.

Based entirely on prepandemic data, both the Surviving Sepsis Campaign and the National Institutes of Health (NIH) COVID-19 Treatment Guidelines recommend HFNC over NIVPP (and do not comment on CPAP) for the treatment of patients with hypoxic respiratory therapy despite low-flow oxygen therapy.[15,16] The authors maintain that there is equipoise regarding whether 1 noninvasive respiratory support strategy is superior for the treatment of patients with COVID-19. And considering the evidence supporting both modalities, the authors recommend that choice of an NIV strategy should be based on comorbidities, patient tolerance, and institutional norms. For example,

CPAP or NIVPP may be preferable to HFNC for patients with COVID-19 and either congestive heart failure or COPD. On the other hand, patients who find NIVPP or CPAP uncomfortable are better suited for treatment with HFNC. Finally, institutional experience and resources must be considered. Over the course of the pandemic many health care systems have developed familiarity and expertise with mostly treating patients with HFNC, CPAP, or NIVPP. Pending the results of the ongoing RENOVATE study (NCT03643939) or future trials, the authors see no reason for these practice patterns to change.[17]

PRONING IN NONINTUBATED PATIENTS WITH CORONAVIRUS DISEASE 2019

Proning in the nonintubated (PINI) refers to the strategy of having hospitalized, nonintubated patients with hypoxic respiratory failure resting in the prone rather than the supine position for extended periods. This strategy is sometimes referred to as "awake" prone ventilation, even though this term is a misnomer because intubated patients could clearly be awake or sedated or asleep whether prone or not; similarly nonintubated patients could be awake or asleep. The proposed mechanisms of benefit of prone ventilation have been best studied for the treatment of intubated patients with ARDS before the SARS-CoV-2 pandemic (see section, "Prone ventilation for intubated patients"). Prepandemic, PINI investigations were limited to case series.[18] A meta-analysis performed by Li and colleagues[19] of 10 clinical trials (n = 1985 patients; in actuality 8 trials were analyzed because 2 trials had no events in either arm) involving patients with COVID-19 receiving PINI compared with supine position ventilation showed a reduction in the need for intubation (risk ratio [RR], 0.84; 95% confidence interval [CI], 0.72–0.97), but did not impact mortality (RR, 1.0; 95% CI, 0.70–1.44). Meta-regression analysis further revealed that PINI only reduced the need for intubation among patients receiving NIV modalities or being treated in the ICU. It should also be noted that the results of this meta-analysis are entirely due to results of a meta-trial (consisting of 6 national, randomized open-label trials) authored by Ehrmann and colleagues[20] (n = 1121), and more specifically patients enrolled in 1 particular national trial (n = 430) who had very different baseline characteristics and were managed differently than patients enrolled at other sites.[21] When the meta-analysis performed by Li and colleagues[19] is repeated excluding this national trial and incorporating the results of a more recent randomized trial performed by Alhazzani and colleagues[22] (n = 400), there is no benefit of PINI on intubation rates (RR, 0.89; 95% CI, 0.77–1.03) (**Fig. 1**). Further complicating the interpretation of PINI clinical studies is that the duration of prone positioning varied across clinical trials. In a more recent prospective, multicenter cohort study of 335 patients in the ICU receiving HFNC (187 with PINI, 148 with nonprone positioning) showed that 6 hours or more of PINI reduced the rate of endotracheal intubation and that 8 hours or more of PINI reduced the risk of hospital mortality.[23] This result makes intuitive sense because the only randomized trial to show a mortality benefit of prone positioning in patients with ARDS receiving mechanical ventilations required that patients receive 16 hours of prone ventilation.[24] On the other hand, rather than a dose response, duration of PINI may actually represent a confounder whereby patients who can tolerate longer sessions of PINI are less severely ill. At present, the NIH COVID-19 Treatment Guidelines recommend a trial of PINI for patient with hypoxemia requiring HFNC and for whom endotracheal intubation is not indicated.[16] Although it is unlikely that PINI is harmful, the benefit of this therapy is not established. If PINI is administered to a patient receiving CPAP, HFNC, or NIVPP the authors suggest that the duration of therapy be extended, ideally lasting 8 hours or more a day.

PINI and the risk of intubation in hospitalized patients with COVID-19

Author	Statistics for each study			Death events/Total		Risk ratio and 95% CI
	Risk ratio	Lower limit	Upper limit	PINI	Control	
Alhazzani et al	0.84	0.65	1.09	70 / 205	79 / 195	
Ehrmann et al[a]	0.90	0.74	1.10	120 / 348	131 / 343	
Fralick et al	1.16	0.36	3.71	6 / 126	5 / 122	
Gad et al	1.00	0.24	4.18	3 / 15	3 / 15	
Garcia et al	0.42	0.08	2.26	2 / 159	4 / 134	
Harris et al	0.97	0.15	6.44	2 / 31	2 / 30	
Jayakumar et al	1.00	0.28	3.63	4 / 30	4 / 30	
Johnson et al	2.00	0.20	19.78	2 / 15	1 / 15	
Rosen et al	1.00	0.53	1.90	12 / 36	13 / 39	
Overall	0.89	0.77	1.03	221 / 965	242 / 923	

0.1 0.2　0.5　1　2　5　10
Favors PINI　　Favors control

Heterogeneity P=0.99; I-squared=0%

Fig. 1. Meta-analysis of 9 randomized trials showing the effect of PINI on the risk of intubation for hospitalized patients with COVID-19. [a]Of note, 5 of 6 national trials from the meta-trial led by Ehrmann and colleagues[20] were included in the analysis.

CLINICAL JUDGMENT SHOULD INFORM THE DECISION TO INTUBATE AND INITIATE MECHANICAL VENTILATION

Early in the pandemic, many health care systems adopted a strategy of early intubation of patients with COVID-19.[25] The rationale for this approach was based on 2 concerns: fear of aerosolizing SARS-CoV-2 with NIV (both NIVPP and HFNC) leading to hospital-acquired COVID-19 and the theoretic risk of patient self-inflicted lung injury.[26,27] The risk of NIV leading to hospital-acquired COVID-19 is not supported by 2 clinical studies.[6,7] And analysis of 245 patients in 11 ICUs showed that early intubation (defined as occurring during the first 2 calendar days of their ICU stay) was associated with increased risk of secondary infection and an increased 60-day mortality risk (hazard ratio [HR], 1.74; 95% CI, 1.07–2.83).[28] Traditionally, clinical data guide the decision to initiate mechanical ventilation in a patient with pneumonia, but clinical judgment dictates the ultimate decision.[29] The authors endorse the use of clinical judgment, rather than an early intubation policy or protocol, when deciding when to intubate a patient with COVID-19.

PATIENTS WITH CORONAVIRUS DISEASE 2019 RECEIVING MECHANICAL VENTILATION: TREATING ACUTE RESPIRATORY DISTRESS SYNDROME

ARDS is diagnosed when a patient has acute respiratory failure, a Pao_2: Fio_2 ratio less than 300 mm Hg, and chest radiography showing bilateral infiltrates in the absence of congestive heart failure.[30] Patients with COVID-19 who clinically deteriorate and require mechanical ventilation almost certainly have ARDS and should be treated with previously proven strategies for patients with non-COVID-19 ARDS. In general, ventilator strategies to support patients with ARDS are designed to minimize the so-called ventilator-induced lung injury caused by the overdistension of ventilated lung units (ie, volutrauma) and the repetitive opening and closing of alveoli during the respiratory cycle (ie, atelectrauma).[31] Since the start of the pandemic there have been no compelling data suggesting that patients with ARDS secondary to SARS-CoV-2 infection should be treated differently than those with prepandemic ARDS in terms of mechanical ventilatory support.

Low Tidal Volume Mechanical Ventilation

In a landmark trial, a low tidal volume (6 mL tidal volume/kg ideal body weight) was shown to reduce mortality compared with a high tidal volume (12 mL tidal volume/kg ideal body weight) for the treatment of ARDS.[32] Thus, 6 mL/kg has become the default tidal volume setting for patients with ARDS; however, clinicians should be mindful to try and minimize the plateau pressure (measured during an inspiratory pause, it is an estimate of the mean alveolar pressure) and driving pressures (computed as the plateau pressure minus positive end expiratory pressure).[33,34] It is generally accepted that the plateau pressure should ideally be less than 32 mm H_2O and that driving pressure should be less than 15 cm H_2O.[34,35]

Prone Ventilation for Intubated Patients

Prone ventilation has a multitude of beneficial effects on the pulmonary system in ARDS, including recruitment of alveoli, improvement in ventilation and perfusion, and lung compliance.[30,36] The PROSEVA study, a multicenter randomized controlled trial involving 466 patients with severe ARDS demonstrated that prone ventilation for 16 h/d compared with ventilation in the supine position improved 28-day mortality (16% vs 32.8%, $P < .001$).[24] It is important to note that a subsequent meta-analysis showed that the mortality benefit of prone ventilation for the treatment of ARDS was only detectable when patients were concomitantly receiving low tidal volume ventilation.[37] Thus, patients with ARDS are best treated with low tidal volume ventilation, while simultaneously receiving prone ventilation.

Paralysis

Chemical paralysis may have a role in ensuring that an individual patient is synchronous with the ventilator and safely maintained in the prone position; however, the routine use of neuromuscular blocking agents has not been consistently shown to improve outcomes in the treatment of patients with ARDS. Paralysis was unlikely to have affected the results of the PROSEVA trial because patients in both study arms were similarly treated with neuromuscular blocking agents (91% of patients receiving prone ventilation and 82% of supine patients). And whereas a study by Papazian and colleagues[38] (n = 340) showed that a 48-hour course of a continuous infusion of a neuromuscular blocking agent increased survival among intubated patients with ARDS, a subsequent, larger trial (n = 1006) by Moss and colleagues was stopped at the second interim analysis due to futility.[39] Thus, use of paralytics should be individualized in ARDS rather than given routinely.[40]

Extracorporeal Membrane Oxygenation as a Rescue Therapy

Despite the use of low tidal volume and prone positioning, patients with ARDS remain susceptible to ventilator-induced lung injury, refractory hypoxemia, and/or refractory hypercapnia. With extracorporeal membrane oxygenation (ECMO), blood is removed from the patient via a large venous catheter, pumped through an extracorporeal membrane in which carbon dioxide is removed and oxygen is delivered, and returned via another large catheter to the right atrium. Patients receiving ECMO therapy are placed on minimal mechanical ventilatory settings eliminating any ventilator-induced lung injury with the hope that lung function will recover over time. Although simple in concept, the actual delivery of ECMO and ECMO-related care requires expertise, costly resources, and is associated with a host of risks and potential complications for an already critically ill patient.[41] Before theSARS-CoV-2 pandemic, in 2 randomized controlled trials, ECMO was not shown to be superior to conventional respiratory care for the treatment of patients with ARDS.[42,43] The Conventional Ventilatory Support versus Extracorporeal Membrane Oxygenation for Severe Adult Respiratory Failure (CESAR) trial (n = 180) was particularly interesting because it showed that patients with ARDS who were *transferred* to a tertiary center specializing in ECMO experienced a 16% survival benefit without severe disability. However, the relative improvement in outcome may have been due to better general care provided at a center of excellence because only 75% of patients in the study arm received ECMO.

Our current understanding of the effectiveness of ECMO for the treatment of ARDS secondary to SARS-CoV-2 is limited in the absence of randomized controlled clinical trials. Retrospective data from one study showed that patients with COVID-19 who were treated with ECMO had an estimated 60-day mortality of 31%, which is similar to ECMO-treated patients before the start of the pandemic.[42,44] In a subsequent, larger trial (n = 4812) that included patients from later in the pandemic, the investigators describe a mortality rate for patients with COVID-19 treated with ECMO of greater than 50%.[45] Possibly the most compelling evidence supporting the use of ECMO in the treatment of COVID-19 can be found in a study performed by Gannon and colleagues[46] that compared the mortality rates of 35 patients who were accepted for transfer by a tertiary center and treated with ECMO, versus 55 patients who were also deemed to be eligible candidates for treatment, but because of hospital capacity strain were not transferred to the tertiary center and subsequently did not receive ECMO. The in-hospital mortality rate for those patients who underwent ECMO was 42.9%, versus 89.1% for those patients who were unable to receive ECMO (adjusted HR, 0.23; 95% CI, 0.12–0.43; $P < .001$). However, the findings of this small, retrospective study must be interpreted cautiously in the context of a health system that may have been overwhelmed during the pandemic.

The authors recommend that patients with COVID-19 who are intubated and failing standard ARDS respiratory supportive strategies be referred for ECMO early in their clinical course especially because determining eligibility varies across centers. Most ECMO programs evaluate patients based on expert opinion in conjunction with established criteria that takes into consideration patient age, body mass index, duration of mechanical ventilation, comorbidities (neurologic function specifically), and extrapulmonary organ dysfunction.[47] The authors further urge clinicians taking care of patients with COVID-19 to engage preferentially with high-volume ECMO centers, because programs with less experience are more likely to have higher mortality rates.[45]

GENERAL CRITICAL CARE SUPPORTIVE CARE

The experience of the SARS-CoV-2 pandemic has served to reinforce the importance of many established supportive measures used to treat all critically ill patients.

Anticoagulation

Rates of deep venous thromboembolism and pulmonary embolism among critically ill patients with COVID-19 are comparable to those among critically ill patients without COVID-19.[48] Moreover, a large (n = 1098) open-label adaptive clinical trial, in which critically ill patients with COVID-19 were randomized to either therapeutic-dose anticoagulation with heparin or pharmacologic thromboprophylaxis, was stopped early for futility.[49] Although not statistically significant, major bleeding occurred more often in patients assigned to receive therapeutic dose anticoagulation compared with patients who were treated with usual care pharmacologic thromboprophylaxis. In light of these data, the authors agree with the NIH COVID-19 Treatment Guidelines recommending pharmacologic thromboprophylaxis and not routine therapeutic-dose anticoagulation for critically ill patients with COVID-19 (NIH).[16]

Fluid Management

There are inherent risks for critically ill patients who are either under or over fluid resuscitated. To date, there are no randomized clinical trials comparing different fluid management strategies for critically ill patients with COVID-19. For the treatment of non-COVID-19-related ARDS, conservative rather than liberal fluid management strategy was shown to increase the number of ventilator-free days (14.6 vs 12.1, $P < .0001$) (a secondary study outcome) albeit without any mortality benefit (the primary study outcome).[50] Considering respiratory failure is the cause or is present in more than 80% of patients who die of COVID-19, the authors recommend a conservative fluid strategy for patients with COVID-19 receiving mechanical ventilation.[51] Estimating the fluid status of a critically ill patient can be challenging; besides daily weight and fluid balance measures, point-of-care ultrasonography can be a useful adjunct to aid in guiding diuretic or fluid resuscitation decisions for the critically ill patient with COVID-19.[52,53]

Minimizing Risk Factors for Delirium

Unfortunately, critically ill patients with COVID-19 have been at high risk for developing delirium, with a reported incidence of greater than 50%.[54,55] In part, this finding may represent an unintended consequence of both the supportive care measures (eg, the frequent use of deep sedation in conjunction with paralytic agents) and hospital infection prevention policies aimed at protecting both health care works and family members and friends of patients. As with all critically ill patients, clinicians should screen all mechanically ventilated patients for delirium using a validated tool such as the The Confusion Assessment method for the ICU (CAM-ICU).[56] Limiting the use of sedative/anxiolytics, especially benzodiazepines, has been the cornerstone of minimizing delirium in the ICU.[57] For example, it may not be necessary to administer neuromuscular blocking agents (and therefore concomitant high-dose sedatives) when patients are undergoing prone ventilation. As previously described, therapeutic paralysis has not been shown to be definitively beneficial in the treatment of patients with ARDS in the prepandemic era; likewise, there are no clinical trials in patients with COVID-19 supporting the routine use of neuromuscular blockade. In an observational study of 156 patients, similar improvement in Pao_2: Fio_2 and O_2Sat: Fio_2 ratios were noted postinitiation of prone ventilation in patients being treated with and without paralysis.[40] Furthermore, there were no adverse events associated with prone positioning performed without neuromuscular blockade. Restrictive hospital visitation policies instituted during the pandemic may also have added to the overall burden of delirium experienced by critically ill patients. Although not consistent, there is prepandemic evidence to suggest that flexible and extended visiting hours can lower the incidence of delirium and anxiety among critically ill patients.[58] Performed during the pandemic, a study comparing rates of delirium among patients with COVID-19 before and after the implementation of an ICU visitor ban did not show a significant increase in the overall incidence of delirium (27.4% vs 30.9%, respectively, $P = .162$); however, a restrictive visitor policy was associated with an increase of hyperactive and mixed subgroups of delirium and high anxiety levels.[59] Thus, evolving hospital visitor policies designed to continue to prevent hospital transmission of SARS-CoV-2 should be tempered by the potential importance of patient-visitor interactions.

SUMMARY

The early adoption of supportive care strategies for the management of ARDS, developed during the prepandemic era, may have been responsible for the improvement in critical care outcomes noted during the early phase (March to May, 2020) of the pandemic. Anecdotally, those of us who have taken care of critically ill patients throughout the pandemic have marveled at how proficient ICU teams of nurses and respiratory therapists have become at routinely repositioning patients with COVID-19, some of whom have chest tubes and are simultaneously receiving continuous renal replacement therapy. In addition to prone ventilation and adherence to low tidal volume ventilation, the expansive use of other measures such as NPPV, and HFNC, have the potential to reduce the need for intubation, if not possibly mortality, for critically ill patients with COVID-19. And although PINI is intriguing, its clinical benefit for patients with COVID-19 has not been established; whether longer durations of therapy (>8 hours) could be beneficial remains to be proven. Finally, the experience of the pandemic has also resulted in recognition of the importance of providing quality critical adjunctive therapies such as deep vein thrombosis prophylaxis, attention to fluid management, and minimizing sedation and neuromuscular blockade for the purpose of reducing the risk of delirium. Despite these early advances, mortality rates among critically ill patients with COVID-19 are largely unchanged over the later phases of the pandemic.[60,61] Although the development of therapeutics to treat patients with severe disease specifically needs to be the primary strategy, supportive care—either by expanding the use of current strategies or developing new approaches—can serve an adjunctive role to improve clinical outcomes for critically ill patients with COVID-19.

CLINICS CARE POINTS

- Lung size does not change with either weight loss or weight gain. Ideal body weight and not actual body weight in kilograms should be used when choosing a low tidal volume for the treatment of mechanically ventilated patients with COVID-19 and ARDS.

- The nomenclature of respiratory supportive care is inherently confusing. NIV, NIPPV, bilevel, and BiPAP (a trade name) are synonymous and describe a system that uses 2 different pressures—IPAP and EPAP. CPAP as the name implies delivers one continuous pressure. HFNC delivers oxygen flow rates ranging from greater than or equal to 15 to 60 LPM as opposed to low-flow or nasal cannula oxygen, which delivers oxygen from 1 to 14 LPM.

- For patients receiving HFNC, the Fio_2 should be titrated based on the patient's pulse oximetry, whereas the flow rate should be titrated based on the clinical assessment of the patient including presence of dyspnea and breathing pattern.

- Not all patients with COVID-19 and ARDS who are intubated and receiving prone ventilation require chemical paralysis; rather, the decision to administer neuromuscular blocking agents should be individualized based on patient safety and ability to maintain synchrony with the ventilator.

- Basic tenants of supportive critical care established before the pandemic remain relevant for the management of patients with severe COVID-19

DISCLOSURE

D.A. Sweeney has nothing to declare. A. Malhotra is funded by the National Institutes of Health. He reports income related to medical education from Livanova, Jazz,

Equillium, and Corvus, unrelated to the content of this manuscript. ResMed provided a philanthropic donation to UC San Diego.

REFERENCES

1. Auld SC, Caridi-Scheible M, Robichaux C, et al. Declines in Mortality Over Time for Critically Ill Adults With Coronavirus Disease 2019. Crit Care Med 2020;48(12): e1382–4.
2. Carbonell R, Urgeles S, Rodriguez A, et al. Mortality comparison between the first and second/third waves among 3,795 critical COVID-19 patients with pneumonia admitted to the ICU: A multicentre retrospective cohort study. Lancet Reg Health Eur 2021;11:100243.
3. Ely EW, Ramanan AV, Kartman CE, et al. Efficacy and safety of baricitinib plus standard of care for the treatment of critically ill hospitalised adults with COVID-19 on invasive mechanical ventilation or extracorporeal membrane oxygenation: an exploratory, randomised, placebo-controlled trial. Lancet Respir Med 2022;10(4):327–36.
4. Group RC, Horby P, Lim WS, et al. Dexamethasone in Hospitalized Patients with Covid-19. N Engl J Med 2021;384(8):693–704.
5. Whittaker R, Brathen Kristofferson A, Valcarcel Salamanca B, et al. Length of hospital stay and risk of intensive care admission and in-hospital death among COVID-19 patients in Norway: a register-based cohort study comparing patients fully vaccinated with an mRNA vaccine to unvaccinated patients. Clin Microbiol Infect 2022;28(6):871–8.
6. Westafer LM, Soares WE 3rd, Salvador D, et al. No evidence of increasing COVID-19 in health care workers after implementation of high flow nasal cannula: A safety evaluation. Am J Emerg Med 2021;39:158–61.
7. Costa W, Miguel JP, Prado FDS, et al. Noninvasive ventilation and high-flow nasal cannula in patients with acute hypoxemic respiratory failure by covid-19: A retrospective study of the feasibility, safety and outcomes. Respir Physiol Neurobiol 2022;298:103842.
8. Confalonieri M, Potena A, Carbone G, et al. Acute respiratory failure in patients with severe community-acquired pneumonia. A prospective randomized evaluation of noninvasive ventilation. Am J Respir Crit Care Med 1999;160(5 Pt 1): 1585–91.
9. Ferrer M, Esquinas A, Leon M, et al. Noninvasive ventilation in severe hypoxemic respiratory failure: a randomized clinical trial. Am J Respir Crit Care Med 2003; 168(12):1438–44.
10. Frat JP, Thille AW, Mercat A, et al. High-flow oxygen through nasal cannula in acute hypoxemic respiratory failure. N Engl J Med 2015;372(23):2185–96.
11. Ospina-Tascon GA, Calderon-Tapia LE, Garcia AF, et al. Effect of High-Flow Oxygen Therapy vs Conventional Oxygen Therapy on Invasive Mechanical Ventilation and Clinical Recovery in Patients With Severe COVID-19: A Randomized Clinical Trial. JAMA 2021;326(21):2161–71.
12. Demoule A, Vieillard Baron A, Darmon M, et al. High-Flow Nasal Cannula in Critically Ill Patients with Severe COVID-19. Am J Respir Crit Care Med 2020;202(7): 1039–42.
13. Grieco DL, Menga LS, Cesarano M, et al. Effect of Helmet Noninvasive Ventilation vs High-Flow Nasal Oxygen on Days Free of Respiratory Support in Patients With COVID-19 and Moderate to Severe Hypoxemic Respiratory Failure: The HENIVOT Randomized Clinical Trial. JAMA 2021;325(17):1731–43.

14. Perkins GD, Ji C, Connolly BA, et al. Effect of Noninvasive Respiratory Strategies on Intubation or Mortality Among Patients With Acute Hypoxemic Respiratory Failure and COVID-19: The RECOVERY-RS Randomized Clinical Trial. JAMA 2022; 327(6):546–58.

15. Alhazzani W, Evans L, Alshamsi F, et al. Surviving Sepsis Campaign Guidelines on the Management of Adults With Coronavirus Disease 2019 (COVID-19) in the ICU: First Update. Crit Care Med 2021;49(3):e219–34.

16. Panel. C-TG. Coronavirus Disease 2019 (COVID-19) treatment Guidelines. National Institutes of Health. Available at: https://www.covid19treatmentguidelines. nih.gov/. Accessed April 7, 2022.

17. High-Flow Nasal Oxygen Cannula Compared to Non-Invasive Ventilation in Adult Patients With AcuTE Respiratory Failure (RENOVATE). Available at: https:// clinicaltrials.gov/ct2/show/NCT03643939. Accessed April 9, 2022.

18. Weatherald J, Solverson K, Zuege DJ, et al. Awake prone positioning for COVID-19 hypoxemic respiratory failure: A rapid review. J Crit Care 2021;61:63–70.

19. Li J, Luo J, Pavlov I, et al. Awake prone positioning for non-intubated patients with COVID-19-related acute hypoxaemic respiratory failure: a systematic review and meta-analysis. Lancet Respir Med 2022. https://doi.org/10.1016/S2213-2600(22) 00043-1.

20. Ehrmann S, Li J, Ibarra-Estrada M, et al. Awake prone positioning for COVID-19 acute hypoxaemic respiratory failure: a randomised, controlled, multinational, open-label meta-trial. Lancet Respir Med 2021;9(12):1387–95.

21. McGuire WC, Pearce AK, Malhotra A. Prone positioning might reduce the need for intubation in people with severe COVID-19. Lancet Respir Med 2021;9(12): e110.

22. Alhazzani W, Parhar KKS, Weatherald J, et al. Effect of Awake Prone Positioning on Endotracheal Intubation in Patients With COVID-19 and Acute Respiratory Failure: A Randomized Clinical Trial. JAMA 2022. https://doi.org/10.1001/jama. 2022.7993.

23. Esperatti M, Busico M, Fuentes NA, et al. Impact of exposure time in awake prone positioning on clinical outcomes of patients with COVID-19-related acute respiratory failure treated with high-flow nasal oxygen: a multicenter cohort study. Crit Care 2022;26(1):16.

24. Guérin C, Reignier J, Richard J-C, et al. Prone Positioning in Severe Acute Respiratory Distress Syndrome. N Engl J Med 2013;368(23):2159–68.

25. Goyal P, Choi JJ, Pinheiro LC, et al. Clinical Characteristics of Covid-19 in New York City. N Engl J Med 2020;382(24):2372–4.

26. Gattinoni L, Chiumello D, Caironi P, et al. COVID-19 pneumonia: different respiratory treatments for different phenotypes? Intensive Care Med 2020;46(6): 1099–102.

27. Haymet A, Bassi GL, Fraser JF. Airborne spread of SARS-CoV-2 while using high-flow nasal cannula oxygen therapy: myth or reality? Intensive Care Med 2020; 46(12):2248–51.

28. Dupuis C, Bouadma L, de Montmollin E, et al. Association Between Early Invasive Mechanical Ventilation and Day-60 Mortality in Acute Hypoxemic Respiratory Failure Related to Coronavirus Disease-2019 Pneumonia. Crit Care Explor 2021;3(1): e0329.

29. Tobin MJ. The criteria used to justify endotracheal intubation of patients with COVID-19 are worrisome. Can J Anaesth 2021;68(2):258–9.

30. Pearce AK, McGuire WC, Malhotra A. Prone Positioning in Acute Respiratory Distress Syndrome. NEJM Evid 2022;1(2). EVIDra2100046.

31. Thompson BT, Chambers RC, Liu KD. Acute Respiratory Distress Syndrome. N Engl J Med 2017;377(6):562–72.

32. Acute Respiratory Distress Syndrome N, Brower RG, Matthay MA, et al. Ventilation with lower tidal volumes as compared with traditional tidal volumes for acute lung injury and the acute respiratory distress syndrome. N Engl J Med 2000; 342(18):1301–8.

33. Amato MBP, Meade MO, Slutsky AS, et al. Driving Pressure and Survival in the Acute Respiratory Distress Syndrome. N Engl J Med 2015;372(8):747–55.

34. Tobin MJ. Culmination of an Era in Research on the Acute Respiratory Distress Syndrome. N Engl J Med 2000;342(18):1360–1.

35. MacIntyre N. Ventilator Management Guided by Driving Pressure: A Better Way to Protect the Lungs? Crit Care Med 2018;46(2):338–9.

36. Guerin C, Albert RK, Beitler J, et al. Prone position in ARDS patients: why, when, how and for whom. Intensive Care Med 2020;46(12):2385–96.

37. Beitler JR, Shaefi S, Montesi SB, et al. Prone positioning reduces mortality from acute respiratory distress syndrome in the low tidal volume era: a meta-analysis. Intensive Care Med 2014;40(3):332–41.

38. Papazian L, Forel JM, Gacouin A, et al. Neuromuscular blockers in early acute respiratory distress syndrome. N Engl J Med 2010;363(12):1107–16.

39. Early Neuromuscular Blockade in the Acute Respiratory Distress Syndrome. N Engl J Med 2019;380(21):1997–2008.

40. Cotton S, Husain AA, Meehan M, et al. A2508 - The Influence of Paralytics on the Safety and Efficacy of Prone Positioning in Covid19 ARDS. presented at: American Thoracic Society; 2021; Session TP48 - TP048 COVID: ARDS clinical studies.

41. Brodie D, Slutsky AS, Combes A. Extracorporeal Life Support for Adults With Respiratory Failure and Related Indications: A Review. JAMA 2019;322(6):557–68.

42. Combes A, Hajage D, Capellier G, et al. Extracorporeal Membrane Oxygenation for Severe Acute Respiratory Distress Syndrome. N Engl J Med 2018;378(21): 1965–75.

43. Peek GJ, Mugford M, Tiruvoipati R, et al. Efficacy and economic assessment of conventional ventilatory support versus extracorporeal membrane oxygenation for severe adult respiratory failure (CESAR): a multicentre randomised controlled trial. Lancet 2009;374(9698):1351–63.

44. Schmidt M, Hajage D, Lebreton G, et al. Extracorporeal membrane oxygenation for severe acute respiratory distress syndrome associated with COVID-19: a retrospective cohort study. Lancet Respir Med 2020;8(11):1121–31.

45. Barbaro RP, MacLaren G, Boonstra PS, et al. Extracorporeal membrane oxygenation for COVID-19: evolving outcomes from the international Extracorporeal Life Support Organization Registry. Lancet 2021;398(10307):1230–8.

46. Gannon WD, Stokes JW, Francois SA, et al. Association Between Availability of ECMO and Mortality in COVID-19 Patients Eligible for ECMO: A Natural Experiment. Am J Respir Crit Care Med 2022. https://doi.org/10.1164/rccm.202110-2399LE.

47. Badulak J, Antonini MV, Stead CM, et al. Extracorporeal Membrane Oxygenation for COVID-19: Updated 2021 Guidelines from the Extracorporeal Life Support Organization. ASAIO J 2021;67(5):485–95.

48. Gallastegui N, Zhou JY, Drygalski AV, et al. Pulmonary Embolism Does Not Have an Unusually High Incidence Among Hospitalized COVID19 Patients. Clin Appl Thromb Hemost 2021;27. 1076029621996471.

49. Investigators R-C, Investigators AC-a, Investigators A, et al. Therapeutic Antico-agulation with Heparin in Critically Ill Patients with Covid-19. N Engl J Med 2021; 385(9):777–89.
50. National Heart L, Blood Institute Acute Respiratory Distress Syndrome Clinical Tri-als N, Wiedemann HP, et al. Comparison of two fluid-management strategies in acute lung injury. N Engl J Med 2006;354(24):2564–75.
51. Kazory A, Ronco C, McCullough PA. SARS-CoV-2 (COVID-19) and intravascular volume management strategies in the critically ill. Proc (Bayl Univ Med Cent) 2020;0(0):1–6.
52. Koratala A, Ronco C, Kazory A. Need for Objective Assessment of Volume Status in Critically Ill Patients with COVID-19: The Tri-POCUS Approach. Cardiorenal Med 2020;10(4):209–16.
53. Thalappillil R, White RS, Tam CW. POCUS to Guide Fluid Therapy in COVID-19. J Cardiothorac Vasc Anesth 2020;34(10):2854–6.
54. Pun BT, Badenes R, Heras La Calle G, et al. Prevalence and risk factors for delirium in critically ill patients with COVID-19 (COVID-D): a multicentre cohort study. Lancet Respir Med 2021;9(3):239–50.
55. Williamson CA, Faiver L, Nguyen AM, et al. Incidence, Predictors and Outcomes of Delirium in Critically Ill Patients With COVID-19. Neurohospitalist 2022; 12(1):31–7.
56. Ely EW, Inouye SK, Bernard GR, et al. Delirium in mechanically ventilated pa-tients: validity and reliability of the confusion assessment method for the intensive care unit (CAM-ICU). JAMA 2001;286(21):2703–10.
57. Pandharipande P, Cotton BA, Shintani A, et al. Prevalence and risk factors for development of delirium in surgical and trauma intensive care unit patients. J Trauma 2008;65(1):34–41.
58. Rosa RG, Tonietto TF, da Silva DB, et al. Effectiveness and Safety of an Extended ICU Visitation Model for Delirium Prevention: A Before and After Study. Crit Care Med 2017;45(10):1660–7.
59. Kim B, Cho J, Park JY, et al. Delirium and Anxiety Outcomes Related to Visiting Policy Changes in the Intensive Care Unit During the COVID-19 Pandemic. Orig-inal Research. Front Aging Neurosci 2022;14. https://doi.org/10.3389/fnagi.2022. 845105.
60. Anesi GL, Jablonski J, Harhay MO, et al. Characteristics, Outcomes, and Trends of Patients With COVID-19-Related Critical Illness at a Learning Health System in the United States. Ann Intern Med 2021;174(5):613–21.
61. Auld SC, Harrington KRV, Adelman MW, et al. Trends in ICU Mortality From Coro-navirus Disease 2019: A Tale of Three Surges. Crit Care Med 2022;50(2):245–55.

Management of Highly Resistant Gram-Negative Infections in the Intensive Care Unit in the Era of Novel Antibiotics

Cornelius J. Clancy, MD*, Minh Hong Nguyen, MD

KEYWORDS

- Antimicrobial resistance • Gram-negative infections • Intensive care unit
- Treatment • Antibiotics

KEY POINTS

- Since 2015, several antibiotics with activity against highly antimicrobial-resistant Gram-negative bacteria have been approved. These antibiotics offer safe and effective alternatives to older drugs such as polymyxins and aminoglycosides, which were previous salvage agents for the treatment of highly antimicrobial-resistant Gram-negative bacterial infections.
- The Infectious Diseases Society of America (IDSA) and European Society for Clinical Microbiology and Infectious Diseases (ESCMID) have recently published guidance and guidelines, respectively, for the treatment of highly resistant Gram-negative bacterial infections. These documents offer recommendations for incorporating new antibiotics into clinical practice.
- To make the best use of new antibiotics, clinicians should understand the microbiology and epidemiology of Gram-negative bacterial infections at their hospitals and in their clinical units. Clinicians and antimicrobial stewardship programs should formulate treatment algorithms that are most appropriate for their practices, which can provide a foundation for treatment decisions in individual patients.

Antimicrobial-resistant (AMR) bacteria and fungi present major challenges to public health globally. According to the Centers for Disease Control and Prevention (CDC), AMR pathogens cause >2.8 million infections and 35,000 deaths per year in the United States (U.S.) from 2012 to 2017.[1] The European Center of Disease and Control estimated that AMR bacteria accounted for 600,000 infections and 27,000 attributable

Department of Medicine, University of Pittsburgh, 867 Scaife Hall, 3550 Terrace Street, Pittsburgh, PA 15203, USA
* Corresponding author.
E-mail address: cjc76@pitt.edu

Infect Dis Clin N Am 36 (2022) 791–823
https://doi.org/10.1016/j.idc.2022.08.004
0891-5520/22/Published by Elsevier Inc.

id.theclinics.com

deaths in Europe in 2015.[2] Almost 70% of these infections and deaths were due to multi-drug-resistant (MDR) Gram-negative bacteria. The Review on Antimicrobial Resistance, commissioned by the United Kingdom government in 2014, projected that AMR infections could cause 10 million deaths annually by 2050, in the absence of coordinated preventive and antibiotic development strategies.[3] The World Health Organization and CDC have identified a number of Gram-negative bacteria as priorities for research and development, including 3rd generation cephalosporin- and carbapenem-resistant Enterobacterales (CRE), MDR-*Pseudomonas aeruginosa*, and carbapenem-resistant *Acinetobacter baumannii* (CRAB).[1,4]

Several antibiotics with activity against MDR Gram-negative bacteria have been approved by the US Food and Drug Administration since 2014. Uptake of these drugs by clinicians has been steady, but sluggish.[5–7] The reasons for the relatively slow uptake are not precisely defined, but factors such as limited clinical trial data specifically for MDR infections and cost likely have contributed.[8] The Infectious Diseases Society of America (IDSA) and European Society of Clinical Microbiology and Infectious Diseases (ESCMID) recently published antibiotic treatment recommendations for Gram-negative bacterial infections in hospitalized patients.[9–11] In part to facilitate rapid dissemination and frequent updates, IDSA recommendations were put forth in guidance documents that were based on comprehensive (but not necessarily systematic) reviews of the literature, clinical experience, and opinion of 6 experts. IDSA guidance focused on infections by AmpC- and extended-spectrum β-lactamase (ESBL)-producing Enterobacterales (which manifest phenotypically as 3rd generation cephalosporin resistance), CRE, MDR-*P. aeruginosa*, CRAB, and *Stenotrophomonas maltophilia*. In contrast, ESCMID issued guidelines that were based on systematic literature review and rigorous GRADE (Grading of Recommendations Assessment, Development, and Evaluation) criteria. They addressed infections by 3rd generation cephalosporin-resistant enterobacterales, CRE, MDR-*P aeruginosa*, and CRAB. An editorial that accompanied ESCMID guidelines offered a succinct summary of similarities and differences between these recommendations and those in the IDSA guidance.[12]

In this article, we will discuss the management of highly resistant Gram-negative bacterial infections in the era of new antibiotics. The discussion will focus in particular on the treatment of intensive care unit (ICU) patients, which is fitting since the pathogens disproportionately infect critically ill hosts. We address the 6 pathogens included in the IDSA guidance documents, since these are the most common and difficult to treat MDR Gram-negative bacteria in ICUs. We will highlight IDSA and ESCMID recommendations, and review background data and rationales used to justify them.

ANTIBIOTICS ACTIVE AGAINST MULTI-DRUG-RESISTANT GRAM-NEGATIVE BACTERIA

Antibiotics with activity against MDR-Gram negative bacteria and their spectra against specific pathogens are shown in **Tables 1** (new agents) and **2** (old agents). Drugs approved by FDA since the end of 2014 include β-lactam/β-lactamase inhibitors (ceftolozane-tazobactam, ceftazidime-avibactam, meropenem-vaborbactam, imipenem-cilastatin-relebactam), a novel aminoglycoside (plazomicin), a novel tetracycline derivative (eravacycline), and a first-in-class cephalosporin-catechol-type siderophore (cefiderocol). Cefiderocol binds to iron via the siderophore and is transported into bacterial cells, where the cephalosporin moiety dissociates, interacts with penicillin-binding protein (PBP)-3, and inhibits cell wall synthesis.[13,14] For the other agents, mechanisms of action are consistent with antibiotic class.

Table 1
Spectra of activity of new antibiotics against MDR gram-negative bacteria *in vitro*.

New agents	ESBL-E	CRE Non-CP	CRE KPC	CRE OXA-48	CRE MBL	DTR-PA	CRAB	Comments
C-T						1		A preferred agent vs. DTR-PA infections; alternative against MDR-PA infections
C-A						2		A preferred agent vs infections by CRE with no carbapenemase, or with KPC and OXA-48; a preferred or alternative agent vs. DTR-PA infections; in combination with aztreonam, it may be a preferred agent against an alternative agent as part of combination vs. *S. maltophilia* infections
M-V								A preferred agent vs. infections by CRE with no carbapenemase, or with KPC
I-R						3		A preferred agent vs. infections by CRE with no carbapenemase, or with KPC; alternative agent vs. DTR-PA infections
PLZ				4	5	6	6	May be alternative agent in selected cases
ERV								May be alternative agent in selected cases
CFD							7	Alternative vs. CRE and DTR-PA infections

Abbreviations: C-A, ceftazidime-avibactam; CFD, cefiderocol; CRAB, carbapenem-resistant *Acinetobacter baumannii*; CRE, carbapenem-resistant Enterobacterales; C-T, ceftolozane-tazobactam; DTR-PA, difficult-to-treat resistance *Pseudomonas aeruginosa*; ERV, eravacycline; ESBL-E, extended-spectrum β-lactamase-producing Enterobacterales; I-R, imipenem-cilastatin-relebactam; KPC, *K. pneumoniae* carbapenemase; MBL, metallo-β-lactamaseMDR, multi-drug resistant; M-V, meropenem-vaborbactam; Non-CP, noncarbapenemase producing; PLZ, plazomicin.

1. Decreased activity against carbapenemase-producing PA; most carbapenem resistance among PA in the United States is not due to carbapenemase production; 2. MICs typically higher than and closer to breakpoint than those of C-T; clinical significance is unknown; 3. Not active against MBL-PA; most carbapenem resistance among PA in the United States is not due to MBL production; 4. Active against majority of OXA-48-producing strains, but increased resistance reported; 5. Not active against a number of New Delhi metallo-β-lactamases; 6. Activity comparable to that of other aminoglycosides; 7. Activity *in vitro*, but performance against CRAB infections in a randomized trial was worse than that of alternative, best available therapy; precise clinical roles of CFD in general await clarification. Red: Not active; Green: Active; Yellow: Intermediate activity.

Table 2
Spectra of activity of old antibiotics against MDR gram-negative bacteria *in vitro*

Old agents	ESBL-E	CRE Non-CP	KPC	OXA-48	MBL	DTR-PA	CRAB	Comments
Poly								Limited by toxicity. May be alternative agent in selected cases
AGs								Limited by toxicity. May be alternative agent in selected cases
AZTR								Combination formulation with avibactam in pipeline
TGC								May be alternative agent in selected cases

Abbreviations: AGs, aminoglycosides; AZTR, aztreonam; CRAB, carbapenem-resistant *Acinetobacter baumannii*; CRE, carbapenem-resistant Enterobacterales; DTR-PA, difficult-to-treat resistance *Pseudomonas aeruginosa*; ESBL-E, extended-spectrum β-lactamase-producing Enterobacterales; KPC, *K. pneumoniae* carbapenemase; MBL, metallo-β-lactamase; MDR, multi-drug resistant; Non-CP, noncarbapenemase producing; Poly, polymyxins; TGC, tigecycline. Red: Not active; Green: Active; Yellow: Intermediate activity.

Treatment of Infections by Multi-Drug-Resistant Gram-Negative Bacteria

Treatment recommendations by IDSA and ESCMID for infections by the MDR Gram-negative bacterial infections mentioned above are summarized in **Table 3**, and discussed by pathogen in the sections later in discussion. Antibiotic dosing recommendations are presented in **Table 4**.

To use IDSA and ESCMID recommendations most effectively and to treat MDR Gram-negative bacterial infections optimally, intensivists should understand microbiology and epidemiology at their hospitals and in their ICUs. Clinicians and antimicrobial stewardship programs should formulate treatment algorithms that are most appropriate for their practices, which can provide a foundation for treatment decisions in individual patients.

Infections by AmpC β-Lactamase Producing Enterobacterales

Background

It is important for intensivists to understand inducible AmpC β-lactamase production, and when to consider it in making treatment decisions. Inducible expression of chromosomal *ampC* genes by certain Enterobacterales can occur in the presence of specific antibiotics, leading to increased minimum inhibitory concentrations (MICs).[15–18] In these situations, an Enterobacterales strain that originally tests as susceptible to the inducing antibiotic may become resistant after treatment is started. This phenomenon may be observed after only a few antibiotic doses.[19] Clinicians should dispense with SPACE or SPICE as acronyms for bacteria at particular risk for inducible AmpC production.[15,19–22] If a mnemonic is to be used, HECK-Yes more accurately captures the bacteria of greatest concern: *Hafnia alvei, Enterobacter cloacae, Citrobacter freundii, Klebsiella* (formerly *Enterobacter*) *aerogenes* and *Yersinia enterocolitica*. The greatest clinical challenges are posed by *E cloacae, C freundii*, and *Klebsiella aerogenes*, which are fairly common ICU pathogens and most likely to become β-lactam resistant.

AmpC induction is most relevant upon exposure of at-risk bacterium to ceftriaxone, ceftazidime, and piperacillin.[15,23–26] More narrow-spectrum β-lactams can be potent AmpC inducers, but the organisms above will generally test nonsusceptible to these agents even at basal *ampC* expression.[27,28] Conversely, ceftriaxone, ceftazidime, and piperacillin are relatively weak inducers,[28] but they are highly susceptible to AmpC hydrolysis.[12,13] Piperacillin can be hydrolyzed even in the presence of tazobactam.[23–26] Emergence of ceftriaxone resistance during treatment has been reported in ~8%-40% of *E cloacae, K aerogenes* or *C freundii* infections.[18,27–31] Therefore, ceftriaxone, ceftazidime and piperacillin -tazobactam are best avoided against infections by these pathogens, even if strains test susceptible to the agents. Data on the emergence of resistance during the treatment of *H alvei* and *Y enterocolitica* infections are more limited,[32–35] but it is advisable in critically ill patients to avoid ceftriaxone, ceftazidime, or piperacillin -tazobactam in favor of another agent that is active *in vitro*. Clinically significant chromosomal *ampC* induction is rare in other bacteria previously thought to be at-risk, such as *Serratia marcescens, Morganella morganii*, and *Providencia species*.[18,29,32] If these pathogens are implicated in infections of critically ill patients, treatment decisions can be guided by susceptibility data.

Treatment

In general, cefepime is the preferred choice for treating critically ill patients infected by bacteria at-risk for chromosomal *ampC* induction, if MIC is ≤ 2 μg/mL. A cefepime MIC ≥4 μg/mL may signal ESBL co-production, in which case responses to the agent are suboptimal.[9,36] In these instances, a carbapenem is generally recommended (assuming susceptibility is demonstrated). Among β-lactams, cefepime has the

Table 3
Recommendations for treatment of MDR gram-negative bacterial infections

Pathogen	IDSA Guidance		ESCMID Guidelines	
	Preferred	Alternative	Preferred	Alternative
AmpC-E	Cefepime (MIC ≤ 2 μg/mL) Carbapenem (cefepime MIC > 4 μg/mL) Cystitis: Nitrofurantoin, TMP-SMX, aminoglycoside	TMP-SMX, Fluoroquinolone	N/A	N/A
ESBL-E (IDSA); 3Ceph-R-E (ESCMID)	Carbapenem cUTI, pyelo: Carbapenems, fluoroquinolones, TMP-SMX Cystitis: Nitrofurantoin, TMP-SMX	If pip-tazo was initiated and there is clinical response, it can be carefully continued Consider oral step-down after response to first-line treatment, preference to fluoroquinolone or TMP-SMX cUTI, pyelo: Aminoglycoside Cystitis: Aminoglycoside	Carbapenem (meropenem, imipenem). Ertapenem can be considered in nonserve BSI, cUTI or pyelo Nonsevere infections: Pip-tazo, amp-sulbactam, fluoroquinolones cUTI, pyelo: Aminoglycoside, IV fosfomycin (not available in US)	Consider oral step-down after response, preference to fluoroquinolone
CRE	No carbapenemase or no data: Ceftaz-avi, meropenem-vabor, imipenem-relebactam KPC: Ceftaz-avi, meropenem-vabor, imipenem-relebactam OXA-48: Ceftaz-avi MBL: Ceftaz-avi and aztreonam combination Nonsevere infections: Consider older agents with activity cUTI, pyelo: Fluoroquinolones, TMP-SMX Cystitis: Fluoroquinolone, TMP-SMX, nitrofurantoin, aminoglycoside, fosfomycin (E. coli only)	No carbapenemase or no data: Meropenem (if ertapenem-R, meropenem-S) KPC: Cefiderocol OXA-48: Cefiderocol MBL: Cefiderocol Nonsevere infections: Fluoroquinolones, TMP-SMX cUTI, pyelo: Meropenem (if ertapenem-R, meropenem-S), ceftaz-avi, meropenem-vabor, imipenem-relebactam, cefiderocol Cystitis: Meropenem (if ertapenem-R, meropenem-S), ceftaz-avi, meropenem-vabor, imipenem-relebactam, cefiderocol	Ceftaz-avibactam, meropenem-vabor MBL: Cefiderocol Nonsevere infections: Consider older agents with activity cUTI, pyelo: Aminoglycoside preferred over tigecycline	

MDR-PA	Active antipseudomonal agent, preference to noncarbapenem if susceptible	Ceftol-tazo, ceftaz-avibactam, imipenem-relebactam	N/A	N/A
DTR-PA	Ceftol-tazo, ceftaz-avibactam, imipenem-relebactam Cystitis: Agents above, aminoglycoside	Cefiderocol Cystitis: Cefiderocol	Ceftol-tazo Nonsevere infections: Old antibiotics with activity	N/A
CRAB	At least 2 active agents, including amp-sulbactam (if active) Mild infections: Monotherapy with active agent may be acceptable	If amp-sulbactam nonsusceptible, can still consider high-dose amp-sulbactam in combination with an active agent	Amp-sulbactam	Other active agent, such as high-dose tigecycline or colistin
S. malto	Combination, with TMP-SMX + minocycline first preference OR TMP-SMX monotherapy, followed by combination if poor response Mild infections: Monotherapy with TMP-SMX, minocycline, tigecycline, levofloxacin or cefiderocol	Other combinations, including ceftaz-avibactam if intolerance or inactivity of other agents	N/A	N/A

Table 4
Dosing of antibiotics for the treatment of MDR gram-negative bacterial infections[a]

Antibiotic	Dosage[b]	Pathogen[c]
Amikacin	20 mg/kg/dose[d] IV x 1 dose, subsequent doses and dosing interval based on pharmacokinetic evaluation Cystitis: 15 mg/kg/dose[d] IV once	AmpC-E, ESBL-E, CRE, DTR-*Pseudomonas aeruginosa*
Ampicillin-sulbactam	9g IV q8h over 4 h OR 27g IV q24 h continuous infusion (high-dose). Mild infections by ampicillin-sulbactam susceptible CRAB: 3g IV q4h	CRAB
Cefepime	2 g IV q8h, infused over 3 h Cystitis: 1 g IV q8h	AmpC-E (cefepime MICs ≤2 mcg/mL)
Cefiderocol	2 g IV q8h, infused over 3 h	CRE, DTR-*P aeruginosa*, CRAB, *Stenotrophomonas maltophilia*
Ceftazidime-avibactam	2.5 g IV q8h, infused over 3 h	CRE, DTR-*P aeruginosa*
Ceftazidime-avibactam and aztreonam	Ceftazidime-avibactam: 2.5 g IV q8h, infused over 3 h PLUS Aztreonam: 2 g IV q8h, infused over 3 h, at the same time as ceftazidime-avibactam	MBL producing CRE, *S maltophilia*
Ceftolozane-tazobactam	3 g IV q8h; infused over 3 h Cystitis: 1.5 g IV q8h, infused over 1 h	DTR-*P aeruginosa*
Ciprofloxacin	ESBL-E or AmpC infections: 400 mg IV q8h-q12 h or 500–750 mg PO q12 h DTR-*P aeruginosa*, pneumonia: 400 mg IV q8h or 750 mg PO q12 h	AmpC-E, ESBL-E
Colistin	Refer to international consensus guidelines on polymyxins[e]	CRE cystitis, DTR-*P aeruginosa* cystitis, CRAB cystitis
Eravacycline	1 mg/kg/dose IV q12 h	CRE, CRAB, *S maltophilia*
Ertapenem	1 g IV q24 h, infused over 30 min	AmpC-E, ESBL-E

		ESBL-E. coli cystitis
Fosfomycin	Cystitis: 3 g PO x 1 dose	ESBL-E. coli cystitis
Gentamicin	7 mg/kg/dose[d] IV x 1 dose, subsequent doses and dosing interval based on pharmacokinetic evaluation; Cystitis: 5 mg/kg/dose[d] IV once	AmpC-E, ESBL-E, CRE, DTR-P aeruginosa
Imipenem-cilastatin	500 mg IV q6h; infused over 3 h; Cystitis: 500 mg IV q6h, infused over 30 min	AmpC-E, ESBL-E, CRE, CRAB (as a component of combination therapy with at least 2 other agents)
Imipenem-cilastatin-relebactam	1.25 g IV q6h, infused over 30 min	CRE, DTR-P aeruginosa
Levofloxacin	750 mg IV/PO q24 h	AmpC-E, ESBL-E, S maltophilia
Meropenem	ESBL-E or AmpC-E infections: 1-2g IV q8h, can consider a 3-h infusion; CRE and CRAB infections: 2g IV q8h, infused over 3 h; Cystitis (standard infusion): 1 g IV q8h	AmpC-E, ESBL-E, CRE, CRAB (as a component of combination therapy with at least 2 other agents)
Meropenem-vaborbactam	4 g IV q8h, infused over 3 h	CRE
Minocycline	200 mg IV/PO q12 h	CRAB, S maltophilia
Nitrofurantoin	Cystitis: Macrocrystal/monohydrate (Macrobid®) 100 mg PO q12 h OR Oral suspension: 50 mg q6h	AmpC-E cystitis, ESBL-E cystitis
Plazomicin	15 mg/kg[d] IV x 1 dose, subsequent doses and dosing interval based on pharmacokinetic evaluation; Cystitis: 15 mg/kg[d] IV x1 dose	AmpC-E, ESBL-E, CRE, DTR-P aeruginosa
Polymyxin B	Refer to international consensus guidelines on polymyxins[e]	DTR-P aeruginosa, CRAB
Tigecycline	200 mg IV x 1 dose, then 100 mg IV q12 h	CRE, CRAB, S maltophilia
Tobramycin	7 mg/kg/dose[d] IV x 1 dose; subsequent doses and dosing interval based on	AmpC-E, ESBL-E, CRE, DTR-P aeruginosa

(continued on next page)

Table 4
(continued)

Antibiotic	Dosage[b]	Pathogen[c]
	pharmacokinetic evaluation Cystitis: 5 mg/kg/dose[d] IV × 1 dose	
Trimethoprim-sulfamethoxazole	8–12 mg/kg/d (trimethoprim component) IV/PO divided q8-12h (consider maximum dose of 960 mg trimethoprim component per day) Cystitis: 160 mg (trimethoprim component) IV/PO q12 h	AmpC-E, ESBL-E, *S maltophilia*

[a] Adapted from IDSA guidance documents. Dosages are for adults, and assume normal renal and hepatic function and that causative bacteria are shown to be susceptible to the given agent.

[b] Dosages that differ for treatment of specific types of infection are highlighted by bolded text.

[c] Pathogens are AmpC-producing Enterobacterales (AmpC-E), extended-spectrum β-lactamase producing Enterobacterales (ESBL-E), carbapenem-resistant Enterobacterales (CRE), *Pseudomonas aeruginosa* with difficult-to-treat resistance (DTR-*P aeruginosa*), carbapenem-resistant *Acinetobacter baumannii* (CRAB), and *Stenotrophomonas maltophilia*.

[d] Use adjusted body weight for patients >120% of ideal body weight for aminoglycoside dosing.

[e] Tsuji BT, et al. International Consensus Guidelines for the Optimal Use of the Polymyxins: Endorsed by the American College of Clinical Pharmacy (ACCP), European Society of Clinical Microbiology and Infectious Diseases (ESCMID), Infectious Diseases Society of America (IDSA), International Society for Anti-infective Pharmacology (ISAP), Society of Critical Care Medicine (SCCM), and Society of Infectious Diseases Pharmacists (SIDP). Pharmacotherapy. 2019; 39(1): 10-39.

advantages of both being a weak AmpC inducer and withstanding hydrolysis.[37–39] Imipenem strongly induces *ampC*, but it and other carbapenems are typically resistant to hydrolysis.[40–42] There are no randomized controlled trials comparing clinical outcomes of patients treated with cefepime versus a carbapenem for AmpC-inducible Enterobacterales infections. However, several observational studies suggest that clinical outcomes are similar.[28,43,44] Case reports of cefepime treatment failures against infections by AmpC-inducible Enterobacterales have led some to recommend against prescribing this agent,[45–47] but the interpretation of these reports is complicated by suboptimal dosing regimens and lack of data on concomitant ESBL production.[48,49]

Fluoroquinolones, aminoglycosides, trimethoprim-sulfamethoxazole (TMP-SMX), tetracycline, or other non–β-lactam antibiotics do not induce *ampC* expression, nor are they substrates for AmpC hydrolysis. The agents may be treatment options in individual cases, including fluoroquinolones and TNP-SMX as possible oral step-down therapy. Intensivists must be aware that oral agents such as doxycycline, amoxicillin-clavulanate, nitrofurantoin, and fosfomycin achieve poor or unreliable serum concentrations, which limits their roles in the treatment of serious infections.[50–54] New β-lactam-β-lactamase inhibitor antibiotics and cefiderocol are more active than piperacillin-tazobactam against bacteria with inducible chromosomal *ampC*, but their use is best reserved for more difficult-to-treat, carbapenem-resistant Gram-negative bacterial infections.

Infections by Extended-Spectrum β-Lactamase-Producing and 3rd Generation Cephalosporin-Resistant Enterobacterales

Background

In the US, the incidence of ESBL Enterobacterales infections increased by 53% from 2012 to 2017.[55] Most clinical microbiology laboratories do not perform routine EBSL testing.[56,57] Instead, ceftriaxone nonsusceptibility (MIC ≥ 2 μg/mL) is commonly used as a marker for possible ESBL production.[58,59] This approach has practical benefits if ESBL testing is not available; however, strains that are not susceptible to ceftriaxone due to other mechanisms may be mis-identified as ESBL producers. ESBLs hydrolyze most penicillins, cephalosporins, and aztreonam. EBSL-producing strains generally remain susceptible to carbapenems. ESBLs do not inactivate non–β-lactam antibiotics, but bla_{KPC}-carrying bacteria often harbor additional genes or gene mutations that mediate resistance to multiple antimicrobials. The most common ESBL Enterobacterales are *Escherichia coli*, *Klebsiella pneumoniae*, *Klebsiella oxytoca*, and *Proteus mirabilis*.[60–62] CTX-M enzymes, particularly CTX-M-15, are the most prevalent ESBLs in the U.S.[61] Other prominent ESBLs include narrow-spectrum TEM and SHV β-lactamases with amino acid substitutions.[63–66]

Treatment of infections outside of the urinary tract

DSA guidance recommended a carbapenem as a preferred treatment of ESBL-Enterobacterales infections outside of the urinary tract. ESCMID guidelines agreed that carbapenem is preferred treatment of severe 3rd generation cephalosporin-resistant-Enterobacterales infections, defined as bloodstream infections (BSIs) or any infection associated with sepsis or septic shock.

Recommendations from both organizations were based on data from the randomized MERINO trial. In MERINO, 30-day mortality rates were significantly lower (4% vs 12%) among patients with BSIs due to ceftriaxone-nonsusceptible *E coli* or *K pneumoniae* (87% confirmed as ESBL carriers) treated with meropenem (1 g intravenously (IV) every 8 hours) than among those who were treated with piperacillin-tazobactam (4.5 g IV every 6 hours).[67] Meropenem was superior despite higher baseline APACHE scores and longer times to appropriate antibiotic therapy in subjects receiving the drug. Potentially counteracting biases were that piperacillin-tazobactam was not administered as prolonged infusion and there was a relatively high rate of piperacillin-tazobactam false susceptibility with automated or strip-gradient testing at study sites. In a re-analysis of data for patients in whom piperacillin-tazobactam susceptibility was confirmed by broth microdilution, the respective mortality rates were 4% and 11% (not statistically significant, although the trend remained strong (95% confidence interval: −1% to 10%)).[68] Another clinical trial (PETERPAN) of meropenem versus piperacillin-tazobactam against cephalosporin-resistant Enterobacterales BSIs is ongoing.[69] Clinical trial data are not available for carbapenems and piperacillin-tazobactam against ESBL-Enterobacterales or ceftriaxone-nonsusceptible infections of nonbloodstream sites.

IDSA guidance did not distinguish between carbapenems. ESMID guidelines endorsed meropenem or imipenem in the settings above, adding ertapenem as an option for BSIs not associated with septic shock. The more conservative recommendation for ertapenem acknowledged that the agent was used in less severe cases or as de-escalation therapy in observational studies of Enterobacterales infections.[11]

In the absence of clinical trial data for nonbloodstream sites, the IDSA panel extrapolated MERINO findings to recommend a carbapenem against all ESBL Enterobacterales infections outside of the urinary tract. Furthermore, they recommended against using piperacillin-tazobactam even for infections by strains testing susceptible *in vitro*, citing MERINO data, potential for ESBL over-expression or presence of multiple β-lactamases, and concerns about the accuracy of piperacillin-tazobactam MIC measurements for ESBL-carrying strains.[68,70–74] The ESCMID panel, in contrast, suggested piperacillin-tazobactam, amoxicillin-clavulanate or a fluoroquinolone for the treatment of nonsevere, ceftriaxone-nonsusceptible infections outside of the bloodstream or urinary tract (see the definition of "severe" infection above). These conditional recommendations were justified based on a stewardship objective of restraining carbapenem use, data from several observational studies, and concerns about the generalizability of MERINO data beyond BSIs.[36,75–88]

Both organizations recommended against using cefepime to treat ESBL or ceftriaxone-nonsusceptible, cefepime-susceptible Enterobacterales infections, as observational studies and a clinical trial subgroup analysis have shown the agent to be inferior or comparable to carbapenems.[89–93] They also indicated that new β-lactam/β-lactamase inhibitors should be reserved for carbapenem-resistant bacterial infections.

Treatment of complicated urinary tract infections or pyelonephritis

IDSA listed fluoroquinolones or TMP-SMX as frontline agents alongside carbapenems for the treatment of cUTIs or pyelonephritis by ESBL Enterobacterales, with once-daily aminoglycosides as an alternative option. ESCMID endorsed once-daily aminoglycosides or IV fosfomycin (not available in the US) against cUTIs by 3rd generation cephalosprin-nonsusceptible Enterobacterales.

In patients treated initially with IV antibiotics for ESBL or 3rd generation cephalosprin-nonsusceptible Enterobacterales infections, including bloodstream and other serious infections, the 2 organizations issued an expert opinion that oral step-down therapy was good practice after appropriate clinical improvement was observed.[94,95] IDSA suggested fluoroquinolones or TMP-SMX. ESCMID suggested fluoroquinolones, older β-lactam/β-lactamase inhibitors, or other agents active against the infecting strain *in vitro*. Due to amoxicillin-clavulanate's unreliable serum levels, IDSA recommended against using this agent for the bloodstream and other serious infections.[96]

Infections by Carbapenem-Resistant Enterobacterales

Background

Carbapenem-resistant Enterobacterales (CRE) are defined by resistance to at least one carbapenem or by the production of a carbapenemase.[97] CRE can be classified as noncarbapenemase-producing or carbapenemase-producing. The former has emerged over the past decade in the US, and presently account for ~40%-60% of CRE infections.[98,99] *K pneumoniae* carbapenemases (KPCs), which can be produced by any Enterobacterales, remain the most common carbapenemases. Other notable carbapenemases include oxacillinases (eg, OXA-48-like) and metallo-β-lactamases (MBLs) such as New Delhi (NDMs), Verona integron-encoded (VIMs) and imipenem-hydrolyzing (IMPs) MBLs.[100,101] Approximately 35% of U.S. CRE strains in 2017 to 19 carried one of these five carbapenemases.[100] Once a strain is identified as CRE, knowledge of carbapenemase production and type of carbapenemase are useful in choosing an optimal antibiotic. At present, however, clinical microbiology laboratories in most U.S. hospitals do not perform phenotypic or genotypic carbapenemase testing.[102]

Treatment of infections by ertapenem-resistant, meropenem-susceptible carbapenem-resistant Enterobacterales

The first step for intensivists treating a CRE-infected patient is to understand the susceptibility of the causative strain to ertapenem and other carbapenems. Most ertapenem-resistant (MIC ≥ 2 μg/mL), meropenem-susceptible (MIC <1 μg/mL) CRE in the US do not produce a carbapenemase.[100,103] Unless a phenotypic or genotypic test for carapenemase is positive, IDSA guidance stated that infections outside of the urinary tract by ertapenem-resistant, meropenem-susceptible CRE can be treated with extended infusion meropenem (see dosing in **Table 4**); if a carbapenemase is detected, a carbapenem should be avoided, even if the strain tests susceptible by MIC. The use of meropenem against meropenem-susceptible CRE infections allows clinicians to reserve a new agent such as ceftazidime-avibactam for infections with fewer treatment options. Meropenem-vaborbactam and imipenem-cilastatin-relebactam are unlikely to provide any benefit beyond that of extended-infusion meropenem against infections by ertapenem-resistant, meropenem-susceptible CRE. ESCMID guidelines did not explicitly address the potential role of extended infusion meropenem against meropenem-susceptible CRE infections. For nonsevere (see definition above) CRE infections; however, they suggested considering, on a case-by-case basis, old antibiotics that are active against the causative strain *in vitro*, a general statement that could encompass meropenem.

Treatment of infections by carbapenemase-producing carbapenem-resistant Enterobacterales

For CRE infections outside of the urinary tract caused by strains for which carbapenemase data are lacking or that are shown to be KPC-producing, IDSA endorsed ceftazidime-avibactam, meropenem-vaborbactam, or imipenem-cilastatin as preferred agents (assuming strains are susceptible *in vitro*). ESCMID endorsed ceftazidime-avibactam or meropenem-vaborbactam for severe CRE infections susceptible to the agents, but deemed data insufficient to reach a conclusion on the role of imipenen-cilastatin-relebactam. Meropenem-vaborbactam and imipenem-cilastatin-relebactam have limited to no activity against CRE that express OXA-48-

like enzymes,[104–106] which makes ceftazidime-avibactam the best choice among new β-lactam/β-lactamase agents for the treatment of infections by such pathogens.

Cefiderocol is likely to be active against most CRE strains producing KPC, OXA-48-like, and other carbapenemases.[107] In a recent trial, clinical cures were achieved in 66% (19/29) and 45% (5/11) of CRE-infected patients treated with cefiderocol and other regimens (mostly polymyxin-based), respectively.[108] IDSA listed cefiderocol as an alternative treatment for carpanemase-producing CRE infections, recommending that it be reserved for infections with fewer therapeutic options.[109]

Ceftazidime-avibactam, meropenem-vaborbactam, and imipenem-cilastatin-relebactam are inactive against MBL-expressing CRE. NDMs and other MBLs do not hydrolyze aztreonam, but the drug is susceptible to AmpC, ESBL, or OXA-48-like enzymes that might also be carried by NDM-producing CRE. Avibactam, however, generally remains effective against the latter β-lactamases. In an observational study of 102 patients with MBL-CRE BSIs, 30-day mortality among patients treated with ceftazidime-avibactam combined with aztreonam was 19%, compared to 44% among those who received other combination regimens (predominantly polymyxin- or tigecycline-based).[109] Cefiderocol is active against MBL-expressing CRE in vitro,[107,110] but observational data for the treatment of MBL-infections are limited.[108] Nevertheless, given the lack of treatment options, IDSA and ESCMID suggest ceftazidime-avibactam and aztreonam combination therapy or cefiderocol monotherapy as preferred regimens against MBL-producing CRE infections.[98,109–115] Ceftazidime-avibactam and aztreonam should be administered simultaneously rather than sequentially.[116]

Treatment of complicated urinary tract infections or pyelonephritis by carbapenem-resistant Enterobacterales

IDSA listed fluoroquinolones or TMP-SMX as frontline agents for the treatment of cUTIs or pyelonephritis by CRE, if susceptibility is demonstrated. ESCMID endorsed aminoglycosides against complicated CRE UTIs. Both organizations recommended against tigecycline monotherapy for BSIs, pneumonia, or UTIs by CRE, due to low serum and urine concentrations and based on a meta-analysis of clinical data for the treatment of pneumonia by Enterobacterales and other bacteria.[117,118] Citing observational and clinical trial data for increased mortality and excess nephrotoxicity with polymyxin-based regimens compared with new β-lactam/β-lactamase regimens, IDSA recommended against using polymyxins.[119–128]

In absence of conclusive data for the clinical benefit of combination antibiotic therapy, IDSA and ESCMID are recommended against this practice, with the possible exception of treating MBL-CRE infections or infections by strains that are only susceptible to polymyxins or aminoglycosides. Intensivists should be aware of increasing reports of emergent resistance to new β-lactam/β-lactamase inhibitors and cefiderocol. To date, ceftazidime-avibactam and merobactam-vaborbactam resistance has been reported in approximately 15% and 3% of CRE infections treated with the respective agents.[119,127,129–133]

Infections by Multi-Drug-Resistant and Difficult-to-Treat Resistance -P. aeruginosa

Background

Multi-drug-resistant -P aeruginosa are defined by nonsusceptibility to at least one antibiotic in at least 3 antibiotic classes to which P aeruginosa are generally susceptible, including penicillins, cephalosporins, fluoroquinolones, aminoglycosides, and carbapenems.[134] DTR-P aeruginosa are a subset of MDR- P aeruginosa, defined by nonsusceptibility to all of the following: piperacillin-tazobactam, ceftazidime, cefepime, aztreonam, meropenem, imipenem-cilastatin, ciprofloxacin, and levofloxacin.[134] MDR- or DTR-*P aeruginosa* typically possess a variety of resistance mechanisms, including decreased expression of outer membrane porins (OprD), hyperproduction of AmpC enzymes, upregulation of efflux pumps, and mutations in PBPs.[135–137] Carbapenemase production is rare in U.S. *P aeruginosa* clinical strains, but it is identified in as many as 20% of carbapenem-resistant *P aeruginosa* in other parts of the world.[138,139]

In international surveillance studies, ~70%-75% of carbapenem resistant-*P aeruginosa* strains are susceptible to cefolozane-tazobactam, ceftazidime-avibactam and imipenem-cilastatin-relebactam *in vitro*.[9] Meropenem-vaborbactam is not active against *P aeruginosa* that are meropenem-resistant. Unlike ceftazidime or imipenem, ceftolozane has independent activity versus carbapenem resistant-*P aeruginosa*. As such, ceftolozane-tazobctam may be somewhat more active than ceftazidime-avibactam and imipenem-cilastatin-relebactam against such strains.[140] Avibactam and relebactam expand ceftazidime and imipenem-cilastatin activity primarily through the inhibition of AmpC, but other resistance mechanisms are unlikely to be impacted.

Cefiderocol is active *in vitro* against the vast majority of carbapenem-nonsusceptible *P aeruginosa* isolates in surveillance studies, although rates may be reduced as the drug is used more widely.[14,141–145] In the CREDIBLE clinical trial, which included 22 unique patients with 29 carbapenem resistant-*P aeruginosa* infections, mortality, clinical cure, and microbiologic response rates were similar among patients treated with cefiderocol and best available treatment (largely colistin-based).[146]

Susceptibility patterns for new agents with potential activity against MDR- and DTR-*P aeruginosa* can vary locally, and intensivists should be aware of data in their units and hospitals. Treatment decisions for infections by these pathogens should be guided by results of susceptibility testing, which may not be routinely performed for new agents in some clinical microbiology labs.

Clinical trial data are scant for cefolozane-tazobactam, ceftazidime-avibactam or imipenem-cilastatin-relebactam against MDR-, carbapenem resistant- or DTR-*P aeruginosa* infections.[9,11] In an observational study of 200 patients with MDR-*P aeruginosa* infections, favorable clinical outcomes were significantly more likely among those treated with ceftolozane-tazobactam than among those receiving a polymyxin- or aminoglycoside-based regimen (81% vs 61%).[147] In a randomized trial of 24 patients with imipenem-nonsusceptible *P aeruginosa* infections, there was a trend toward favorable clinical responses being more common with imipenem-cilastatin-relebactam than imipenem-cilastatin plus colistin (81% vs 63%).[122] Pooling data for MDR-*P aeruginosa* infections from 5 randomized trials, investigators reported clinical response rates of 57% (32/57) and 54% (21/39) for patients treated with ceftazidime-avibactam and older antibiotic regimens, respectively.[148] Interpretation of these results was complicated by ceftazidime-avibactam nonsusceptibility in one-third of strains.

Treatment

For infections by MDR-*P aeruginosa* that do not manifest DTR, clinicians can choose among antibiotics that retain susceptibility. IDSA guidance endorsed an active β-lactam administered as high-dose continuous infusion; if the causative strain is susceptible to an old, noncarbapenem β-lactam, such an agent is preferred over a carbapenem. ESCMID agreed that the use of an older, active agent represents good clinical practice, even if definitive clinical data for the superiority of one drug or class over another are lacking. A new β-lactam/β-lactamase agent is considered a less desirable treatment option when other active antibiotics, in particular β-lactams, are available, in keeping with stewardship principles.

IDSA and ESCMID recommended ceftolozane-tazobactam as a first-choice agent against DTR-*P aeruginosa* infections. IDSA also listed ceftazidime-avibactam or imipenem-cilastatin-relebactam as preferred options, but ESCMID deemed clinical data insufficient at present to recommend these drugs.

The role of cefiderocol in treating DTR-*P aeruginosa* infections is unclear. IDSA listed cefiderocol as an alternative treatment option for DTR-*P aeruginosa* infections outside of the urinary tract, if the use of new β-lactam-β-lactamase inhibitors is precluded by inactivity, intolerance, or unavailability. For less severe DTR-*P aeruginosa* cUTIs or pyelonephritis, once-daily aminoglycosides might also be a reasonable alternative treatment; clinical data for such regimens are limited.

Data on the value of combination antibiotic therapy or nebulized antibiotics against MDR- and DTR-*P aeruginosa* infections for improving clinical outcomes or suppressing resistance are inconclusive. IDSA recommended against routinely using such regimens. In cases for which none of the preferred antibiotics are active, IDSA suggested that an aminoglycoside (assuming susceptibility is demonstrated) might be combined with agent for which MIC is closest to the resistance breakpoint. ESCMID noted that recommendations cannot be made for or against combination therapy. If polymyxins or aminoglycosides are used against nonsevere carbapenem-resistant *P aeruginosa* infections, ESCMID recommended that they be given with another agent that is active *in vitro*.

Infections by Carbapenem-Resistant *Acinetobacter baumannii*

Background

The acronym CRAB refers to infections by *A baumannii* and other species within the *baumannii* and *calcoaceticus* complexes.[149] Carbapenem resistance is multifactorial, stemming from OXA-24/40-like carbapenemases, OXA-23-like carbapenemases, MBLs and/or additional serine carbapenemases.[150] CRAB isolates are invariably resistant to antibiotics in addition to carbapenems. Multiple β-lactamases are often produced. Aminoglycosides, including plazomicin, are generally inactivated by modifying enzymes or 16S rRNA methyltransferases. Fluoroquinolone resistance is mediated by the upregulation of efflux pumps. A unique feature of *A baumannii* is that up to 50% of strains are susceptible to sulbactam, a competitive β-lactamase inhibitor.[151–153] In high doses, sulbactam saturates *A baumannii* PBP1 and PBP3, exerting antibacterial activity *in vitro* and in animal models. Sulbactam resistance is likely primarily driven by PBP mutations. Sulbactam is available as a stand-alone agent in some parts of the world, but it must be administered as ampicillin-sulbactam in North America and Europe. Clavulanate and other nonsulbactam β-lactamase inhibitors are not active against CRAB.

Several studies, mostly of retrospective observational design, compared *in vitro* active antibiotics for the treatment of CRAB infections, in particular pneumonia. Due to variability and limitations of the studies, there are at best low-certainty data for advantages with any regimen. At least five observational and small randomized trials have reported that ampicillin-sulbactam or sulbactam (alone or in combination with another antibiotic) were superior or comparable to polymyxins (mostly colistin) in patients with susceptible CRAB ventilator-associated pneumonia, healthcare-associated pneumonia and assorted infections.[11] In five other retrospective observational studies, sulbactam-containing regimens, for the most part, were also superior or comparable to tigecyline-containing regimens.[11] Meta-analyses of observational studies and clinical trials that included 1835 and 2118 CRAB-infected patients found that sulbactam-containing regimens were associated with lowest mortality among treatment options, as well as significantly less nephrotoxicity than treatment that included colistin.[154,155]

Conclusions cannot be drawn from four comparative studies of polymyxins vs. tigecycline, due to the use of various antibiotic combinations and dosing regimens.[11] The CREDIBLE trial compared cefiderocol and best available therapy (BAT, most commonly polymyxin-based regimens) for the treatment of carbapenem-resistant Gram-negative bacterial infections. Among patients with CRAB infections, mortality rates at 28 days were 49% (21/42) and 17% (3/17) in cefiderocol and BAT groups, respectively.

At least seven clinical trials have evaluated the role of combination antibiotic therapy.[156–161] Only one trial showed an outcome benefit with combination treatment, but this was also the only study that included high-dose ampicillin-sulbactam in the combination arm (4 g ampicillin and 2 g sulbactam IV every 6 hours).[162]

Treatment
IDSA and ESCMID made general treatment recommendations for CRAB infections, which do not distinguish between types of infections. The organizations agreed on some basic principles. For infections by sulbactam-susceptible CRAB, they endorsed ampicillin-sulbactam as the preferred agent. IDSA indicated that antibiotic monotherapy may be considered against nonsevere CRAB infections. However, both IDSA and ESCMID endorsed combination therapy with at least 2 active antibiotics against moderate-severe CRAB infections. Unvalidated rationales for this recommendation, as stated by IDSA, were that there is no gold standard therapeutic regimen for CRAB infections, patients are typically severely ill, many infections (and pneumonia in particular) are associated with high bacterial burdens, and emergence of resistance during treatment is common. IDSA and ESCMID recommended against combining meropenem with polymyxin (without a third agent), based on data from 2 clinical trials.[10,11,156,157] When meropenem is used, it should be given as high dose, extended infusion; imipenem can be used as an alternative carbapenem. If using high-dose ampicillin-sulbactam and carbapenem, clinicians should be mindful of potential for additive β-lactam neurotoxicity. Finally, both organizations recommend against treatment with cefiderocol or rifampin, unless the use of other agents is precluded by lack of therapeutic response or intolerance.

For CRAB infections that are resistant to sulbactam, IDSA suggested that high-dose ampicillin-sulbactam might still be used in combination with an active agent; this recommendation is not supported by clinical data, but rather based on the potential for sulbactam to saturate altered PBPs.[10] ESCMID recommended using active antibiotics, but noted that evidence was insufficient to recommend specific agents.[11]

IDSA preferred minocycline among tetracyclines against susceptible CRAB infections, citing longstanding clinical experience with the drug; high-dose tigecycline was listed as an alternative. ESCMID, in contrast, indicated that high-dose tigecycline was the preferred tetracycline. Neither organization issued a recommendation for or against eravacycline, citing a need for clinical data. Rifamycins were not recommended, due to lack of clinical effectiveness in studies to date and concern for toxicity and drug interactions.

IDSA did not feel that data supported the use of nebulized antibiotics as part of combination regimens, and expressed concern about unequal drug distribution in infected lungs and bronchoconstriction (as reported in 10%–20% of patients receiving aerosolized antibiotics).[109]

Infections by S. maltophilia

Sarzynski SH et al. [Trimethoprim-Sulfamethoxazole versus Levofloxacin for Stenotrophomonas maltophilia Infections: A Retrospective Comparative Effectiveness Study of Electronic Health Records from 154 US Hospitals. Open Forum Infect Dis. 2022 Jan 17;9(2):ofab644. PMID: 35097154.] and please describe the impact on the evidence base and recommendations for S. maltophilia management.

Background

Like *A baumannii. S. maltophilia* is both a colonizer and a cause of opportunistic infections in critically ill patients.[163] *S maltophilia* strains typically carry a wide array of antibacterial resistance genes and resistance-conferring gene mutations.[164] L1 MBLs and L2 serine β-lactamases render most β-lactams ineffective against *S maltophilia*.[163] The former hydrolyzes penicillins, cephalosporins, and carbapenems, but not aztreonam; the latter has extended cephalosporin activity and ability to hydrolyze aztreonam. *S maltophilia* are intrinsically resistant to aminoglycosides due to chromosomal acetyltransferase enzymes.[165] Strains can accumulate multidrug efflux pumps that reduce the activity of fluoroquinolones and tetracyclines, and they harbor chromosomal *Smqnr* genes that further diminish fluoroquinolone effectiveness.[163,166] Intensivists should also recognize that antibiotic susceptibility testing of *S maltophilia* is problematic. The Clinical and Laboratory Standards Institute (CLSI) has established MIC interpretive criteria against *S maltophilia* for TMP-SMX, ticarcillin-clavulanate, ceftazidime, cefiderocol, levofloxacin, minocycline, and chloramphenicol. Confidence in MIC interpretive criteria is undermined by concerns about the reproducibility of results, limited pharmacokinetic-pharmacodynamic (PK-PD) data used to assign breakpoints for most agents, and insufficient data on correlations between MICs and clinical outcomes.[167,168]

TMP-SMX is long recognized by clinicians as first-line therapy for *S maltophilia* infections. More than 90% of *S maltophilia* strains are susceptible to TMP-SMX in surveillance studies.[169,170] Baseline susceptibility of *S maltophilia* to levofloxacin and minocycline range from ~30%-80% and ~70 to 90%, respectively, in various studies.[171,172] In time-kills studies, fluoroquinolones did not exert sustained inhibition of *S maltophilia* growth.[173–175] Modeling also suggested that fluoroquinolone monotherapy may not achieve appropriate PK-PD target attainment for *S maltophilia* infections.[173] Emergence of fluoroquinolone resistance during the treatment of patients is well-described.[171,172,176,177]

Tigecycline activity appears similar to slightly lower than that of minocycline *in vitro*.[169,173,178–181] Data for eravacycline are limited, but MICs in general were low in studies to date. Omadacycline has limited *in vitro* activity against *S maltophilia* relative to other tetracycline derivatives.[178]

Cefiderocol is active against almost 100% of *S maltophilia*, including strains resistant to other agents.[141,182–184] The drug was potent using simulated human dosing in neutropenic thigh and lung mouse models of *S maltophilia* infection, and results correlated with *in vitro* efficacy under iron-depleted conditions.[185–192] Only 30% to 40% of *S maltophilia* strains are susceptible to ceftazidime using CLSI interpretive criteria, due to expression of L1 and L2 β-lactamases.[185–191,193] The combination of ceftazidime-avibactam and aztreonam may overcome L1 and L2 β-lactamases.[185–191] The addition of avibactam to ceftazidime does not meaningfully enhance the latter's activity against *S maltophilia*.

A validated gold standard antibiotic or combination regimen against *S maltophilia* infections is not identified, and robust comparative effectiveness studies among commonly used agents are lacking. Even for TMP-SMX, rigorous clinical data are scant. In the largest study of TMP-SMX treatment, mortality at 14 days was 25% among 91 patients with *S maltophilia* BSIs.[193] In a recent systematic review and meta-analysis of 663 patients in 7 retrospective cohorts and 7 case-control studies, mortality rates were 26% and 33% among those treated with fluoroquinolone and TMP-SMX, respectively (OR 0.62, 95% CI 0.39–0.99). These data are difficult to interpret because studies were observational, outcomes for specific fluoroquinolones and TMP-SMX did not differ, and criteria to distinguish colonization from disease were not stated clearly. In a sub-group analysis of bacteremic patients, significant differences in mortality were not observed for those receiving fluoroquinolone or TMP-SMX. More recently, a retrospective review of observational data from 1581 patients with positive S maltophilia blood or lower respiratory cultures at 154 US hospitals between 2005 and 2017 found comparable mortality among those treated with levofloxacin or TMP-SMX.[194] Mortality was lower for patients treated empirically with levofloxacin rather than TMP-SMX, and lower among those with positive lower respiratory cultures. In small observational studies, outcomes were similar for patients with a variety of S maltophilia infections treated with TMP-SMX vs. minocycline or tigecycline.[10,195,196] These studies were limited by selection bias, small sample sizes, heterogeneity in host and microbial data, and the use of additional active agents in some patients. At present, clinical data for cefiderocol and the combination of ceftazidime-avibactam and aztreonam are cursory.

Treatment

For moderate-severe S maltophilia infections, IDSA guidance recommended one of the 3approaches: combination therapy, with a preference for TMP-SMX and minocycline; initiation of TMP-SMX monotherapy, and addition of a second agent if clinical improvement is not observed; or the combination of ceftazidime-avibactam and aztreonam, if there is intolerance or inactivity of TMP-SMX and minocycline.

For mild infections, IDSA proposed TMP-SMX, minocycline, levofloxacin, or cefiderocol monotherapy as acceptable treatment options, with preference assigned to TMP-SMX and minocycline. Minocycline was endorsed over tigecycline based on slightly more favorable in vitro data, the presence of CLSI interpretive breakpoints, availability of an oral formulation, and better tolerability. IDSA recommended against the use of ceftazidime. Although fluoroquinolones were suggested as potential monotherapy for mild infections, the panel preferred these agents in combination regimens (preferably with TMP-SMX) based on time-kill and PK modeling data. Because susceptibility criteria are not established for ciprofloxacin and moxifloxacin and based on observational clinical data, levofloxacin was the preferred fluoroquinolone.[194] As for IDSA guidance against other AMR Gram-negative infections, recommendations for treatment will be updated regularly to incorporate new data.[194]

SUMMARY

IDSA and ESCMID recommendations are based on up-to-date reviews of the literature. Clinical data for the treatment of MDR Gram-negative bacterial infections will continue to emerge. Moreover, several agents in the antibiotic development pipeline with activity against bacteria reviewed above, including CRAB, are poised to be approved in the not-too-distant future. IDSA identified the dissemination of timely clinical practice guidelines and guidance as a top strategic priority, recognizing that extended time periods between updates of documents limited their utility. Plans are for IDSA guidance on the treatment of Gram-negative bacterial infections to be updated regularly as new data emerge, with revised documents posted on the society website. A first update of the guidance for ESBL Enterobacterales, CRE, and DTR-P aeruginosa infections was recently released.

Neither IDSA nor ESCMID addressed the empiric treatment of patients in whom MDR Gram-negative bacterial infections might be suspected. This is a complex issue, for which conclusive data to guide recommendations are lacking and best practices are dependent on local conditions. It is unclear what threshold likelihood of resistance to a given first-choice antibiotic justifies the empiric use of an alternative agent. Clinicians and stewardship programs will need to make their own determinations in this regard and devise treatment algorithms based on microbiology and epidemiology in their hospitals. In the future, professional societies should consider offering guidance on empiric treatment, setting forth principles that can be adapted in various clinical settings.

CLINICS CARE POINTS

- The key to optimal treatment of MDR Gram-negative bacterial infections is understanding local epidemiology and microbiology.
- New resources to guide management of MDR Gram-negative infections are IDSA Treatment Guidance documents, available and regularly updated on-line, and ESCMID Guidelines.
- IDSA Guidance and EXCMID Guidelines are largely in agreement, with the most pronounced differences in treatment of ESBL-producing Gram-negative bacterial infections. In part, these differences reflect varying interpretations of MERINO clinical trial data, and variations in local epidemiology and antibiotic availability.
- Clinicians can assess data on their own, and use the Guidance and Guideline documents as references for devising best approaches in their practices.

DISCLOSURE

The authors have nothing to disclose.

REFERENCES

1. Centers for Disease Control and Prevention. Antibiotic Resistance Threats in the United States, 2019. Available at: https://www.cdc.gov/drugresistance/pdf/threats-report/2019-ar-threats-report-508.pdf.
2. Tacconelli E, Carrara E, Savoldi A, et al. Discovery, research, and development of new antibiotics: The WHO priority list of antibiotic-resistant bacteria and tuberculosis. Lancet Infect Dis 2018;18:318–27.
3. O'Neill J. Review on Antimicrobial Resistance Tackling drug-resistant infections globally: Final report and recommendations. AMR Review website. 2016. Available at:https://amrreview.org/#:~:text=%E2%80%9CThe%20Review%20on%20Antimicrobial%20Resistance,actions%20to%20tackle%20it%20internationally. . Accessed 2022 July 13.
4. World Health Organization. WHO Publishes List of Bacteria for Which New Antibiotics are Urgently Needed. 2017. Available from. http://www.who.int/mediacentre/news/releases/2017/bacteria-antibiotics-needed/en/ [Last accessed on 2022 July 13.
5. Clancy CJ, Potoski BA, Buehrle D, et al. Estimating the Treatment of Carbapenem-Resistant Enterobacteriaceae Infections in the United States Using Antibiotic Prescription Data. Open Forum Infect Dis 2019;6(8):ofz344.
6. Clancy CJ, Nguyen MH. Estimating the size of the United States market for new antibiotics with activity against carbapenem-resistant Enterobacteriaceae. Antimicrob Agents Chemother 2019;63(12):e01733-19.

7. Strich JR, Ricotta E, Warner S, et al. Pharmacoepidemiology of ceftazidime-avibactam use: a retrospective cohort anlaysis of 210 US hospitals. Clin Infect Dis 2020;72(4):611–21.

8. Clancy CJ, Nguyen MH. Buying Time: The AMR Action Fund and the State of Antibiotic Development in the United States 2020. Open Forum Infect Dis 2020;7(11):ofaa464.

9. Tamma PD, Aitken SL, Bonomo RA, et al. Infectious Diseases Society of America Guidance on the Treatment of Extended-Spectrum beta-lactamase Producing Enterobacterales (ESBL-E), Carbapenem-Resistant Enterobacterales (CRE), and Pseudomonas aeruginosa with Difficult-to-Treat Resistance (DTR-P. aeruginosa). Clin Infect Dis 2021;72(7):e169–83.

10. Tamma PD, Aitken SL, Bonomo RA, et al. Infectious Diseases Society of America Guidance on the Treatment of AmpC β-lactamase producing Enterobacterales, Carbapenem-resistant Acinetobacter baumainnii, and Stenotrophomas maltophilia infections. Clin Infect Dis 2022;74(12):2089–114.

11. Paul M, Carrara E, Retamar P, et al. European Society of Clinical Microbiology and Infectious Diseases (ESCMID) guidelines for the treatment of infections caused by multidrug-resistant Gram-negative bacilli (endorsed by European Society of Intensive Care Medicine). Clin Microbiol Infect 2022;28:521–47.

12. Lawandi A, Yek C, Kadri SS. IDSA guidance and ESCMID guidelines: complementary approaches toward a care standard for MDR Gram-negative infections. Clin Microbiol Infect 2022;28(4):465–9.

13. McCreary EK, Heil EL, Tamma PD. New Perspectives on Antimicrobial Agents: Cefiderocol. Antimicrob Agents Chemother 2021;65(8):e0217120.

14. Ito A, Sato T, Ota M, et al. *In Vitro* Antibacterial Properties of Cefiderocol, a Novel Siderophore Cephalosporin, against Gram-Negative Bacteria. Antimicrob Agents Chemother 2018;62(1):e01454-17.

15. Tamma PD, Doi Y, Bonomo RA, et al. Antibacterial Resistance Leadership G. A Primer on AmpC beta-Lactamases: Necessary Knowledge for an Increasingly Multidrug-resistant World. Clin Infect Dis 2019;69(8):1446–55.

16. Eliopoulos GM. Induction of beta-lactamases. J Antimicrob Chemother 1988; 22(Suppl A):37–44.

17. Bennett PM, Chopra I. Molecular basis of beta-lactamase induction in bacteria. Antimicrob Agents Chemother 1993;37(2):153–8.

18. Jacobson KL, Cohen SH, Inciardi JF, et al. The relationship between antecedent antibiotic use and resistance to extended-spectrum cephalosporins in group I beta-lactamase-producing organisms. Clin Infect Dis 1995;21(5):1107–13.

19. Lindberg F, Westman L, Normark S. Regulatory components in Citrobacter freundii ampC beta-lactamase induction. Proc Natl Acad Sci U S A 1985; 82(14):4620–4.

20. Underwood S, Avison MB. Citrobacter koseri and Citrobacter amalonaticus isolates carry highly divergent beta-lactamase genes despite having high levels of biochemical similarity and 16S rRNA sequence homology. J Antimicrob Chemother 2004;53(6):1076–80.

21. Petrella S, Clermont D, Casin I, et al. Novel class A beta-lactamase Sed-1 from Citrobacter sedlakii: genetic diversity of beta-lactamases within the Citrobacter genus. Antimicrob Agents Chemother 2001;45(8):2287–98.

22. Matsen JM, Blazevic DJ, Ryan JA, et al. Characterization of indole-positive Proteus mirabilis. Appl Microbiol 1972;23(3):592–4.

23. Papp-Wallace KM, Bethel CR, Caillon J, et al. Beyond Piperacillin-Tazobactam: Cefepime and AAI101 as a Potent beta-Lactam-beta-Lactamase Inhibitor Combination. Antimicrob Agents Chemother 2019;63(5):e00105–19.

24. Endimiani A, Doi Y, Bethel CR, et al. Enhancing resistance to cephalosporins in class C beta-lactamases: impact of Gly214Glu in CMY-2. Biochemistry 2010; 49(5):1014–23.

25. Drawz SM, Papp-Wallace KM, Bonomo RA. New beta-lactamase inhibitors: a therapeutic renaissance in an MDR world. Antimicrob Agents Chemother 2014;58(4):1835–46.

26. Bush K, Bradford PA. Interplay between beta-lactamases and new beta-lactamase inhibitors. Nat Rev Microbiol 2019;17(5):295–306.

27. Hilty M, Sendi P, Seiffert SN, et al. Characterisation and clinical features of Enterobacter cloacae bloodstream infections occurring at a tertiary care university hospital in Switzerland: is cefepime adequate therapy? Int J Antimicrob Agents 2013;41(3):236–49.

28. Tamma PD, Girdwood SC, Gopaul R, et al. The use of cefepime for treating AmpC beta-lactamase-producing Enterobacteriaceae. Clin Infect Dis 2013; 57(6):781–8.

29. Choi SH, Lee JE, Park SJ, et al. Emergence of antibiotic resistance during therapy for infections caused by Enterobacteriaceae producing AmpC beta-lactamase: implications for antibiotic use. Antimicrob Agents Chemother 2008; 52(3):995–1000.

30. Chow JW, Fine MJ, Shlaes DM, et al. Enterobacter bacteremia: clinical features and emergence of antibiotic resistance during therapy. Ann Intern Med 1991; 115(8):585–90.

31. Kaye KS, Cosgrove S, Harris A, et al. Risk factors for emergence of resistance to broad-spectrum cephalosporins among Enterobacter spp. Antimicrob Agents Chemother 2001;45(9):2628–30.

32. Kohlmann R, Bahr T, Gatermann SG. Species-specific mutation rates for ampC derepression in Enterobacterales with chromosomally encoded inducible AmpC beta-lactamase. J Antimicrob Chemother 2018;73(6):1530–6.

33. Liu C, Wang X, Chen Y, et al. Three Yersinia enterocolitica AmpD Homologs Participate in the Multi-Step Regulation of Chromosomal Cephalosporinase, AmpC. Front Microbiol 2016;7:1282.

34. Seoane A, Francia MV, Garcia Lobo JM. Nucleotide sequence of the ampC-ampR region from the chromosome of Yersinia enterocolitica. Antimicrob Agents Chemother 1992;36(5):1049–52.

35. Girlich D, Naas T, Bellais S, et al. Heterogeneity of AmpC cephalosporinases of Hafnia alvei clinical isolates expressing inducible or constitutive ceftazidime resistance phenotypes. Antimicrob Agents Chemother 2000;44(11):3220–3.

36. Tamma PD, Rodriguez-Bano J. The Use of Noncarbapenem beta-Lactams for the Treatment of Extended-Spectrum beta-Lactamase Infections. Clin Infect Dis 2017;64(7):972–80.

37. Hancock RE, Bellido F. Antibacterial in vitro activity of fourth generation cephalosporins. J Chemother 1996;8(Suppl 2):31–6.

38. Negri MC, Baquero F. In vitro selective concentrations of cefepime and ceftazidime for AmpC beta-lactamase hyperproducer Enterobacter cloacae variants. Clin Microbiol Infect 1999;5(Suppl 1):S25–8.

39. Harris PN, Wei JY, Shen AW, et al. Carbapenems versus alternative antibiotics for the treatment of bloodstream infections caused by Enterobacter, Citrobacter

or Serratia species: a systematic review with meta-analysis. J Antimicrob Chemother 2016;71(2):296–306.

40. Sanders CC, Bradford PA, Ehrhardt AF, et al. Penicillin-binding proteins and induction of AmpC beta-lactamase. Antimicrob Agents Chemother 1997;41(9): 2013–5.

41. Weber DA, Sanders CC. Diverse potential of beta-lactamase inhibitors to induce class I enzymes. Antimicrob Agents Chemother 1990;34(1):156–8.

42. Livermore DM, Oakton KJ, Carter MW, et al. Activity of ertapenem (MK-0826) versus Enterobacteriaceae with potent beta-lactamases. Antimicrob Agents Chemother 2001;45(10):2831–7.

43. Siedner MJ, Galar A, Guzman-Suarez BB, et al. Cefepime vs other antibacterial agents for the treatment of Enterobacter species bacteremia. Clin Infect Dis 2014;58(11):1554–63.

44. Tan SH, Ng TM, Chew KL, et al. Outcomes of treating AmpC-producing Enterobacterales bacteraemia with carbapenems vs. non-carbapenems. Int J Antimicrob Agents 2020;55(2):105860.

45. Barnaud G, Benzerara Y, Gravisse J, et al. Selection during cefepime treatment of a new cephalosporinase variant with extended-spectrum resistance to cefepime in an Enterobacter aerogenes clinical isolate. Antimicrob Agents Chemother 2004;48(3):1040–2.

46. Song W, Moland ES, Hanson ND, et al. Failure of cefepime therapy in treatment of Klebsiella pneumoniae bacteremia. J Clin Microbiol 2005;43(9):4891–4.

47. Limaye AP, Gautom RK, Black D, et al. Rapid emergence of resistance to cefepime during treatment. Clin Infect Dis 1997;25(2):339–40.

48. Charrel RN, Pages JM, De Micco P, et al. Prevalence of outer membrane porin alteration in beta-lactam-antibiotic-resistant Enterobacter aerogenes. Antimicrob Agents Chemother 1996;40(12):2854–8.

49. Fung-Tomc JC, Gradelski E, Huczko E, et al. Differences in the resistant variants of Enterobacter cloacae selected by extended-spectrum cephalosporins. Antimicrob Agents Chemother 1996;40(5):1289–93.

50. Procter and Gamble Pharmaceuticals, Inc. MACROBID - nitrofurantoin monohydrate and nitrofurantoin, macrocrystalline capsule [package insert]. Available at: www.accessdata.fda.gov/drugsatfda_docs/label/2009/020064s019lbl.pdf. Accessed October 24, 2022.

51. U.S. Food and Drug Administration. MONUROL (fosfomycin tromethamine) SACHET [package insert]. Available at: www.accessdata.fda.gov/drugsatfda_docs/label/2008/050717s005lbl.pdf. Accessed 5 August 2020.

52. Huttner A, Kowalczyk A, Turjeman A, et al. Effect of 5-Day Nitrofurantoin vs Single-Dose Fosfomycin on Clinical Resolution of Uncomplicated Lower Urinary Tract Infection in Women: A Randomized Clinical Trial. JAMA 2018;319(17): 1781–9.

53. Agwuh KN, MacGowan A. Pharmacokinetics and pharmacodynamics of the tetracyclines including glycylcyclines. J Antimicrob Chemother 2006;58(2): 256–65.

54. Fox MT, Melia MT, Same RG, et al. A Seven-Day Course of TMP-SMX May Be as Effective as a Seven-Day Course of Ciprofloxacin for the Treatment of Pyelonephritis. Am J Med 2017;130(7):842–5.

55. Jernigan JA, Hatfield KM, Wolford H, et al. Multidrug-Resistant Bacterial Infections in U.S. Hospitalized Patients, 2012-2017. N Engl J Med 2020;382(14): 1309–19.

56. Robberts FJ, Kohner PC, Patel R. Unreliable extended-spectrum beta-lactamase detection in the presence of plasmid-mediated AmpC in Escherichia coli clinical isolates. J Clin Microbiol 2009;47(2):358–61.

57. Clinical and Laboratory Standards Institute. M100: performance standards for antimicrobial susceptibility testing. 31st edition. Wayne (PA): Clinical and Laboratory Standards Institute; 2021.

58. Tamma PD, Humphries RM. PRO: Testing for ESBL production is necessary for ceftriaxone-non-susceptible Enterobacterales: perfect should not be the enemy of progress. JAC Antimicrob Resist 2021;3(2):dlab019.

59. Mathers AJ, Lewis JS, CON 2nd. Testing for ESBL production is unnecessary for ceftriaxone-resistant Enterobacterales. JAC Antimicrob Resist 2021;3(2): dlab020.

60. Tamma PD, Sharara SL, Pana ZD, et al. Molecular Epidemiology of Ceftriaxone Non-Susceptible Enterobacterales Isolates in an Academic Medical Center in the United States. Open Forum Infect Dis 2019;6(8):ofz353.

61. Haidar G, Philips NJ, Shields RK, et al. Ceftolozane-Tazobactam for the Treatment of Multidrug-Resistant Pseudomonas aeruginosa Infections: Clinical Effectiveness and Evolution of Resistance. Clin Infect Dis 2017;65(1):110–20.

62. Tamma PD, Smith TT, Adebayo A, et al. Prevalence of bla CTX-M Genes in Gram-Negative Bloodstream Isolates across 66 Hospitals in the United States. J Clin Microbiol 2021;59(6):e00127-21.

63. Bush K, Bradford PA. Epidemiology of beta-Lactamase-Producing Pathogens. Clin Microbiol Rev 2020;33(2):e00047-e19.

64. Bush K, Jacoby GA. Updated functional classification of beta-lactamases. Antimicrob Agents Chemother 2010;54(3):969–76.

65. Castanheira M, Farrell SE, Krause KM, et al. Contemporary diversity of beta-lactamases among Enterobacteriaceae in the nine U.S. census regions and ceftazidime-avibactam activity tested against isolates producing the most prevalent beta-lactamase groups. Antimicrob Agents Chemother 2014;58(2):833–8.

66. Castanheira M, Simner PJ, Bradford PA. Extended-spectrum beta-lactamases: an update on their characteristics, epidemiology and detection. JAC Antimicrob Resist 2021;3(3):dlab092.

67. Harris PNA, Tambyah PA, Lye DC, et al. Effect of Piperacillin-Tazobactam vs Meropenem on 30-Day Mortality for Patients With E coli or Klebsiella pneumoniae Bloodstream Infection and Ceftriaxone Resistance: A Randomized Clinical Trial. JAMA 2018;320(10):984–94.

68. Henderson A, Paterson DL, Chatfield MD, et al. Association between minimum inhibitory concentration, beta-lactamase genes and mortality for patients treated with piperacillin/tazobactam or meropenem from the MERINO study. Clin Infect Dis 2020;73(11):e3842–50.

69. Harris PN, Yin M, Jureen R, et al. Comparable outcomes for beta-lactam/beta-lactamase inhibitor combinations and carbapenems in definitive treatment of bloodstream infections caused by cefotaxime-resistant Escherichia coli or Klebsiella pneumoniae. Antimicrob Resist Infect Control 2015;4:14.

70. Livermore DM, Andrews JM, Hawkey PM, et al. Are susceptibility tests enough, or should laboratories still seek ESBLs and carbapenemases directly? J Antimicrob Chemother 2012;67(7):1569–77.

71. Zhou M, Wang Y, Liu C, et al. Comparison of five commonly used automated susceptibility testing methods for accuracy in the China Antimicrobial Resistance Surveillance System (CARSS) hospitals. Infect Drug Resist 2018;11: 1347–58.

72. Paterson DL, Henderson A, Harris PNA. Current evidence for therapy of ceftriaxone-resistant Gram-negative bacteremia. Curr Opin Infect Dis 2020; 33(1):78–85.
73. Livermore DM, Day M, Cleary P, et al. OXA-1 beta-lactamase and non-susceptibility to penicillin/beta-lactamase inhibitor combinations among ESBL-producing Escherichia coli. J Antimicrob Chemother 2019;74(2):326–33.
74. Wang R, Cosgrove SE, Tschudin-Sutter S, et al. Cefepime Therapy for Cefepime-Susceptible Extended-Spectrum beta-Lactamase-Producing Entero-bacteriaceae Bacteremia. Open Forum Infect Dis 2016;3(3):ofw132.
75. Rodríguez-Baño J, Navarro MD, Retamar P, et al. Extended-Spectrum Beta-Lactamases-Red Espanola de Investigacion en Patologia Infecciosa/Grupo de Estudio de Infeccion Hospitalaria G. beta-Lactam/beta-lactam inhibitor combinations for the treatment of bacteremia due to extended-spectrum beta-lacta-mase-producing Escherichia coli: a post hoc analysis of prospective cohorts. Clin Infect Dis 2012;54(2):167–74.
76. Ng TM, Khong WX, Harris PN, et al. Empiric Piperacillin-Tazobactam versus Car-bapenems in the Treatment of Bacteraemia Due to Extended-Spectrum Beta-Lactamase-Producing Enterobacteriaceae. PLoS One 2016;11(4):e0153696.
77. Tamma PD, Han JH, Rock C, et al. Carbapenem therapy is associated with improved survival compared with piperacillin-tazobactam for patients with extended-spectrum beta-lactamase bacteremia. Clin Infect Dis 2015;60(9): 1319–25.
78. Tsai HY, Chen YH, Tang HJ, et al. Carbapenems and piperacillin/tazobactam for the treatment of bacteremia caused by extended-spectrum beta-lactamase-producing Proteus mirabilis. Diagn Microbiol Infect Dis 2014;80(3):222–6.
79. Dizbay M, Ozger HS, Karasahin O, et al. Treatment efficacy and superinfection rates in complicated urinarytract infections treated with ertapenem or piperacil-lin tazobactam. Turk J Med Sci 2016;46(6):1760–4.
80. Seo YB, Lee J, Kim YK, et al. Randomized controlled trial of piperacillin-tazobactam, cefepime and ertapenem for the treatment of urinary tract infection caused by extended-spectrum beta-lactamase-producing Escherichia coli. BMC Infect Dis 2017;17(1):404.
81. Yoon YK, Kim JH, Sohn JW, et al. Role of piperacillin/tazobactam as a carbapenem-sparing antibiotic for treatment of acute pyelonephritis due to extended-spectrum beta-lactamase-producing Escherichia coli. Int J Antimi-crob Agents 2017;49(4):410–5.
82. Sharara SL, Amoah J, Pana ZD, et al. Is Piperacillin-Tazobactam Effective for the Treatment of Pyelonephritis Caused by ESBL-producing Organisms? Clin Infect Dis 2019;71(8):e331–7.
83. Nasir N, Ahmed S, Razi S, et al. Risk factors for mortality of patients with ceftri-axone resistant E. coli bacteremia receiving carbapenem versus beta lactam/ beta lactamase inhibitor therapy. BMC Res Notes 2019;12(1):611.
84. Xiao T, Yang K, Zhou Y, et al. Risk factors and outcomes in non-transplant pa-tients with extended-spectrum beta-lactamase-producing Escherichia coli bacteremia: a retrospective study from 2013 to 2016. Antimicrob Resist Infect Control 2019;8:144.
85. Ko JH, Lee NR, Joo EJ, et al. Appropriate non-carbapenems are not inferior to carbapenems as initial empirical therapy for bacteremia caused by extended-spectrum beta-lactamase-producing Enterobacteriaceae: a propensity score weighted multicenter cohort study. Eur J Clin Microbiol Infect Dis 2018;37(2): 305–11.

86. Meini S, Laureano R, Tascini C, et al. Clinical outcomes of elderly patients with bloodstream infections due to extended-spectrum beta-lactamase-producing Enterobacteriaceae in an Italian Internal Medicine ward. Eur J Intern Med 2018;48:50–6.

87. Ofer-Friedman H, Shefler C, Sharma S, et al. Carbapenems Versus Piperacillin-Tazobactam for Bloodstream Infections of Nonurinary Source Caused by Extended-Spectrum Beta-Lactamase-Producing Enterobacteriaceae. Infect Control Hosp Epidemiol 2015;36(8):981–5.

88. Bitterman R, Paul M, Leibovici L, et al. PipEracillin Tazobactam Versus mERoPE-Nem for Treatment of Bloodstream Infections Caused by Cephalosporin-resistant Enterobacteriaceae (PETERPEN). Available at: https://clinicaltrials.gov/ct2/show/NCT03671967. Accessed 16 September 2021.

89. Chopra T, Marchaim D, Veltman J, et al. Impact of cefepime therapy on mortality among patients with bloodstream infections caused by extended-spectrum-beta-lactamase-producing Klebsiella pneumoniae and Escherichia coli. Antimicrob Agents Chemother 2012;56(7):3936–42.

90. Zanetti G, Bally F, Greub G, et al. Cefepime versus imipenem-cilastatin for treatment of nosocomial pneumonia in intensive care unit patients: a multicenter, evaluator-blind, prospective, randomized study. Antimicrob Agents Chemother 2003;47(11):3442–7.

91. Burgess DS, Hall RG 2nd. In vitro killing of parenteral beta-lactams against standard and high inocula of extended-spectrum beta-lactamase and non-ESBL producing Klebsiella pneumoniae. Diagn Microbiol Infect Dis 2004;49(1):41–6.

92. Kim SA, Altshuler J, Paris D, et al. Cefepime versus carbapenems for the treatment of urinary tract infections caused by extended-spectrum beta-lactamase-producing enterobacteriaceae. Int J Antimicrob Agents 2018;51(1):155–8.

93. Lepeule R, Leflon-Guibout V, Vanjak D, et al. Clinical spectrum of urine cultures positive for ESBL-producing Escherichia coli in hospitalized patients and impact on antibiotic use. Med Mal Infect 2014;44(11–12):530–4.

94. Tamma PD, Conley AT, Cosgrove SE, et al. Association of 30-Day Mortality With Oral Step-Down vs Continued Intravenous Therapy in Patients Hospitalized With Enterobacteriaceae Bacteremia. JAMA Intern Med 2019;179(3):316–23.

95. Punjabi C, Tien V, Meng L, et al. Oral Fluoroquinolone or Trimethoprim-sulfamethoxazole vs. beta-lactams as Step-Down Therapy for Enterobacteriaceae Bacteremia: Systematic Review and Meta-analysis. Open Forum Infect Dis 2019;6(10):ofz364.

96. GlaxoSmithKline. AUGMENTIN® (amoxicillin/clavulanate potassium): Powder for Oral Suspension and Chewable Tablets [Package Insert]. Available at: https://www.accessdata.fda.gov/drugsatfda_docs/label/2008/050575s037550597s044050725s025050726s019lbl.pdf. Accessed 14 September 2021.

97. Centers for Disease Control and Prevention. Facility Guidance for Control of Carbapenem-resistant Enterobacteriaceae (CRE): November 2015 Update - CRE Toolkit, 2015. Available at: https://www.cdc.gov/hai/pdfs/cre/cre-guidance-508.pdf.

98. Sabour S, Huang Y, Bhatnagar A, et al. Detection and Characterization of Targeted Carbapenem-Resistant Healthcare-Associated Threats: Findings from The Antibiotic Resistance Laboratory Network, 2017 to 2019. Antimicrob Agents Chemother 2021;65:e0110521.

99. van Duin D, Arias CA, Komarow L, et al. Molecular and clinical epidemiology of carbapenem-resistant Enterobacterales in the USA (CRACKLE-2): a prospective cohort study. Lancet Infect Dis 2020;20(6):731–41.
100. Aitken SL, Tarrand JJ, Deshpande LM, et al. High Rates of Nonsusceptibility to Ceftazidime-avibactam and Identification of New Delhi Metallo-beta-lactamase Production in Enterobacteriaceae Bloodstream Infections at a Major Cancer Center. Clin Infect Dis 2016;63(7):954–8.
101. Senchyna F, Gaur RL, Sandlund J, et al. Diversity of resistance mechanisms in carbapenem-resistant Enterobacteriaceae at a health care system in Northern California, from 2013 to 2016. Diagn Microbiol Infect Dis 2019;93(3):250–7.
102. Tamma PD, Simner PJ. Phenotypic Detection of Carbapenemase-Producing Organisms from Clinical Isolates. J Clin Microbiol 2018;56(11):e01140-18.
103. Spiliopoulou I, Kazmierczak K, Stone GG. In vitro activity of ceftazidime/avibactam against isolates of carbapenem-non-susceptible Enterobacteriaceae collected during the INFORM global surveillance programme (2015-17). J Antimicrob Chemother 2020;75(2):384–91.
104. Castanheira M, Doyle TB, Collingsworth TD, et al. Increasing frequency of OXA-48-producing Enterobacterales worldwide and activity of ceftazidime/avibactam, meropenem/vaborbactam and comparators against these isolates. J Antimicrob Chemother 2021;76(12):3125–34.
105. Castanheira M, Doyle TB, Kantro V, et al. Meropenem-Vaborbactam Activity against Carbapenem-Resistant Enterobacterales Isolates Collected in U.S. Hospitals during 2016 to 2018. Antimicrob Agents Chemother 2020;64(2): e01951-19.
106. Pfaller MA, Huband MD, Mendes RE, et al. In vitro activity of meropenem/vaborbactam and characterisation of carbapenem resistance mechanisms among carbapenem-resistant Enterobacteriaceae from the 2015 meropenem/vaborbactam surveillance programme. Int J Antimicrob Agents 2018;52(2):144–50.
107. Tamma PD, Hsu AJ. Defining the Role of Novel beta-Lactam Agents That Target Carbapenem-Resistant Gram-Negative Organisms. J Pediatr Infect Dis Soc 2019;8(3):251–60.
108. Sandri AM, Landersdorfer CB, Jacob J, et al. Population pharmacokinetics of intravenous polymyxin B in critically ill patients: implications for selection of dosage regimens. Clin Infect Dis 2013;57(4):524–31.
109. Dobias J, Denervaud-Tendon V, Poirel L, et al. Activity of the novel siderophore cephalosporin cefiderocol against multidrug-resistant Gram-negative pathogens. Eur J Clin Microbiol Infect Dis 2017;36(12):2319–27.
110. Humphries RM, Yang S, Hemarajata P, et al. First Report of Ceftazidime-Avibactam Resistance in a KPC-3-Expressing Klebsiella pneumoniae Isolate. Antimicrob Agents Chemother 2015;59(10):6605–7.
111. Biagi M, Wu T, Lee M, et al. Searching for the Optimal Treatment for Metallo- and Serine-beta-Lactamase Producing Enterobacteriaceae: Aztreonam in Combination with Ceftazidime-avibactam or Meropenem-vaborbactam. Antimicrob Agents Chemother 2019;63(12):e01426-19.
112. Sieswerda E, van den Brand M, van den Berg RB, et al. Successful rescue treatment of sepsis due to a pandrug-resistant, NDM-producing Klebsiella pneumoniae using aztreonam powder for nebulizer solution as intravenous therapy in combination with ceftazidime/avibactam. J Antimicrob Chemother 2020;75(3): 773–5.
113. Benchetrit L, Mathy V, Armand-Lefevre L, et al. Successful treatment of septic shock due to NDM-1-producing Klebsiella pneumoniae using ceftazidime/

avibactam combined with aztreonam in solid organ transplant recipients: report of two cases. Int J Antimicrob Agents 2020;55(1):105842.

114. Falcone M, Daikos GL, Tiseo G, et al. Efficacy of Ceftazidime-avibactam Plus Aztreonam in Patients With Bloodstream Infections Caused by Metallo-beta-lactamase-Producing Enterobacterales. Clin Infect Dis 2021;72(11):1871–8.

115. Lodise TP, Smith NM, O'Donnell N, et al. Determining the optimal dosing of a novel combination regimen of ceftazidime/avibactam with aztreonam against NDM-1-producing Enterobacteriaceae using a hollow-fibre infection model. J Antimicrob Chemother 2020;75(9):2622–32.

116. De la Calle C, Rodriguez O, Morata L, et al. Clinical characteristics and prognosis of infections caused by OXA-48 carbapenemase-producing Enterobacteriaceae in patients treated with ceftazidime-avibactam. Int J Antimicrob Agents 2019;53(4):520–4.

117. Eckmann C, Montravers P, Bassetti M, et al. Efficacy of tigecycline for the treatment of complicated intra-abdominal infections in real-life clinical practice from five European observational studies. J Antimicrob Chemother 2013;68(Suppl 2): ii25–35.

118. Chen Z, Shi X. Adverse events of high-dose tigecycline in the treatment of ventilator-associated pneumonia due to multidrug-resistant pathogens. Medicine (Baltimore) 2018;97(38):e12467.

119. Shields RK, Nguyen MH, Chen L, et al. Ceftazidime-Avibactam Is Superior to Other Treatment Regimens against Carbapenem-Resistant Klebsiella pneumoniae Bacteremia. Antimicrob Agents Chemother 2017;61(8):e00883-17.

120. van Duin D, Lok JJ, Earley M, et al. Colistin Versus Ceftazidime-Avibactam in the Treatment of Infections Due to Carbapenem-Resistant Enterobacteriaceae. Clin Infect Dis 2018;66(2):163–71.

121. Wunderink RG, Giamarellos-Bourboulis EJ, Rahav G, et al. Effect and Safety of Meropenem-Vaborbactam versus Best-Available Therapy in Patients with Carbapenem-Resistant Enterobacteriaceae Infections: The TANGO II Randomized Clinical Trial. Infect Dis Ther 2018;7(4):439–55.

122. Motsch J, Murta de Oliveira C, Stus V, et al. RESTORE-IMI 1: A Multicenter, Randomized, Double-blind Trial Comparing Efficacy and Safety of Imipenem/Relebactam vs Colistin Plus Imipenem in Patients With Imipenem-nonsusceptible Bacterial Infections. Clin Infect Dis 2020;70(9):1799–808.

123. Karaiskos I, Daikos GL, Gkoufa A, et al. Ceftazidime/avibactam in the era of carbapenemase-producing Klebsiella pneumoniae: experience from a national registry study. J Antimicrob Chemother 2021;76(3):775–83.

124. Hakeam HA, Alsahli H, Albabtain L, et al. Effectiveness of ceftazidime-avibactam versus colistin in treating carbapenem-resistant Enterobacteriaceae bacteremia. Int J Infect Dis 2021;109:1–7.

125. Caston JJ, Lacort-Peralta I, Martin-Davila P, et al. Clinical efficacy of ceftazidime/avibactam versus other active agents for the treatment of bacteremia due to carbapenemase-producing Enterobacteriaceae in hematologic patients. Int J Infect Dis 2017;59:118–23.

126. Alraddadi BM, Saeedi M, Qutub M, et al. Efficacy of ceftazidime-avibactam in the treatment of infections due to Carbapenem-resistant Enterobacteriaceae. BMC Infect Dis 2019;19(1):772.

127. Tumbarello M, Trecarichi EM, Corona A, et al. Efficacy of Ceftazidime-Avibactam Salvage Therapy in Patients With Infections Caused by Klebsiella pneumoniae Carbapenemase-producing K. pneumoniae. Clin Infect Dis 2019;68(3):355–64.

128. Shields RK, Chen L, Cheng S, et al. Emergence of Ceftazidime-Avibactam Resistance Due to Plasmid-Borne blaKPC-3 Mutations during Treatment of Carbapenem-Resistant Klebsiella pneumoniae Infections. Antimicrob Agents Chemother 2017;61(3):e02097-16.

129. Shields RK, Potoski BA, Haidar G, et al. Clinical Outcomes, Drug Toxicity, and Emergence of Ceftazidime-Avibactam Resistance Among Patients Treated for Carbapenem-Resistant Enterobacteriaceae Infections. Clin Infect Dis 2016; 63(12):1615–8.

130. Shields RK, McCreary EK, Marini RV, et al. Early experience with meropenem-vaborbactam for treatment of carbapenem-resistant Enterobacteriaceae infections. Clin Infect Dis 2019;71(3):667–71.

131. Shields RK, Iovleva A, Kline EG, et al. Clinical evolution of AmpC-mediated ceftazidime-avibactam and cefiderocol resistance in Enterobacter cloacae complex following exposure to cefepime. Clin Infect Dis 2020;71(10):2713–6.

132. Shields RK, Nguyen MH, Chen L, et al. Pneumonia and Renal Replacement Therapy Are Risk Factors for Ceftazidime-Avibactam Treatment Failures and Resistance among Patients with Carbapenem-Resistant Enterobacteriaceae Infections. Antimicrob Agents Chemother 2018;62(5):e02497-17.

133. Alosaimy S, Lagnf AM, Morrisette T, et al. Real-world, Multicenter Experience With Meropenem-Vaborbactam for Gram-Negative Bacterial Infections Including Carbapenem-Resistant Enterobacterales and Pseudomonas aeruginosa. Open Forum Infect Dis 2021;8(8):ofab371.

134. Kadri SS, Adjemian J, Lai YL, et al. Difficult-to-Treat Resistance in Gram-negative Bacteremia at 173 US Hospitals: Retrospective Cohort Analysis of Prevalence, Predictors, and Outcome of Resistance to All First-line Agents. Clin Infect Dis 2018;67(12):1803–14.

135. Magiorakos AP, Srinivasan A, Carey RB, et al. Multidrug-resistant, extensively drug-resistant and pandrug-resistant bacteria: an international expert proposal for interim standard definitions for acquired resistance. Clin Microbiol Infect 2012;18(3):268–81.

136. Lister PD, Wolter DJ, Hanson ND. Antibacterial-resistant Pseudomonas aeruginosa: clinical impact and complex regulation of chromosomally encoded resistance mechanisms. Clin Microbiol Rev 2009;22(4):582–610.

137. Wolter DJ, Lister PD. Mechanisms of beta-lactam resistance among Pseudomonas aeruginosa. Curr Pharm Des 2013;19(2):209–22.

138. Karlowsky JA, Kazmierczak KM, de Jonge BLM, et al. In Vitro Activity of Aztreonam-Avibactam against Enterobacteriaceae and Pseudomonas aeruginosa Isolated by Clinical Laboratories in 40 Countries from 2012 to 2015. Antimicrob Agents Chemother 2017;61(9):e00472-17.

139. Karlowsky JA, Kazmierczak KM, Bouchillon SK, et al. In Vitro Activity of Ceftazidime-Avibactam against Clinical Isolates of Enterobacteriaceae and Pseudomonas aeruginosa Collected in Asia-Pacific Countries: Results from the INFORM Global Surveillance Program, 2012 to 2015. Antimicrob Agents Chemother 2018;62(7):e02569-17.

140. Buehrle DJ, Shields RK, Chen L, et al. Evaluation of the In Vitro Activity of Ceftazidime-Avibactam and Ceftolozane-Tazobactam against Meropenem-Resistant Pseudomonas aeruginosa Isolates. Antimicrob Agents Chemother 2016;60(5):3227–31.

141. Rolston KVI, Gerges B, Shelburne S, et al. Activity of Cefiderocol and Comparators against Isolates from Cancer Patients. Antimicrob Agents Chemother 2020;64(5):e01955-19.

142. Falagas ME, Skalidis T, Vardakas KZ, et al. Activity of cefiderocol (S-649266) against carbapenem-resistant Gram-negative bacteria collected from inpatients in Greek hospitals. J Antimicrob Chemother 2017;72(6):1704–8.

143. Golden AR, Adam HJ, Baxter M, et al. *In Vitro* Activity of Cefiderocol, a Novel Siderophore Cephalosporin, against Gram-Negative Bacilli Isolated from Patients in Canadian Intensive Care Units. Diagn Microbiol Infect Dis 2020;97(1): 115012.

144. Hackel MA, Tsuji M, Yamano Y, et al. *In Vitro* Activity of the Siderophore Cephalosporin, Cefiderocol, against Carbapenem-Nonsusceptible and Multidrug-Resistant Isolates of Gram-Negative Bacilli Collected Worldwide in 2014 to 2016. Antimicrob Agents Chemother 2018;62(2):e01968-17.

145. Karlowsky JA, Hackel MA, Tsuji M, et al. *In Vitro* Activity of Cefiderocol, a Siderophore Cephalosporin, Against Gram-Negative Bacilli Isolated by Clinical Laboratories in North America and Europe in 2015-2016: SIDERO-WT-2015. Int J Antimicrob Agents 2019;53(4):456–66.

146. Bassetti M, Echols R, Matsunaga Y, et al. Efficacy and safety of cefiderocol or best available therapy for the treatment of serious infections caused by carbapenem-resistant Gram-negative bacteria (CREDIBLE-CR): a randomised, open-label, multicentre, pathogen-focused, descriptive, phase 3 trial. Lancet Infect Dis 2021;21(2):226–40.

147. Pogue JM, Kaye KS, Veve MP, et al. Ceftolozane/Tazobactam vs Polymyxin or Aminoglycoside-based Regimens for the Treatment of Drug-resistant Pseudomonas aeruginosa. Clin Infect Dis 2020;71(2):304–10.

148. Stone GG, Newell P, Gasink LB, et al. Clinical activity of ceftazidime/avibactam against MDR Enterobacteriaceae and Pseudomonas aeruginosa: pooled data from the ceftazidime/avibactam Phase III clinical trial programme. J Antimicrob Chemother 2018;73(9):2519–23.

149. Vijayakumar S, Biswas I, Veeraraghavan B. Accurate identification of clinically important Acinetobacter spp.: an update. Future Sci OA 2019;5(6):FSO395.

150. Bonomo RA, Szabo D. Mechanisms of multidrug resistance in Acinetobacter species and Pseudomonas aeruginosa. Clin Infect Dis 2006;43(Suppl 2): S49–56.

151. Penwell WF, Shapiro AB, Giacobbe RA, et al. Molecular mechanisms of sulbactam antibacterial activity and resistance determinants in Acinetobacter baumannii. Antimicrob Agents Chemother 2015;59(3):1680–9.

152. McLeod SM, Shapiro AB, Moussa SH, et al. Frequency and Mechanism of Spontaneous Resistance to Sulbactam Combined with the Novel beta-Lactamase Inhibitor ETX2514 in Clinical Isolates of Acinetobacter baumannii. Antimicrob Agents Chemother 2018;62(2):e01576-17.

153. Krizova L, Poirel L, Nordmann P, et al. TEM-1 beta-lactamase as a source of resistance to sulbactam in clinical strains of Acinetobacter baumannii. J Antimicrob Chemother 2013;68(12):2786–91.

154. Liu J, Shu Y, Zhu F, et al. Comparative efficacy and safety of combination therapy with high-dose sulbactam or colistin with additional antibacterial agents for multiple drug-resistant and extensively drug-resistant Acinetobacter baumannii infections: A systematic review and network meta-analysis. J Glob Antimicrob Resist 2021;24:136–47.

155. Jung SY, Lee SH, Lee SY, et al. Antimicrobials for the treatment of drug-resistant Acinetobacter baumannii pneumonia in critically ill patients: a systemic review and Bayesian network meta-analysis. Crit Care 2017;21(1):319.

156. Yilmaz GR, Guven T, Guner R, et al. Colistin alone or combined with sulbactam or carbapenem against A. baumannii in ventilator-associated pneumonia. J Infect Dev Ctries 2015;9(5):476–85.
157. Paul M, Daikos GL, Durante-Mangoni E, et al. Colistin alone versus colistin plus meropenem for treatment of severe infections caused by carbapenem-resistant Gram-negative bacteria: an open-label, randomised controlled trial. Lancet Infect Dis 2018;18(4):391–400.
158. Sirijatuphat R, Thamlikitkul V. Preliminary study of colistin versus colistin plus fosfomycin for treatment of carbapenem-resistant Acinetobacter baumannii infections. Antimicrob Agents Chemother 2014;58(9):5598–601.
159. Durante-Mangoni E, Signoriello G, Andini R, et al. Colistin and rifampicin compared with colistin alone for the treatment of serious infections due to extensively drug-resistant Acinetobacter baumannii: a multicenter, randomized clinical trial. Clin Infect Dis 2013;57(3):349–58.
160. Aydemir H, Akduman D, Piskin N, et al. Colistin vs. the combination of colistin and rifampicin for the treatment of carbapenem-resistant Acinetobacter baumannii ventilator-associated pneumonia. Epidemiol Infect 2013;141(6):1214–22.
161. Park HJ, Cho JH, Kim HJ, et al. Colistin monotherapy versus colistin/rifampicin combination therapy in pneumonia caused by colistin-resistant Acinetobacter baumannii: A randomised controlled trial. J Glob Antimicrob Resist 2019;17: 66–71.
162. Makris D, Petinaki E, Tsolaki V, et al. Colistin versus Colistin Combined with Ampicillin-Sulbactam for Multiresistant Acinetobacter baumannii Ventilator-associated Pneumonia Treatment: An Open-label Prospective Study. Indian J Crit Care Med 2018;22(2):67–77.
163. Brooke JS. Stenotrophomonas maltophilia: an emerging global opportunistic pathogen. Clin Microbiol Rev 2012;25(1):2–41.
164. Trifonova A, Strateva T. Stenotrophomonas maltophilia - a low-grade pathogen with numerous virulence factors. Infect Dis (Lond) 2019;51(3):168–78.
165. Okazaki A, Avison MB. Aph(3')-IIc, an aminoglycoside resistance determinant from Stenotrophomonas maltophilia. Antimicrob Agents Chemother 2007; 51(1):359–60.
166. Gordon NC, Wareham DW. Novel variants of the Smqnr family of quinolone resistance genes in clinical isolates of Stenotrophomonas maltophilia. J Antimicrob Chemother 2010;65(3):483–9.
167. Khan A, Pettaway C, Dien Bard J, et al. Evaluation of the Performance of Manual Antimicrobial Susceptibility Testing Methods and Disk Breakpoints for Stenotrophomonas maltophilia. Antimicrob Agents Chemother 2021;65:e02631-20.
168. Khan A, Arias CA, Abbott A, et al. Evaluation of the Vitek 2, Phoenix and Microscan for Antimicrobial Susceptibility Testing of Stenotrophomonas maltophilia. J Clin Microbiol 2021;59:e0065421.
169. Wei C, Ni W, Cai X, et al. Evaluation of Trimethoprim/Sulfamethoxazole (SXT), Minocycline, Tigecycline, Moxifloxacin, and Ceftazidime Alone and in Combinations for SXT-Susceptible and SXT-Resistant Stenotrophomonas maltophilia by In Vitro Time-Kill Experiments. PLoS One 2016;11(3):e0152132.
170. Al-Jasser AM. Stenotrophomonas maltophilia resistant to trimethoprim-sulfamethoxazole: an increasing problem. Ann Clin Microbiol Antimicrob 2006; 5:23.
171. Cho SY, Kang CI, Kim J, et al. Can levofloxacin be a useful alternative to trimethoprim-sulfamethoxazole for treating Stenotrophomonas maltophilia bacteremia? Antimicrob Agents Chemother 2014;58(1):581–3.

172. Baek JH, Kim CO, Jeong SJ, et al. Clinical factors associated with acquisition of resistance to levofloxacin in Stenotrophomonas maltophilia. Yonsei Med J 2014; 55(4):987–93.

173. Wei C, Ni W, Cai X, et al. A Monte Carlo pharmacokinetic/pharmacodynamic simulation to evaluate the efficacy of minocycline, tigecycline, moxifloxacin, and levofloxacin in the treatment of hospital-acquired pneumonia caused by Stenotrophomonas maltophilia. Infect Dis (Lond) 2015;47(12):846–51.

174. Grillon A, Schramm F, Kleinberg M, Jehl F. Comparative Activity of Ciprofloxacin, Levofloxacin and Moxifloxacin against Klebsiella pneumoniae, Pseudomonas aeruginosa and Stenotrophomonas maltophilia Assessed by Minimum Inhibitory Concentrations and Time-Kill Studies. PLoS One 2016;11(6):e0156690.

175. Ba BB, Feghali H, Arpin C, et al. Activities of ciprofloxacin and moxifloxacin against Stenotrophomonas maltophilia and emergence of resistant mutants in an in vitro pharmacokinetic-pharmacodynamic model. Antimicrob Agents Chemother 2004;48(3):946–53.

176. Nys C, Cherabuddi K, Venugopalan V, et al. Clinical and Microbiologic Outcomes in Patients with Monomicrobial Stenotrophomonas maltophilia Infections. Antimicrob Agents Chemother 2019;63(11):e00788-19.

177. Bonfiglio G, Cascone C, Azzarelli C, et al. Levofloxacin in vitro activity and time-kill evaluation of Stenotrophomonas maltophilia clinical isolates. J Antimicrob Chemother 2000;45(1):115–7.

178. Biagi M, Tan X, Wu T, et al. Activity of Potential Alternative Treatment Agents for Stenotrophomonas maltophilia Isolates Nonsusceptible to Levofloxacin and/or Trimethoprim-Sulfamethoxazole. J Clin Microbiol 2020;58(2):e01603-19.

179. Looney WJ, Narita M, Muhlemann K. Stenotrophomonas maltophilia: an emerging opportunist human pathogen. Lancet Infect Dis 2009;9(5):312–23.

180. Farrell DJ, Sader HS, Jones RN. Antimicrobial susceptibilities of a worldwide collection of Stenotrophomonas maltophilia isolates tested against tigecycline and agents commonly used for S. maltophilia infections. Antimicrob Agents Chemother 2010;54(6):2735–7.

181. Giamarellos-Bourboulis EJ, Karnesis L, Galani I, et al. In vitro killing effect of moxifloxacin on clinical isolates of Stenotrophomonas maltophilia resistant to trimethoprim-sulfamethoxazole. Antimicrob Agents Chemother 2002;46(12): 3997–9.

182. Biagi M, Vialichka A, Jurkovic M, et al. Activity of Cefiderocol Alone and in Combination with Levofloxacin, Minocycline, Polymyxin B, or Trimethoprim-Sulfamethoxazole against Multidrug-Resistant Stenotrophomonas maltophilia. Antimicrob Agents Chemother 2020;64(9):e00559-20.

183. Hsueh SC, Lee YJ, Huang YT, et al. In vitro activities of cefiderocol, ceftolozane/ tazobactam, ceftazidime/avibactam and other comparative drugs against imipenem-resistant Pseudomonas aeruginosa and Acinetobacter baumannii, and Stenotrophomonas maltophilia, all associated with bloodstream infections in Taiwan. J Antimicrob Chemother 2019;74(2):380–6.

184. Yamano Y. In Vitro Activity of Cefiderocol Against a Broad Range of Clinically Important Gram-negative Bacteria. Clin Infect Dis 2019;69(Suppl 7):S544–51.

185. Chen IH, Kidd JM, Abdelraouf K, et al. Comparative In Vivo Antibacterial Activity of Human-Simulated Exposures of Cefiderocol and Ceftazidime against Stenotrophomonas maltophilia in the Murine Thigh Model. Antimicrob Agents Chemother 2019;63:e01558-19.

186. Biagi M, Lamm D, Meyer K, et al. Activity of Aztreonam in Combination with Avibactam, Clavulanate, Relebactam, and Vaborbactam against Multidrug-

Resistant Stenotrophomonas maltophilia. Antimicrob Agents Chemother 2020; 64(12):e00297-20.

187. Mojica MF, Papp-Wallace KM, Taracila MA, et al. Avibactam Restores the Susceptibility of Clinical Isolates of Stenotrophomonas maltophilia to Aztreonam. Antimicrob Agents Chemother 2017;61(10):e00777-17.

188. Hand E, Davis H, Kim T, et al. Monotherapy with minocycline or trimethoprim/sulfamethoxazole for treatment of Stenotrophomonas maltophilia infections. J Antimicrob Chemother 2016;71(4):1071–5.

189. Lin Q, Zou H, Chen X, et al. Avibactam potentiated the activity of both ceftazidime and aztreonam against S. maltophilia clinical isolates in vitro. BMC Microbiol 2021;21(1):60.

190. Sader HS, Duncan LR, Arends SJR, et al. Antimicrobial Activity of Aztreonam-Avibactam and Comparator Agents When Tested against a Large Collection of Contemporary Stenotrophomonas maltophilia Isolates from Medical Centers Worldwide. Antimicrob Agents Chemother 2020;64(11):e01433-20.

191. Emeraud C, Escaut L, Boucly A, et al. Aztreonam plus Clavulanate, Tazobactam, or Avibactam for Treatment of Infections Caused by Metallo-beta-Lactamase-Producing Gram-Negative Bacteria. Antimicrob Agents Chemother 2019; 63(5):e00010-19.

192. Mojica MF, Ouellette CP, Leber A, et al. Successful Treatment of Bloodstream Infection Due to Metallo-beta-Lactamase-Producing Stenotrophomonas maltophilia in a Renal Transplant Patient. Antimicrob Agents Chemother 2016;60(9): 5130–4.

193. Muder RR, Harris AP, Muller S, et al. Bacteremia due to Stenotrophomonas (Xanthomonas) maltophilia: a prospective, multicenter study of 91 episodes. Clin Infect Dis 1996;22(3):508–12.

194. Sarzynski SH, Warner S, Sun J, et al. Trimethoprim-Sulfamethoxazole Versus Levofloxacin for Stenotrophomonas maltophilia Infections: A Retrospective Comparative Effectiveness Study of Electronic Health Records from 154 US Hospitals. Open Forum Infect Dis 2022;9(2):ofab644.

195. Jacobson S, Junco Noa L, Wallace MR, et al. Clinical outcomes using minocycline for Stenotrophomonas maltophilia infections. J Antimicrob Chemother 2016;71(12):3620.

196. Grillon A, Schramm F, Kleinberg M, et al. Comparative Activity of Ciprofloxacin, Levofloxacin and Moxifloxacin against Klebsiella pneumoniae, Pseudomonas aeruginosa and Stenotrophomonas maltophilia Assessed by Minimum Inhibitory Concentrations and Time-Kill Studies. PLoS One 2016;11(6):e0156690.

Management of Unique Pneumonias Seen in the Intensive Care Unit

Brooke K. Decker, MD[a],*, LaToya A. Forrester, MPH, CIC[a],
David K. Henderson, MD[a]

KEYWORDS

- Pneumonia • Nosocomial • Health care–associated infections • Legionella

KEY POINTS

- Regions, hospitals, and individual hospital floors may have a unique and clinically significant microbiota; knowledge of this local antibiogram may improve clinical care.
- Empirical therapy should be converted to targeted therapy as soon as possible to limit potentially harmful exposure to overly broad-spectrum antimicrobials.
- Infection prevention surveillance definitions are designed to be standardized and sensitive, although they may not perfectly overlap with clinical disease.
- Robust, prospective surveillance detects signals early and may lead to identification of reservoirs of resistant or waterborne pathogens that can be remediated to prevent future infections.

INTRODUCTION

Severe infections may require intensive care unit (ICU) admission. Even when admitted for noninfectious reasons, the clinical course of critically ill patients may be complicated by the acquisition of infection. A 2017 prevalence study conducted at 1150 centers in 88 countries estimated the incidence of suspected or proven infections among ICU patients to be about 54%.[1] In the United States between the years 2006 and 2010, approximately 19% of adults hospitalized with pneumonia were admitted to the ICU and 13% required assisted ventilation.[2] The Centers for Disease Control and Prevention (CDC) 2020 National and State Healthcare-Associated Infections Progress Report noted an overall 35% increase in ventilator-associated events (VAE) between 2019 and 2020.[3] The marked increase in VAE strongly aligns with the 2019 SARS-CoV-2 pandemic; however, as earlier data suggest, additional factors may contribute to the development of cases of pneumonia in patients who require ICU-level care.

[a] Hospital Epidemiology Service, NIH Clinical Center, 10 Center Drive MSC 1214, Bethesda, MD 20892, USA
* Corresponding author.
E-mail address: Brooke.decker@nih.gov

Infect Dis Clin N Am 36 (2022) 825–837
https://doi.org/10.1016/j.idc.2022.07.003
0891-5520/22/Published by Elsevier Inc.

id.theclinics.com

This article explores some unusual and complex pneumonias, focusing on hospital-acquired infections, and highlights certain unusual microorganisms that have unique clinical significance. In addition, this article addresses diagnostic and treatment considerations in the critically ill patient population. Establishing a conceptual understanding of pneumonia and its epidemiology is an important first step in understanding what makes some ICU-based infections unusual and complex. Pneumonia will be defined both clinically and in a standardized surveillance definition.

DEFINITION

Pneumonia is perhaps most simply described as an acute infection of the lungs.[4] The Infectious Disease Society of America (IDSA) and the America Thoracic Society (ATS) define pneumonia as the presence of both (1) a new lung infiltrate and (2) signs of acute infection, including fever, purulent sputum, leukocytosis, or hypoxia.[5] As is the case for the term "fever," pneumonia" is an infectious process that is not homogeneous but a group of distinct syndromes with separate epidemiologies, pathogenesis, clinical courses, and outcomes. Pneumonia is the most common cause of hospital admission for US adults, with about 1.5 million adults seeking care for pneumonia every year and more than 40,000 resulting deaths.[6] The World Health Organization noted that pneumonia accounts for 14% of all deaths of children younger than 5 years, a devastating (pre-SARS-CoV-2) 740,180 deaths in 2019.[7] Pneumonia is additionally classified by the setting in which the infection was most likely acquired (community- vs health care–associated) as well as causative microorganisms (viral, bacterial, fungal). Understanding the definitional differences between community-acquired pneumonia (CAP) and health care–associated pneumonia (HCAP) is necessary both from diagnostic and empirical treatment standpoints and also to ensure prompt identification and remediation of factors associated with in-hospital morbidity and mortality. **Fig. 1** outlines the rubric used to classify patients presenting on admission with a diagnosis of pneumonia (CAP) versus those who potentially acquired pneumonia during hospitalization (HAP). A retired category of pneumonia, HCAP, included exposure to the health care environment, hypothesizing increased risk for different or resistant organisms.[8] This category was subsequently discontinued, as causative organisms were closely aligned with CAP, and patient outcomes worsened with broader antibiotic treatment prescribed to cover projected (but not demonstrated) resistant pathogens.[9] A subset of HAP known as ventilator-associated pneumonia (VAP) represents the most dangerous extreme, affecting the most vulnerable of hospitalized patients.

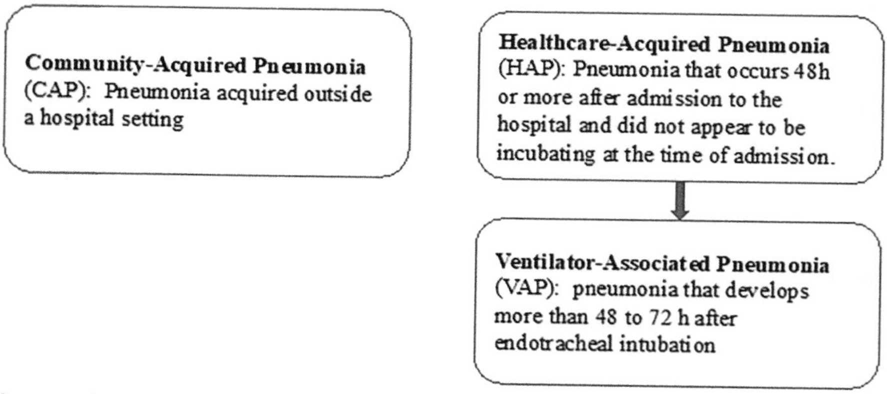

Community-Acquired Pneumonia (CAP): Pneumonia acquired outside a hospital setting

Healthcare-Acquired Pneumonia (HAP): Pneumonia that occurs 48h or more after admission to the hospital and did not appear to be incubating at the time of admission.

Ventilator-Associated Pneumonia (VAP): pneumonia that develops more than 48 to 72 h after endotracheal intubation

Fig. 1. Definition of community-acquired versus health care–acquired pneumonia.

HAP, including VAP, represents the second most common health care–associated infection in the United States.[10] VAP is defined as pneumonia that develops more than 48 to 72 hours after endotracheal intubation.[11] Establishing an impartial definition for VAP can be challenging because many conditions that develop in critically ill patients possess similar signs and symptoms. Specifically, ventilated patients often have infiltrates detected on chest radiology that have noninfectious causes. Without objective interpretation of radiological evidence of pneumonia (eg, infiltrates vs opacities vs volume overload), creating a standardized surveillance definition is challenging. Similarly, the creation of interventional strategies such as preventative bundles depends on an accurate and specific definition. This picture can be further clouded by the fact that, in addition to being associated with lung infection, purulent secretions may be secondary to inflammation of the trachea and bronchi. Finally, a noted increase in white cell count and fever can indicate sepsis not associated with the respiratory system.[12] To provide a more objective approach to the identification of VAP, in 2013, CDC shifted its surveillance focus from VAP to VAE for adult patients. The redefined VAE rubric was designed to eliminate the subjective interpretation found within the original VAP definition by broadening the focus to capture pneumonia as well as complications associated with mechanical ventilation that are also a source of considerable morbidity and mortality in ICU patients.[13] The new definition eliminated reliance on radiographic evidence and interpretation, and instead the new VAE algorithm outlines a baseline period of stability or improvement of a patient's oxygenation on the ventilator. A sustained increase in fraction of inspired oxygen (Fio_2) or PEEP may indicate a ventilator-associated condition (VAC). At the point of identification of a VAC, the reviewer looks for the introduction or change in antimicrobial therapy, white cell count, or temperature to meet criteria for infection-related ventilator-associated complications (IVAC). For VAE that meet the criteria for IVAC, further evaluation to determine if a possible ventilator-associated pneumonia is present includes evidence of purulent respiratory secretions or microbiological specimens positive for organisms compatible with lower respiratory infection. **Fig. 2** provides a summary of the key components of the VAE algorithm. Although this algorithm is objective and designed such that surveillance and reporting of cases in even a large medical center can be accomplished by nonclinicians, it is not without pitfalls. Only about 40% of clinically diagnosed VAPs meet VAE criteria.[13] Because of their complex and more severely ill patient populations, many academic centers and large, critical access hospitals feel they are treated inequitably by this change in definition. Moreover, at the time of the implementation of the adult VAE algorithm, insufficient data were available to develop a pediatric VAE definition. In 2015, CDC developed and implemented a pediatric VAE definition, based primarily on a study that demonstrated that events defined by changes in Fio_2 and mean airway pressure were associated with increases in patient's length of stay.[14]

Given the significant morbidity and mortality associated with a pneumonia diagnosis and the need to reduce or prevent health care–associated infections, clear, objective, standardized criteria identifying pneumonia trends within a population are necessary. The clinical definition is subjective and considers all available diagnostic data unique to that patient. In the United States, pneumonia categorized by surveillance definitions are tracked via the CDC via the National Healthcare Tracking System (National Healthcare Safety Network [NHSN]) surveillance system. Aggregated data are used to establish preventative strategies and guidelines for reducing the mortality and morbidity associated with pneumonia and can be used as a marker of quality and linked to reimbursements. At times, discrepancies are identified between the surveillance definitions and the clinical diagnosis agreed on by the clinicians providing care.[15] In these

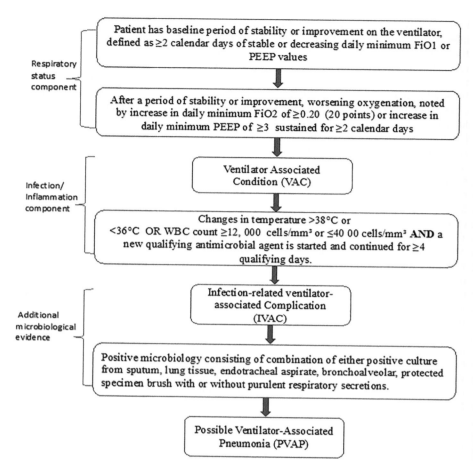

Fig. 2. VAE definition algorithm summary as of January 2022. (*Adapted from* Centers for Disease Control and Prevention. National Healthcare Safety Network (NHSN). Ventilator-associated Events (VAE): Chapter 10: Ventilator-Associated Event (VAE) Protocol – January 2022. Available at https://www.cdc.gov/nhsn/pdfs/pscmanual/10-vae_final.pdf.)

cases, the surveillance definition should not override the clinical judgment associated with the diagnosis, management, and treatment of a singular patient with pneumonia. Similarly, clinical judgment should not be used as a justification for underreporting an infection meeting the NHSN surveillance criteria, as failing to report these infections violates Medicare laws and regulations.

The causative agents of pneumonia can vary, including environmental and chemical irritants (air pollution, smoking), aspiration (foreign substances entering the lungs), device-related (prolonged mechanical ventilation), and, more commonly, by microorganisms. For the context of this article, the authors focus on microorganisms as the causative agent.

MICROBIAL CAUSES OF PNEUMONIA

Pneumonia can be caused by viruses, bacteria, fungi, and even some parasites. In the United States, the most common causes of viral pneumonia are influenza, respiratory syncytial virus (RSV), and SARS-CoV-2. The most common cause of bacterial pneumonia is *Streptococcus pneumoniae* (pneumococcus).[16] In critically ill patients, more than 50% of health care–acquired pneumonia and ventilator-associated pneumonia are caused by multidrug-resistant (MDR) organisms, regardless of duration of hospitalization, and previous antibiotic use was the most significant risk factor.[17] Fungal pneumonias are often associated with severe immunosuppression but occasionally occur in immunocompetent hosts (eg, Histoplasma and Coccidioides pneumonias).

DIAGNOSTIC TESTING

Empirical antibiotic treatment should not be delayed in patients who have sepsis and evidence of infection. Early acquisition of diagnostic specimens, including sputum or lower respiratory tract cultures and blood cultures, should be obtained, ideally, before antibiotic initiation or changes to ensure optimal sensitivity in all hospitalized patients with pneumonia. Identifying the cause of pneumonia may help narrow or tailor therapy to the causative organism, improving outcomes while limiting adverse events and supporting antimicrobial stewardship. Routine culture is effective in identifying the most common bacterial causes of pneumonia and is the most appropriate first step. Further diagnostic testing, molecular testing (including multiplex testing platforms), pathogen-specific tests such as Legionella urinary antigen, and special media requiring respiratory cultures (Legionella, mycobacteria, fungal, and so forth) should be obtained in ICU patients with undifferentiated pneumonia after routine cultures or with risk factors that make unusual pneumonia more likely. Legionella cultures are recommended for all hospital-associated pneumonia and all severe pneumonias. Identifying organisms of public health concern may serve to identify a remediable outbreak and prevent further cases.[5] Some organisms, including resistant organisms, *Mycoplasma pneumoniae*, *Mycobacterium tuberculosis*, and viral respiratory infections are transmitted person to person. Transmission-based precautions should be implemented with a transmissible diagnosis, preventing exposures to other patients or staff.[18] Noninvasive sampling techniques such as endotracheal aspiration as well as more invasive techniques including bronchoalveolar or gastric lavage and protected or blind bronchial sampling can also be considered, especially in hospital-acquired pneumonia,[19] but they should be interpreted with caution, considering the risk of upper airway contamination and uncertain specificity. Moreover, not prematurely assuming the pathogen growing in culture is the one responsible for the patient's illness is important, especially if the pathogen is not a typical cause of respiratory infection, such as Candida[20] or Enterococcus.[21] These organisms are more likely to colonize hospitalized patient's respiratory tracts than cause pneumonia, and the search should continue for a more likely causative organism when they are isolated.

During influenza season it is reasonable to perform viral polymerase chain reaction (PCR) for influenza; antigen testing for influenza is not recommended in critically ill patients due to the lower sensitivity of this modality and the potential to miss cases that might benefit from appropriate therapy such as oseltamivir.[22] During the SARS-CoV-2 pandemic, ruling out COVID-19 has been an appropriate first step in the diagnosis of severe pneumonia. Other appropriate viral testing, including multiplex PCR platforms, may serve to identify common respiratory pathogens and, even if no treatments are available, serve to support discontinuation of unnecessary antimicrobial agents. Clinicians must be aware of the limitations of the multiplex system being used, as different panels test for different sets of organisms, and antimicrobial sensitivities to the organisms on the panel also may differ from one panel to the next. Additional pathogen-specific testing should be tailored to current endemic trends, regional and/or risk factor–associated pathogens (such as hantavirus, ebolavirus, fungal, and so forth). A reasonable approach includes starting with the most likely tests and appropriate empirical treatments and pursuing further and less probable causes if initial studies are not revealing.

Bacterial Pathogens

Gram-negative pathogens frequently associated with outbreaks include Carbapenemase-producing Enterobacterales, MDR Pseudomonas, Acinetobacter baumannii, and Stenotrophomonas; however, more unusual pathogens may be a more significant concern to a particular hospital or unit. Having a close relationship with the hospital infection prevention team and openly collaborating and sharing information with that team are essential for successful management of these pathogens. Although infection prevention is responsible for designating what does or does not meet criteria for ventilator-associated pneumonia, the astute clinician should always inquire about what pathogens are implicated. Understanding this level of detail will assist in identifying trends and may provide a more finely tuned assessment of pathogens of interest to the practicing clinician.

Carbapenemase-producing Enterobacterales are gram-negative, fermenting bacteria that test resistant to at least one carbapenem antibiotic (ertapenem, meropenem, doripenem, or imipenem) or produce carbapenemase. Other organisms including Pseudomonas may also carry carbapenemases, and the organisms can broadly be called carbapenemase-producing organisms (CPO). Patients admitted to the ICU may harbor CPO on admission or may acquire CPO due to transmission from health care worker hands or the environment during their stay. CPO colonization is associated with increased length of stay and mortality.[23] Surveillance screening and molecular diagnostics may assist in identifying CPO colonized patients before a clinical specimen is detected, which would allow more rapid organism-based isolation precautions to be instituted.[24] For patients with known CPO colonization who develop evidence of infection, empirical therapy should cover colonizing pathogenic organisms, but if a susceptible pathogen is isolated, deescalation of antibiotics should be prompt, as overly broad antibiotics can negatively affect mortality.[25]

Among ICU patients diagnosed with VAP, infection with Stenotrophomonas was significantly associated with severe critical illness as measured by Sequential Organ Failure Assessment (SOFA) score greater than 2 and exposure to broad spectrum antibiotics such as carbapenems. Concerningly, effective antibiotic coverage did not improve mortality, and diagnosis of Stenotrophomonas was associated with greater 60-day mortality in these patients.[26]

Atypical Pathogens

The term "atypical pneumonia" was first coined in the preantibiotic period in 1938 to distinguish these milder cases from the more typical and lethal lobar infections.[27] Since that time, it has been used to generally refer to pneumonias wherein the imaging findings are more diffuse, the organisms are not readily identifiable with routine methods, or those that may require specific treatments.[27] The most commonly identified atypical pneumonia organisms are Legionella, Mycoplasma pneumoniae, and Chlamydophila pneumoniae.

Of the atypical pneumonias that occur in health care settings, Legionellosis, first identified as the cause of a 16% fatal pneumonia associated with the 1976 American Legion Convention in Philadelphia is the most feared atypical pneumonia.[28] Waterborne Legionella bacteria are the cause of outbreaks of severe and mortal illness.

As a waterborne pathogen, Legionella can be mitigated, but prevention may necessitate large facility expenditures in buildings that have established biofilms and a history of nosocomial cases. The Veterans Affairs administration implemented a comprehensive Legionella prevention program in 2014 and has demonstrated significant reductions in both health care–associated Legionella pneumonia[29] and water positivity[30] after program implementation. The most important way to prevent nosocomial Legionellosis is to ensure patients are tested for Legionella when hospital-associated pneumonia is detected, regardless of severity. Identifying cases will lead to evaluation and remediation of health care sources of Legionella bacteria, potentially preventing future infections. Current guidelines recommend testing all severe pneumonia and all hospital-associated pneumonia for Legionella. Depending on local prevalence, it may be appropriate to test other types of CAP for Legionella. Available laboratory modalities for the detection of Legionella include antigen testing of urine and PCR or culture of respiratory samples. Understanding the type of testing available in your hospital laboratory as well as the limitations of this testing technique will help avoid missing the diagnosis. The most widely available urinary antigen test only detects Serogroup 1, which is the most common cause of human disease; however, more than 16% of cases are due to other serogroups or species.[31] Detection of hospital-associated Legionella must result in prompt, exhaustive investigation of hospital water sources, preventive strategies implemented, and any potential sources remediated. The source of community-acquired Legionella pneumonia may be harder to identify and remediate, but identification and remediation of these sources provides significant public health benefit.

The most common agent used to treat Legionella is azithromycin, at least in part because many cases of Legionella are likely undiagnosed and successfully treated with outpatient community–acquired pneumonia therapy, although the ideal treatment would be longer than what is currently recommended for undifferentiated CAP. Fluoroquinolones and doxycycline are also effective therapies. Treatment of atypical pneumonia should not be withheld in the setting of risk factors for torsades de Pointes such as prolonged heart rate–corrected QT interval. Doxycycline provides adequate coverage without the same risk as macrolides and fluoroquinolones.[32] Additional antibiotics with activity, although rarely used, include clarithromycin and quinupristin/dalfopristin.[33] Although the literature has suggested a potential fluoroquinolone benefit over other treatments,[34] a recent large systematic review showed no difference between fluoroquinolone or macrolide treatment.[35]

Mycoplasma pneumonia is a contagious, endemic, and epidemic upper and lower respiratory infection. M pneumoniae has been incriminated in outbreaks in congregate settings and in health care workers.[36] This organism is not identified on routine sputum culture, and will be missed if not specifically looked for, but is estimated to cause 20% to 40% of epidemic bacterial pneumonias. Infections are commonly relatively mild and self-limited, but Mycoplasma can present as potentially severe and sometimes deadly pneumonia. Identifying this organism in real time requires molecular testing or specialized culture media and incubation times; in addition, specialized culture and serology can be used to confirm the diagnosis, although answers will often not arrive in time to assist in clinical decision-making. M pneumoniae is not susceptible to even broad-spectrum antibiotics typically prescribed for typical bacterial infections, and unless atypical organisms are specifically targeted with the use of macrolides, fluoroquinolones, or tetracyclines, the patient may fail to improve. Without appropriate diagnostic testing, Mycoplasma-caused pneumonia may be missed altogether. In keeping with trends in antimicrobial overuse and resistance, macrolide-resistant M pneumoniae has been increasingly reported in some areas.[37]

Viral Pathogens

Before the SARS-CoV-2 pandemic, improved detection using multiplex PCR assays suggested that up to 50% of lower respiratory tract infection requiring ICU care may have a viral cause.[38] During outbreaks such as the SARS-CoV-2 pandemic, or influenza season, specific testing of respiratory or nasopharyngeal specimens for a suspected virus is the most judicious use of testing resources. Clinicians practicing during the COVID-19 pandemic are unlikely to neglect viral causes of severe pneumonia. Before COVID-19, MERS-CoV and SARS-CoV-1 were causes of severe viral pneumonia associated with more limited spread of novel coronaviruses. In addition to SARS-CoV-2, influenza is a frequent cause of severe pneumonia occurring seasonally in the winter months with a higher mortality in the extremes of age, those with comorbid health conditions, and those who are pregnant. Influenza vaccination attenuates risk, and a history of vaccine avoidance should increase the pretest suspicion of this vaccine-preventable illness.[38] Pandemic, novel, or sometimes called Avian influenzas are a significant concern and may be responsible for a future pandemic.[39] Outside of pandemic spread, less efficient zoonotic transmission may occur in persons who have risk factors such as those involved in farming or hunting.[40] These novel influenza strains may be detected by PCR and multiplex PCR testing platforms but may be reported as "Influenza A, untypable." Awareness of the PCR platform being used and its limitations are critical to understanding the potential implications of untyped influenzas (if you are accustomed to receiving a type). If novel influenza is suspected, airborne isolation rather than droplet isolation should be initiated,[18] and further consultation with the state or local health department or, in some instances, with the CDC may be necessary to obtain further identification. The rapid identification of influenza and administration of antiviral neuraminidase inhibitor treatment (within 48 hours of symptom onset) have been shown to improve outcome.[41] RSV, Rhinovirus, human metapneumovirus, and parainfluenza virus are potential causes of severe pneumonia (often in immunologically compromised patients) that may be detected by multiplex studies. If these organisms are found, the most helpful intervention may be to discontinue broad spectrum antibiotic therapy in order to reduce the risk of adverse events.[25] Adenovirus is another viral cause of severe respiratory illness that has been implicated in health care outbreaks of severe pneumonia.[42] Enterovirus D68 is an epidemic cause of severe pneumonias and was associated with a 2014 outbreak of severe pneumonia with associated rare neurologic complications.[43] Mimivirus has been isolated from hospitalized patients with severe and ventilator-associated pneumonias.[44] This fascinating, giant virus is known to inhabit contaminated potable water from which, similar to Legionella, it infects waterborne environmental acanthamoeba.[45] Commercial testing and treatments are not available for Mimivirus. Other pathogens the authors are currently unable to detect can cause clinically significant infections and seems highly likely, so further study is warranted.

Fungal pneumonias are most commonly seen in patients with significant immunosuppression, but ICU stay and the relative immunosuppression of critical illness as well as iatrogenic immunosuppression with steroids given in this context can increase the risk of fungal infection. Mold infections are a dangerous complication of severe COVID-19 infection,[46] and a similarly increased risk was seen with H1N1 infections.[47] Before the COVID-19 pandemic invasive Aspergillus infection complicated the courses of 0.3% to 5% of ICU patients and 12% of ventilator-associated pneumonias.[48] Increased suspicion and targeted testing for mold infection is warranted in cases of severe viral pneumonia, corticosteroid treatment, and decompensated cirrhosis.[49] Treatment with azole antifungal agents such as voriconazole or isavuconazole is the mainstay of Aspergillus treatment. Liposomal amphotericin may be necessary in settings of endemic mycosis and resistant molds.[46]

EMPIRICAL TREATMENT

Critically ill patients manifesting evidence of a new infectious process require empirical antibiotic therapy, targeted to the most likely cause of their infections. The frequency of different pathogens may vary from institution, by region and seasonally. Considering such local insights when selecting empirical therapy is critical to success. The most common pathogens isolated from nosocomial pneumonia in the ICU are gram-negative aerobes (64%), and the most commonly reported pathogens were *Staphylococcus aureus* and *Pseudomonas aeruginosa*.[21,50] Current guidelines would suggest treatment with a β-lactam antibiotic plus a macrolide (or fluoroquinolone) if the patient has risk factors for pseudomonas and/or plus vancomycin if the patient has risk factors for methicillin-resistant *Staphylococcus aureus* (MRSA) for severe CAP. Risk factors associated with MRSA or Pseudomonas infection in this setting include prior isolation of MRSA or Pseudomonas or hospitalization in the last 60 days that included parenteral antibiotic treatment.[5] Pseudomonas infection is seen more likely in patients who are ventilated.[21] In patients for whom the QT elongation risk makes prescription of macrolides or fluoroquinolones risky, treatment of atypical organisms can be accomplished with doxycycline instead.[32] Empirical treatment of HAP or VAP should include broad spectrum anti-MRSA (if >10%–20% of unit isolates are methicillin-resistant) and antipseudomonal coverage. For VAP, a second gram-negative agent such as a fluoroquinolone or aminoglycoside may be indicated depending on the patient's risk factors for drug resistance or if the resistance level is greater than 10% to the first agent in the local flora (as represented in the hospital antibiogram).[19] In addition to tailoring your empirical regimen to the local antibiogram, additional consideration of local factors associated with unique pneumonias should be made, most specifically for Legionella.[32] Being aware of any local outbreaks and including empirical coverage targeting hospital-specific pathogens, especially in the setting of an outbreak or endemic resistant pathogen, is a critical success factor.[9] Empirical treatment provided should be promptly narrowed when culture data support such narrowing (eg, stopping vancomycin if gram-negative organisms are isolated or if MRSA swabs are negative),[51] discontinuing double-coverage when, or narrowing broad-spectrum coverage as soon as, an organism is identified to be susceptible to a narrow spectrum agent.

SUMMARY

ICU patients are frequently infected on presentation and are vulnerable to hospital acquisition of infections. Regions, hospitals, and individual hospital floors may have a unique and clinically significant microbiota. Awareness of the local hospital antibiogram and situational awareness of epidemic or endemic pathogens should guide testing and empirical therapy. Empirical therapy should be converted to targeted therapy as soon as possible to limit potentially harmful exposure to overly broad spectrum antimicrobials. Infection prevention surveillance definitions are designed to be standardized and sensitive, although they may not perfectly overlap with clinical disease. Robust, prospective surveillance detects signals early and may lead to identification of reservoirs of resistant or waterborne pathogens that can be remediated to prevent future infections.

CLINICS CARE POINTS

- Treatment with atypical pneumonia is important, especially when cultures are unrevealing in a clinical situation consistent with pneumonia.
- Doxycycline provides adequate coverage for atypical pneumonia, and does not exacerbate prolonged QTc.
- Once an organism is identified, antibiotic therapy should be rapidly targeted to the narrowest effected spectrum to reduce the risk of antibiotic-associated adverse events, including the selection of resistant organisms.

DISCLOSURE

Ms L.A. Forrester, Dr B. Decker, and Dr D.K. Henderson have no commercial or financial conflicts of interest, and this article was not supported by any funding source.

REFERENCES

1. Vincent JL, Sakr Y, Singer M, et al. Prevalence and Outcomes of Infection Among Patients in Intensive Care Units in 2017. JAMA 2020;323(15):1478–87.
2. Storms AD, Chen JF, Jackson LA, et al. Rates and risk factors associated with hospitalization for pneumonia with ICU admission among adults. Bmc Pulm Med 2017;17:208.
3. 2020 National and State Healthcare-Associated Infections Progress Report Last Updated: October 26, 2021. Available at: https://www.cdc.gov/hai/data/portal/progress-report.html. Accessed August 11, 2022.
4. Quinton LJ, Walkey AJ, Mizgerd JP. Integrative Physiology of Pneumonia. Physiol Rev 2018;98(3):1417–64.
5. Metlay JP, Waterer GW, Long AC, et al. Diagnosis and Treatment of Adults with Community-acquired Pneumonia. An Official Clinical Practice Guideline of the American Thoracic Society and Infectious Diseases Society of America. Am J Respir Crit Care Med 2019;200(7):e45–67.
6. Pneumonia. Available at: https://www.cdc.gov/dotw/pneumonia/index.html. Last updated: October 8, 2021, viewed 8/11/227. Last updated 11 November 2021, viewed 8/11/2214. Last updated January 1, 2021, viewed 8/11/2216. Last updated October 22, 2020, viewed 8/11/22.
7. Pneumonia. Available at: https://www.who.int/news-room/fact-sheets/detail/pneumonia.
8. Tablan O, Anderson L, Besser R, et al. Guidelines for preventing health-care–associated pneumonia, 2003: recommendations of CDC and the Healthcare Infection Control Practices Advisory Committee. MMWR Recomm Rep 2004;53(RR03):1–36.
9. Kalil AC, Metersky ML, Klompas M, et al. Executive Summary: Management of Adults With Hospital-acquired and Ventilator-associated Pneumonia: 2016 Clinical Practice Guidelines by the Infectious Diseases Society of America and the American Thoracic Society. Clin Infect Dis 2016;63(5):575–82.
10. Koenig SM, Truwit JD. Ventilator-associated pneumonia: diagnosis, treatment, and prevention. Clin Microbiol Rev 2006;19(4):637–57.
11. Kalanuria AA, Ziai W, Mirski M. Ventilator-associated pneumonia in the ICU. Crit Care 2014;18(2):208.

12. He Q, Wang W, Zhu SC, et al. The epidemiology and clinical outcomes of ventilator-associated events among 20,769 mechanically ventilated patients at intensive care units: an observational study. Crit Care 2021;25(1).
13. Klompas M. Ventilator-Associated Events: What They Are and What They Are Not. Respir Care 2019;64(8):953–61.
14. Ventilator-associated Events (VAE). Available at: https://www.cdc.gov/nhsn/psc/vae/index.html.
15. Klompas M. Is a ventilator-associated pneumonia rate of zero really possible? Curr Opin Infect Dis 2012;25(2):176–82.
16. Causes of Pneumonia. Available at: https://www.cdc.gov/pneumonia/causes.html.
17. Verhamme KM, De Coster W, De Roo L, et al. Pathogens in early-onset and late-onset intensive care unit-acquired pneumonia. Infect Control Hosp Epidemiol 2007;28(4):389–97.
18. Appendix A. Available at: https://www.cdc.gov/infectioncontrol/guidelines/isolation/appendix/index.html.
19. Kalil AC, Metersky ML, Klompas M, et al. Management of Adults With Hospital-acquired and Ventilator-associated Pneumonia: 2016 Clinical Practice Guidelines by the Infectious Diseases Society of America and the American Thoracic Society. Clin Infect Dis 2016;63(5):e61–111.
20. Meersseman W, Lagrou K, Spriet I, et al. Significance of the isolation of Candida species from airway samples in critically ill patients: a prospective, autopsy study. Intensive Care Med 2009;35(9):1526–31.
21. Richards MJ, Edwards JR, Culver DH, et al. Nosocomial infections in medical intensive care units in the United States. National Nosocomial Infections Surveillance System. Crit Care Med 1999;27(5):887–92.
22. Chow EJ, Doyle JD, Uyeki TM. Influenza virus-related critical illness: prevention, diagnosis, treatment. Crit Care 2019;23(1):214.
23. Dautzenberg MJD, Wekesa AN, Gniadkowski M, et al. The association between colonization with carbapenemase-producing enterobacteriaceae and overall ICU mortality: an observational cohort study. Crit Care Med 2015;43(6):1170–7.
24. Kim DK, Kim HS, Pinto N, et al. Xpert CARBA-R Assay for the Detection of Carbapenemase-Producing Organisms in Intensive Care Unit Patients of a Korean Tertiary Care Hospital. Ann Lab Med 2016;36(2):162–5.
25. Pickens CI, Wunderink RG. Principles and Practice of Antibiotic Stewardship in the ICU. Chest 2019;156(1):163–71.
26. Saied WI, Merceron S, Schwebel C, et al. Ventilator-associated pneumonia due to Stenotrophomonas maltophilia: Risk factors and outcome. J Infect 2020;80(3):279–85.
27. Forgie S, Marrie TJ. Healthcare-associated atypical pneumonia. Semin Respir Crit Care Med 2009;30(1):67–85.
28. Fraser DW, Tsai TR, Orenstein W, et al. Legionnaires' disease: description of an epidemic of pneumonia. N Engl J Med 1977;297(22):1189–97.
29. Gamage SD, Ambrose M, Kralovic SM, et al. Legionnaires Disease Surveillance in US Department of Veterans Affairs Medical Facilities and Assessment of Health Care Facility Association. JAMA Netw Open 2018;1(2):e180230.
30. Ambrose M, Kralovic SM, Roselle GA, et al. Implementation of Legionella Prevention Policy in Health Care Facilities: The United States Veterans Health Administration Experience. J Public Health Manag Pract 2020;26(2):E1–11.
31. Yu VLPJ, Pastoris MC, Stout JE, et al. Distribution of Legionella species and serogroups isolated by culture in patients with sporadic community-acquired legionellosis: an international collaborative survey. J Infect Dis 2002;186(1):127–8.

32. Phin N, Parry-Ford F, Harrison T, et al. Epidemiology and clinical management of Legionnaires' disease. Lancet Infect Dis 2014;14(10):1011–21.
33. Stout JE, Arnold B, Yu VL. Activity of azithromycin, clarithromycin, roxithromycin, dirithromycin, quinupristin/dalfopristin and erythromycin against Legionella species by intracellular susceptibility testing in HL-60 cells. J Antimicrob Chemother 1998;41(2):289–91.
34. Garcia-Vidal C, Sanchez-Rodriguez I, Simonetti AF, et al. Levofloxacin versus azithromycin for treating legionella pneumonia: a propensity score analysis. Clin Microbiol Infect 2017;23(9):653–8.
35. Jasper AS, Musuuza JS, Tischendorf JS, et al. Are Fluoroquinolones or Macrolides Better for Treating Legionella Pneumonia? A Systematic Review and Meta-analysis. Clin Infect Dis 2021;72(11):1979–89.
36. Murray HW, Tuazon C. Atypical pneumonias. Med Clin North Am 1980;64(3):507–27.
37. Waites KB, Xiao L, Liu Y, et al. Mycoplasma pneumoniae from the Respiratory Tract and Beyond. Clin Microbiol Rev 2017;30(3):747–809.
38. Nguyen C, Kaku S, Tutera D, et al. Viral Respiratory Infections of Adults in the Intensive Care Unit. J Intensive Care Med 2016;31(7):427–41.
39. Kain T, Fowler R. Preparing intensive care for the next pandemic influenza. Crit Care 2019;23(1):337.
40. St Charles KM, Ssematimba A, Malladi S, et al. Avian Influenza in the U.S. Commercial Upland Game Bird Industry: An Analysis of Selected Practices as Potential Exposure Pathways and Surveillance System Data Reporting. Avian Dis 2018;62(3):307–15.
41. Muthuri SG, Venkatesan S, Myles PR, et al. Effectiveness of neuraminidase inhibitors in reducing mortality in patients admitted to hospital with influenza A H1N1pdm09 virus infection: a meta-analysis of individual participant data. Lancet Respir Med 2014;2(5):395–404.
42. Klinger JR, Sanchez MP, Curtin LA, et al. Multiple cases of life-threatening adenovirus pneumonia in a mental health care center. Am J Respir Crit Care Med 1998;157(2):645–9.
43. Midgley CM, Jackson MA, Selvarangan R, et al. Severe respiratory illness associated with enterovirus D68 - Missouri and Illinois, 2014. MMWR Morb Mortal Wkly Rep 2014;63(36):798–9.
44. Colson P, Aherfi S, La Scola B, et al. The role of giant viruses of amoebas in humans. Curr Opin Microbiol 2016;31:199–208.
45. Rayamajhee B, Dinesh Subedi D, Peguda HK, et al. A Systematic Review of Intracellular Microorganisms within Acanthamoeba to Understand Potential Impact for Infection. Pathogens 2021;10(2):225.
46. Koehler PBM, Chakrabarti A, Chen SCA, et al. European Confederation of Medical Mycology; International Society for Human Animal Mycology; Asia Fungal Working Group; INFOCUS LATAM/ISHAM Working Group; ISHAM Pan Africa Mycology Working Group; European Society for Clinical Microbiology; Infectious Diseases Fungal Infection Study Group; ESCMID Study Group for Infections in Critically Ill Patients; Interregional Association of Clinical Microbiology and Antimicrobial Chemotherapy; Medical Mycology Society of Nigeria; Medical Mycology Society of China Medicine Education Association; Infectious Diseases Working Party of the German Society for Haematology and Medical Oncology; Association of Medical Microbiology; Infectious Disease Canada. : Defining and managing COVID-19-associated pulmonary aspergillosis: the 2020 ECMM/ISHAM consensus criteria for research and clinical guidance. Lancet Infect Dis 2021;21(6):e149–62.

47. Wauters J, Baar I, Meersseman P, et al. Invasive pulmonary aspergillosis is a frequent complication of critically ill H1N1 patients: a retrospective study. Intensive Care Med 2012;38(11):1761–8.
48. Chen F, Danyal Qasir D, Morris AC. Invasive Pulmonary Aspergillosis in Hospital and Ventilator-Associated Pneumonias. Semin Respir Crit Care Med 2022;43(2):234–42.
49. Kluge S, Strauß R, Kochanek M, et al. Aspergillosis: Emerging risk groups in critically ill patients. Med Mycol 2021;60(1):myab064.
50. Sader HS, Castanheira M, Ryan Arends SJ, et al. Geographical and temporal variation in the frequency and antimicrobial susceptibility of bacteria isolated from patients hospitalized with bacterial pneumonia: results from 20 years of the SENTRY Antimicrobial Surveillance Program (1997-2016). J Antimicrob Chemother 2019;74(6):1595–606.
51. Mergenhagen KASK, Wattengel BA, Lesse AJ, et al. Determining the Utility of Methicillin-Resistant Staphylococcus aureus Nares Screening in Antimicrobial Stewardship. Clin Infect Dis 2020;71(5):1142–8.

Management of Common Postoperative Infections in the Surgical Intensive Care Unit

Staci T. Aubry, MD[a], Lena M. Napolitano, MD, FACS, FCCP, MCCM[a],*

KEYWORDS

- Surgical ICU • Surgical infections • Source control • Postoperative infections
- Bacteremia

KEY POINTS

- Postoperative infections in the SICU include intra-abdominal infections (cholecystitis/cholangitis, diverticlulitis, colitis, pancreatitis, peritonitis), soft tissue infections (necrotizing and non-necrotizing, surgical site infections), and hospital-acquired infections (catheter-associated urinary tract infections [CAUTI], central line-associated bloodstream infections [CLABSIs], and pneumonia [ventilator-associated pneumonia [VAP] and hospital-acquired pneumonia [HAP]). Respiratory, abdominal, and bloodstream infections are most common in SICU patients.

- Adequate "source control" (elimination of a focus of invasive infection by drainage, debridement, and/or device removal) is required for optimal treatment of surgical infections, in addition to early appropriate broad-spectrum antimicrobial therapy to cover all potential causative pathogens. In SICU patients, surgical source control is required in most patients (75%), with percutaneous drainage performed in 25%.

- Current guidelines recommend obtaining microbiologic specimens during all source control procedures, related to increased MDRO pathogens, and the important goal to ensure appropriate antimicrobial treatment based on identified causative pathogens. Determination of whether the patient has MDRO risk factors is important in choosing optimal empirical antimicrobial therapy for postoperative SICU infections. Definitive pathogen identification is required for appropriate deescalation of antibiotics.

- Optimal duration of antimicrobial therapy is 4 days for treatment of intra-abdominal infection with adequate source control in non-ICU patients (STOP-IT trial), but this trial had few ICU patients. In postoperative ICU patients (n = 249) with postoperative IAI with adequate source control and adequate empirical antimicrobial therapy, the DURAPOP trial confirmed no difference of 8- versus 15-day antibiotic therapy.

- Based on the results of recent randomized trials, 7 days is emerging as the optimal duration of antimicrobial therapy for uncomplicated gram-negative bacteremia rather than a duration of 14 days, but adequate source control must be achieved.

Continued

[a] Acute Care Surgery, Surgical Critical Care, Department of Surgery, University of Michigan Health System, Room 1C421 University Hospital, 1500 East Medical Center Drive, Ann Arbor, MI 48109-0033, USA
* Corresponding author.
E-mail address: lenan@umich.edu

Infect Dis Clin N Am 36 (2022) 839–859
https://doi.org/10.1016/j.idc.2022.07.005
0891-5520/22/© 2022 Elsevier Inc. All rights reserved.

id.theclinics.com

Continued

- Infections that are difficult to eradicate include fracture-related infections (FRI), osteomyelitis with orthopedic implants, mesh infections, and cardiac implantable electrophysiological device (CIED) infections. Most will require additional surgery for removal of all infected prosthetic material for adequate source control.

INTRODUCTION

Postoperative infection and sepsis in the surgical intensive care unit (SICU) are common problems, and can be the reason for SICU admission or can be acquired during the SICU stay. Both diagnosis and management of infection and sepsis in the SICU can be complex, related to the surgical procedures performed, patient comorbidities (ie, immunosuppression related to solid organ transplant patients), and resistant pathogens. Importantly, the need for "source control" of many postoperative infections can pose specific challenges and significant complexity in patient management. Postoperative infections in the SICU are associated with increased morbidity, mortality, and resource utilization, and therefore a strong focus on infection preventive strategies is warranted.

Epidemiology of Infections in Surgical Intensive Care Unit Patients

In the Sepsis Occurrence in Acutely Ill Patients (SOAP) study, which included 44% (n = 1388) surgical patients across 198 intensive care units (ICUs) in 24 European countries, the lung was the most common site of infection (68%), followed by the abdomen (22%), blood (20%), and urinary tract (14%).[1] Sepsis was confirmed in 43% of surgical patients, and was more common in emergency versus elective surgical patients. However, specific infections were not assessed separately in the surgical patient cohort.

A large multicenter China study of 3665 surgical patient SICU admissions reported that abdominal infections (72%) were more common than lung infections (53%), and gram-negative bacteria isolates were most common.[2] Polymicrobial (44%) and fungal (28%) infections were also common. In the SOAP study, gram-positive bacteria (mainly *Streptococcus*) and *Escherichia coli* were more frequent isolates in surgical patients.

Similar findings were reported in the Extended Prevalence of Infection in Intensive Care (EPIC II and III) observational point prevalence studies in which 64% of infections were respiratory in origin and 20% intra-abdominal, and ICU-acquired infections were 21%. The EPIC II study included data from 2007 (n = 13,796) from 1265 ICUs from 75 countries and reported that 51% of ICU patients had infections with a hospital mortality rate of 33%.[3] Surgical patients comprised the majority (72%) of the study cohort, with elective surgical (23.3%), emergent surgical (38.5%), and trauma (9.9%) patients. Emergency surgical patients had the highest infection prevalence (45.6%) compared with elective (12.9%) and trauma (9.0%) patients. Multivariate regression analysis confirmed that admission after emergency surgery or trauma was independently associated with higher risk of infection.

Larger data collection (n = 15,202) from 2017 in the EPIC III Trial across 88 countries including 1150 ICUs reported an infection rate of 54% with a 30% mortality. The most common site of infection was respiratory (60%), followed by abdominal (18%) and bloodstream (15%).[4] Surgical patients comprised 45.4% of the study cohort, with

21% elective, 16.8% emergent, and 7.6% trauma. Infection was more common in emergency surgery (62%) and trauma patients (46%) compared with elective surgery (27%) patients. In all these studies, the ICU mortality rate of infected patients was much higher (more than double in some) than that of infected patients.

Approach to Diagnosis of Infection in Surgical Intensive Care Unit Patients

In the SICU, the approach to diagnosis of infection relies heavily on the patient and surgical procedure characteristics. Furthermore, evaluation must include assessment for possible ICU-acquired infections (central line-associated bloodstream infections [CLABSIs], catheter-associated urinary tract infections [CAUTIs], ventilator-associated pneumonia [VAP]) or surgery-related infections. Patients in the SICU with longer ICU length of stay will be at much higher risk for ICU-acquired infections, and preventive strategies are of paramount importance.

It is challenging to make a definitive diagnosis of postoperative infection in SICU patients, because many surgical patients have fever postoperatively. In a single-institution prospective study, clinical diagnosis differentiated infected and noninfected patients with only 61.5% accuracy (sensitivity 60.3%; specificity 64.4%; $P = 0.0049$) and physician concordance was poor ($\kappa = 0.33$). Prediction of the infectious source was correct only 60% of the time. Culture and objective data and SICU antibiotic protocols led to an overall 78% appropriate initiation of antibiotics versus 48% when treatment was based on clinical evaluation alone.[5]

Detailed assessment of all potential sources of infection with clinical examination, pan-culture, laboratory and procalcitonin measurement, and appropriate diagnostic imaging is warranted. Additional important considerations in infection diagnostic evaluation include postoperative day presentation and the type of surgery that was performed. The approach to a patient on postoperative days 0 to 1 is different than days 5 to 7. The early postoperative period signs of altered mental status, fever, and leukocytosis may be related to postoperative inflammation from the surgical procedure versus a systemic inflammatory response to a surgical source control procedure. The patient who has infectious signs and symptoms on day 5 to 7 postoperatively may prompt diagnostic imaging and empirical antibiotics due to concern for pneumonia, postoperative abscess, anastomotic leak, or surgical site infection (SSI) (superficial, deep, or organ/space).

During initial evaluation, patient risk factors must also be considered. Patients with increased risk for infections because of immunosuppression (ie, transplant patients), comorbidities, prior use of antibiotics, and existing known multidrug-resistant organisms (MDROs) must have treatment plans that take these factors into account. Empirical antibiotics for treatment of postoperative infections must be adjusted if MDRO risk factors are present.

Empirical and Definitive Management of Postoperative Infections in the Surgical Intensive Care Unit

Antimicrobial therapy

Just as for treatment of general ICU patients with possible infection, early appropriate empirical antibiotics must be administered as diagnostic strategies to confirm infection are initiated.[6] Empirical intravenous (IV) antibiotics should cover all possible causative pathogens of the presumed infection site, because inadequate empirical antimicrobial therapy is associated with increased mortality.[7] For patients with sepsis, every hour delay of antibiotics is associated with increased mortality. The 2021 Surviving Sepsis Guidelines[8] recommend initiation of empirical antibiotics within 1 hour in patients with septic shock. Determination of whether the patient has MDRO risk factors (**Table 1**) is important in choosing optimal empirical antimicrobial therapy for postoperative infections.

Pathogen identification of the postoperative infection is very important. Once all culture results are available for review, deescalation of antimicrobial therapy may be considered, and cessation of all unnecessary antibiotics is required. Definitive antimicrobial management and optimal duration of antibiotic therapy must be established at this time; this may require a concomitant assessment of abscess drain output (character and amount) and need for additional diagnostic follow-up radiologic imaging, that is, computed tomographic (CT) imaging to determine whether postoperative abscess has fully resolved.

The use of real-time dashboards, medical data, and microbiology systems can allow intensivists to optimize antibiotics in ICU patients. ICU dashboards (**Fig. 1**) can provide the ability to comprehensively review information of patient characteristics, health care-associated infections, antimicrobial resistance patterns, antibiograms in the ICU, and adherence to protocols of care and guidelines to achieve optimal patient outcomes.

Source control therapy

Definitive management of postoperative surgical infections may require "source control," with either percutaneous or surgical approach. National guidelines[9,10] recommend that source control should be achieved urgently in patients with sepsis and septic shock. In patients with intra-abdominal infections (IAIs), source control should be achieved within 24 hours of the diagnosis. Delayed and inadequate source control are both independently associated with worse outcome.

In a study of 353 SICU patients with severe IAIs, surgical source control was required in 75% of patients, with 25% requiring percutaneous procedures (mostly in biliary and pancreatic IAI). Complete source control was achieved in only 67% of patients, and 50% required multiple source control procedures. Inadequate source control was associated with persistent organ failure and worse outcome.[11]

Table 1
Risk factors for MDRO infection in ICU patients

Predictors	At ICU admission	During the ICU stay
Patient features	Comorbid illness/immunosuppression/ recent hospital and/or ICU stay	Higher severity of acute illness/Invasive interventions
Type of infection	Hospital-acquired > health care-associated > community-acquired	ICU-acquired > others
Antimicrobial selection pressure	Prior antibiotics[a]/antifungals	Antibiotics[a]/antifungals in the ICU
Colonization status	Previously documented colonization with MDRB	In-ICU acquisition of MDRB
Local epidemiology	Epidemiology of MDRB in community/ hospital/areas recently traveled to	Local epidemiology of MDRB in the ICU
Infection prevention measures	Poor hygiene practices in hospital	Poor hygiene practices in the ICU

Abbreviation: MDRB, multidrug-resistant bacteria.
[a] Especially if agents with broad-spectrum and/or potent activity against intestinal anaerobes.
From Timsit, JF., Bassetti, M., Cremer, O. et al. Rationalizing antimicrobial therapy in the ICU: a narrative review. Intensive Care Med 45, 172–189 (2019); with permission.

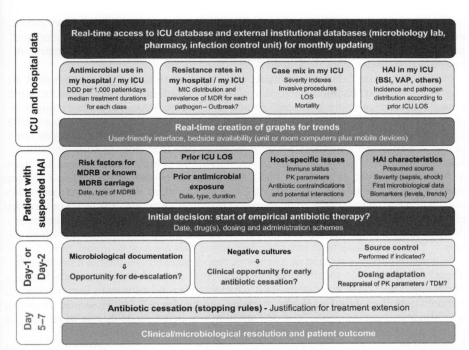

Fig. 1. An ICU dashboard to optimize antibiotics and treatment for IAI in ICU patients. BSI, bloodstream infection; IAI, intra-abdominal infections; LOS, length of stay; MDRB, multidrug-resistant bacteria. DDD, defined daily doses; HAI, hospital-acquired infections, MIC, minimum inhibitory concentration, PK, pharmacokinetics, TDM, therapeutic drug monitoring. (*From* Timsit, JF., Bassetti, M., Cremer, O. et al. Rationalizing antimicrobial therapy in the ICU: a narrative review. Intensive Care Med 45, 172–189 (2019). https://doi.org/10. 1007/s00134-019-05520-5; with permission.)

Current guidelines recommend obtaining microbiologic specimens during all source control procedures, related to increased prevalence of MDRO pathogens, and the important goal of ensuring appropriate antimicrobial treatment based on identified causative pathogens.

Intensive care unit-acquired postoperative infections in the surgical intensive care unit

Postoperative SICU patients may require mechanical ventilation, central venous catheters, arterial lines, and urinary catheters, and are therefore at risk for ICU-acquired infections (CLABSIs, CAUTIs, and VAP). These patients are also at risk for *Clostridium difficile* infection given the need for perioperative antibiotics to reduce the risk of SSI.[12] Prevention, diagnosis, and treatment of these ICU-acquired infections are no different than those in medical ICU patients, and national/international guidelines are helpful in standardization of practice.[13–15]

Specific Postoperative Infections in the Surgical Intensive Care Unit

Intra-abdominal infections

The classification of IAIs is either "uncomplicated" or "complicated." Uncomplicated IAIs are contained in the gastrointestinal tract, such as cholecystitis or appendicitis, with no evidence of extension beyond the hollow viscus. These patients typically do not require critical care. However, complicated IAI occurs when the infection travels into the peritoneal space, beyond the hollow viscus, causing abscess formation and peritonitis. These patients often require management in the SICU. Complicated IAI mortality rate ranges from 20% to 40%.[16]

Peritonitis can be defined as primary, secondary, or tertiary. Primary peritonitis is due to spontaneous bacterial peritonitis, or due to indwelling catheters, either for peritoneal dialysis or ventriculoperitoneal shunts for hydrocephalus. Secondary peritonitis is caused by a perforated hollow viscus (appendicitis, diverticulitis) and is the most common complicated IAI. Depending on the source of peritonitis, the mortality rate varies. A perforated colon has a higher mortality rate than perforated appendicitis. Notably, secondary peritonitis related to postoperative complication, such as anastomotic leak or missed enterotomy, has a mortality rate of greater than 30%. Tertiary peritonitis is due to infection recurrence either due to impaired host defense or inadequate source control; this is most common in patients who are critically ill or have a compromised immune system. To qualify as tertiary peritonitis, recurrent infection must occur more than 48 hours after perceived source control of secondary peritonitis.[17] These infections tend to harbor pathogens that are multidrug resistant.[18]

Abdominal sepsis is defined as a systemic response to an IAI, and the mortality rate of abdominal sepsis is much higher than that of IAI alone.[19] The Complicated Intra-Abdominal Infections Observational (CIAO) study (from 68 centers in Europe over a 6-month period) reported an overall mortality rate for IAIs of 7.5%. However, patients with abdominal sepsis or septic shock at admission had a mortality rate of 32.4%.[20]

Diagnosis of intra-abdominal infections

CT is the most useful imaging study for diagnosis of IAIs. However, for patients with possible IAIs who are critically ill requiring mechanical ventilation, vasopressors, or continuous renal replacement therapy, transportation to CT is not always possible or safe. Other possible useful bedside adjuncts include plain radiograph or ultrasound imaging, but the sensitivity and specificity when compared with CT are much lower. In patients who are severely critically ill, bedside abdominal exploration can be considered for diagnosis.

Duration of antibiotics for intra-abdominal infections

Controversy still exists regarding the optimal duration of antibiotics in patients with complicated IAIs (**Table 2**), especially those who are critically ill. The Study to Optimize Peritoneal Infection Therapy (STOP-IT) randomized trial aimed to determine the optimal duration of antibiotics after adequate source control, either via surgical intervention or via percutaneous drainage. Four days of antibiotic therapy was not inferior to longer courses (2 days beyond resolution of signs/symptoms of infection) for the end points of SSI, recurrent IAIs, or death.[21] Treatment failure in the trial was associated with steroids, higher APACHE scores, colonic sources of IAIs, and hospital-acquired infections. The patients with increasing treatment failure had increasing number of risk factors, but the duration of antibiotic therapy was not a factor in treatment failure.[22] Limitations of the STOP-IT trial were a small number of critically ill patients and the exclusion of patients who required an open abdomen approach.

The DURAPOP trial (multicenter, randomized)[23,24] compared the efficacy of 8- versus 15-day antibiotic therapy in critically ill ICU patients (n = 249) with postoperative IAIs in 21 French ICUs. Patients with adequate source control and adequate empirical antimicrobial therapy within 24 hours of the surgical source control procedure were randomized on postoperative day 8 to no additional antibiotics or long-course therapy. No differences were identified in 45-day mortality (11% 8-day vs

Table 2
Guideline recommendations for duration of antimicrobial therapy for IAI

Guideline	Complicated IAI	Uncomplicated IAI
IDSA (2010)	4–7 d	24 h postcholecystectomy with acute cholecystitis contained in gallbladder viscera
SIS (2017)	24 h for traumatic bowel perforations operated on within 12 h and for gastroduodenal perforations operated on within 24 h	24 h postoperatively in nonperforated, acute, or gangrenous cholecystitis
	4 d (96 h) with adequate source control procedure	Same as cIAI
	Consider limit of 5–7 d in established IAI and no source control procedure	Same as cIAI
	Consider limit of 7 d for secondary bacteremia with source control and patient no longer bacteremic	Reassessment for source control recommended in 5–7 d when full antimicrobial therapy is not achieved
WSES (2017)	3–5 d with adequate source control procedure	Postoperative antimicrobial therapy unnecessary in definitive source control
	Diagnostic investigation for uncontrolled infection or treatment failure with signs of peritonitis or systemic infection beyond 5–7 d of antimicrobial treatment	
TG18 (2018)	Not applicable	24 h postcholecystectomy for community-acquired grades I–II cholecystitis
		4–7 d for gallbladder perforation, emphysema, or necrosis noted during cholecystectomy, and for grades I–III cholangitis with source control
		2 wk for grades I–III cholangitis and cholecystitis with gram-positive cocci bacteremia

Abbreviations: cIAI, Complicated Intra-abdominal Infection; IDSA, Infectious Diseases Society of America; SIS, Surgical Infection Society; TG18, Tokyo Guidelines 2018; WSES, World Society of Emergency Surgery.

Data from Solomkin JS, Mazuski JE, Bradley JS, et al. Diagnosis and management of complicated intra-abdominal infection in adults and children: guidelines by the Surgical Infection Society and the Infectious Diseases Society of America. Clin Infect Dis. 2010;50:133-164; Mazuski JE, Tessier JM, May AK, et al. The Surgical Infection Society revised guidelines on the management of intra-abdominal infection. Surg Infect (Larchmt). 2017;18:1-76; Gomi H, Solomkin JS, Schlossberg D, et al. Tokyo Guidelines 2018: antimicrobial therapy for acute cholangitis and cholecystitis. J Hepatobiliary Pancreat Sci. 2018;25:3-16; and Sartelli M, Chichom-Mefire A, Labricciosa FM, et al. The management of intra-abdominal infections from a global perspective: 2017 WSES guidelines for management of intra-abdominal infections. World J Emerg Surg. 2017;12:29.

15% 15-day), ICU/hospital length of stay, emergence of multidrug resistant bacteria, or reoperation rate.

In patients with IAIs with inadequate source control, the 2017 Surgical Infection Society (SIS) Guidelines recommend "no more than 5 to 7 days of antimicrobial therapy be provided to patients with established IAI in who definitive source control is not performed. We suggest that clinical parameters, including fever, leukocytosis, and adequacy of gastrointestinal function, be assessed periodically to determine whether antimicrobial therapy can be discontinued sooner. We suggest that patients that do not respond fully to antimicrobial therapy within 5 to 7 days be reassessed for failure of source control, and consideration for potential source control intervention."

What is the optimal antibiotic duration in patients with IAIs with bacteremia? There are no large randomized trials for guidance in this specific situation. The current SIS Guidelines recommendation is "that most patients with secondary bacteremia because of IAI who have undergone adequate source control and are no longer bacteremic can have antimicrobial therapy discontinued after 7 days." The major exception to this is those with *Staphylococcus aureus* bacteremia, who should be treated for a minimum of 14 days with IV antibiotics.

Specific intra-abdominal infections (biliary, diverticulitis, pancreatitis)
The 3 most common IAIs in the ICU in both postoperative and medical patients are biliary infections (cholecystitis and cholangitis) diverticulitis, and pancreatitis. In surgical patients who have had prior laparotomy and bowel resection, the most common IAIs are complications of their initial operative procedure, including intra-abdominal abscess (organ/space SSI), anastomotic leak, and enterocutaneous fistulae.

Biliary infections
In the surgical ICU, the more severe biliary infections are encountered. These infections include emphysematous cholecystitis, or complications of acute cholecystitis, such as perforation of the gallbladder leading to abscess or peritonitis, and cholangitis. These infections are typically caused by aerobic, enteric, gram-negative bacilli and aerobic gram-positive organisms. Emphysematous cholecystitis with gas in the gallbladder wall is caused by clostridial organisms.

Cholangitis presents as a pentad of symptoms, including jaundice, fever, tenderness in the right upper quadrant, hyperbilirubinemia, and elevated white blood cell count. Ultrasonography reveals dilation of the common bile duct. In patients with severe cholangitis (cholangitis with other organ dysfunction), urgent (<24 hours) biliary drainage, usually by endoscopic retrograde cholangiopancreatography, is recommended in addition to IV antibiotics. For acute cholangitis, antibiotic duration should be for 4 to 7 days beyond definitive source control. For patients with pericholecystic abscess or perforation, antibiotics should be continued until clinical evidence of infection has resolved with normal white blood cell count, improved abdominal pain, and afebrile.

Diverticulitis
Diverticulitis can be uncomplicated or complicated. Uncomplicated is often managed in general care or as an outpatient. Antibiotic treatment can be used selectively rather than routinely in immunocompetent patients with mild acute uncomplicated diverticulitis. Antibiotic treatment is now strongly advised in immunocompromised patients.[25]

Complicated diverticulitis can often be managed with antibiotics alone if there are no signs of sepsis and the abscess is less than 4 cm in size on CT imaging. When abscesses are greater than 4 cm, percutaneous drainage can successfully resolve 80% of patients with a low risk of complication or need for reintervention.[26]

The mortality rate for patients with diverticulitis with Hinchey III is reported as 6% but increases greatly to 35% for fecal peritonitis (Hinchey IV). When a patient has peritonitis or sepsis from diverticulitis, SICU admission and surgical intervention may be required. Surgery may also be required if patients do not improve with antibiotics and percutaneous drainage. Surgical options include Hartmann procedure (sigmoid resection with end colostomy) or sigmoid resection with colorectal anastomosis with or without a loop ileostomy. A systematic review and meta-analysis comparing Hartmann procedure with colectomy with primary anastomosis in patients with Hinchey class III or IV colonic diverticulitis (n = 1066) found that primary anastomosis was associated with significantly higher stoma reversal rates, reduced reversal-related morbidity, but no differences in overall mortality, morbidity, or reintervention rates after the index procedure.[27]

Furthermore, laparoscopic peritoneal lavage with subsequent surgical resection if indicated had lower surgical morbidity and hospital length of stay compared with the primary resection and anastomosis group. The 2019 EAES/SAGES Diverticulitis Guidelines[28] recommend "Lavage may be considered in selected Hinchey III patients by surgeons with appropriate expertise and the ability to closely watch for and manage complications. The lower stoma rate should be weighed against the higher risk of complications and re-intervention."

In cases of septic shock due to perforated diverticulitis and peritonitis, with ongoing hemodynamic instability not responsive to fluid resuscitation and requiring vasopressors, an initial damage control surgery may be the optimal initial operative procedure for prompt IAI definitive source control. An open abdomen approach is maintained, and after hemodynamic stabilization a second operative intervention is undertaken, and is associated with a high rate of primary intestinal anastomosis and abdominal closure (**Fig. 2**).[29,30]

Pancreatitis

The severity of pancreatitis is identified by the presence of necrosis, infection, and associated systemic signs of illness. Patients in the surgical ICU with pancreatitis are typically those showing signs of organ dysfunction. The first step to management is fluid resuscitation to prevent pancreatic necrosis, imaging to assess severity and pancreatic necrosis, early nutritional support, and consideration of endoscopic retrograde cholangiopancreatography if biliary origin.

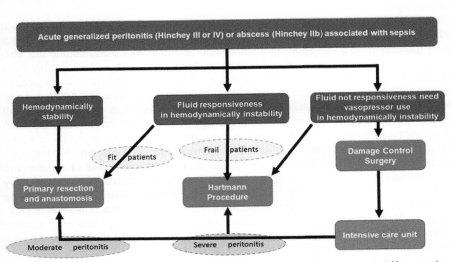

Fig. 2. Treatment algorithm for patients with diverticular perforation and diffuse peritonitis. (*From* Cirocchi R, Sapienza P, Anania G, et al. State-of-the-art surgery for sigmoid diverticulitis. Langenbecks Arch Surg. 2022;407(1):1-14. https://doi.org/10.1007/s00423-021-02288-5; under CC BY 4.0.)

Approximately 30% of patients with pancreatitis may develop pancreatic necrosis. Antibiotics and percutaneous drainage are not recommended in cases of severe acute or noninfected necrotizing pancreatitis.[31] For documented infected pancreatic necrosis, therapeutic antibiotics and drainage are both recommended.[32] Empirical broad-spectrum antibiotics should be initiated and narrowed after percutaneous drainage and pathogen identification.[33]

Optimal management for infected pancreatic necrosis is the "step-up" approach including percutaneous catheter drainage, followed by a second drain as needed. If adequate drainage is not achieved, then a minimally invasive necrosectomy is the next step. When compared with open necrosectomy, the minimally invasive necrosectomy had reduced rates of the primary composite end point (12% vs 50%, including major complications [new-onset multiple organ failure or multiple systemic complications, perforation of a visceral organ or enterocutaneous fistula, or bleeding] or death). Mortality was not significantly different.[34,35] The long-term follow-up of patients in the PANTER trial confirmed the "step-up approach" for necrotizing pancreatitis was superior to open necrosectomy, without increased risk of reinterventions.[36]

The recent POINTER trial[37,38] examined whether earlier, nonoperative drainage was beneficial for patients with infected pancreatic necrosis. Immediate (within 24 hours after diagnosis of infection) antibiotics and image-guided percutaneous or endoscopic drainage was compared with postponed drainage until development of walled-off pancreatic necrosis. No mortality difference was noted, and postponed drainage was associated with fewer invasive interventions and decreased need for surgical necrosectomy. So drainage is best delayed until the development of walled off necrosis, which most commonly occurs 30 days after onset.

When initial percutaneous drainage procedures demonstrate lack of clinical improvement, the next steps (**Fig. 3**) include video-assisted retroperitoneal debridement, minimally invasive retroperitoneal pancreatectomy, transluminal direct endoscopic necrosectomy, and more recently laparoscopic transgastric necrosectomy.[39]

Pulmonary infections

Hospital-acquired pneumonia or VAP[13] are the most common pulmonary infections in postoperative SICU patients, and are covered elsewhere in this issue. Pleural infections (parapneumonic effusion, empyema, infected bronchopleural fistula) are also common and can be the result of pneumonia, hemothorax, chest trauma, bacterial seeding of preexisting effusion or hemothorax, or spread from other sources (esophagus, mediastinitis, subdiaphragmatic abscess). Diagnostic imaging (ultrasonography, CT scan) and thoracentesis are helpful in diagnosis. The mainstay of management is appropriate antibiotics and drainage (pleural source control). Duration of antimicrobial therapy is widely variable depending on the adequacy of source control, because loculated pleural effusions and empyema are common.[40] Chest tube drainage size is still controversial, but smaller-bore chest tubes (14F or smaller) are more popular even in the presence of loculated effusions or purulence due to safety and patient comfort. However, no randomized controlled trials have been done comparing small- with large-bore chest tubes. If chest tube drainage alone is not sufficient for source control, other treatment options should be considered, including intrapleural therapy with tissue plasminogen activator (TPA) and dornase, or surgical decortication via video-assisted thoracoscopy or thoracotomy.[41]

Bacteremia

Current treatment guidelines recommend a treatment duration of 14 days of antimicrobial therapy for bacteremia. Both surveys and observational studies have reported that

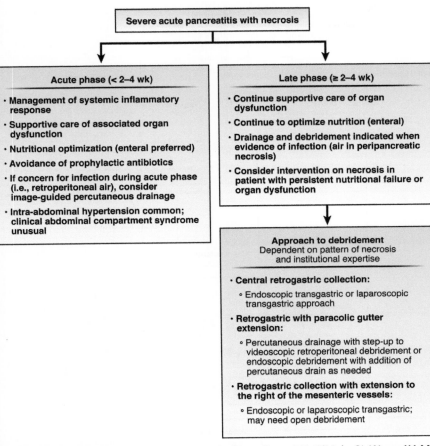

Fig. 3. Management of necrotizing pancreatitis. (*From* Baron TH, DiMaio CJ, Wang AY, Morgan KA. American Gastroenterological Association Clinical Practice Update: Management of Pancreatic Necrosis. Gastroenterology. 2020 Jan;158(1):67-75.e1. https://doi.org/10.1053/j.gastro.2019.07.064.)

actual treatment durations for bacteremia are at least 14 days, and sometimes longer. Longer courses of antibiotics increase risk for adverse effects, drive emergence of resistance, and lead to increased hospital length of stay and higher costs. Recent data from 2 published multicenter randomized trials support that antibiotic duration for gram-negative bacteremia in hospitalized noncritically ill patients with signs of early response to treatment can be reduced from the standard of 14 days to 7 days to limit antibiotic exposure with no negative impact on patient outcome.

In a 2-year multicenter Swiss trial of 500 adults with gram-negative bacteremia,[42,43] patients were randomized at day 5 of antibiotic therapy to individualized C-reactive protein (CRP)-guided treatment duration, fixed 7-day duration, or fixed 14-day duration (control group). In the CRP-guided group, antibiotic therapy was discontinued when serum CRP level (measured every 1–2 days) had decreased 75% from peak value and the patient had been afebrile for 48 hours. Clinical failure at day 30 (defined as recurrent bacteremia, suppurative complication, or restart of antibiotics) occurred in 2.4% (4 of 164) of the CRP group (median antibiotic duration, 7 days, range 5–

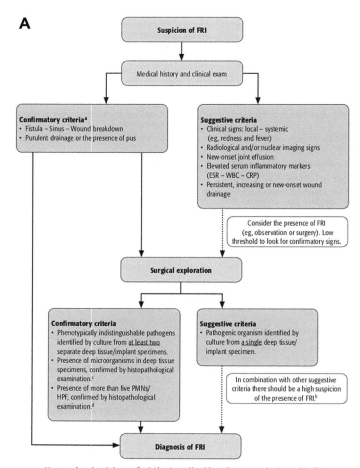

A

Suspicion of FRI

Medical history and clinical exam

Confirmatory criteria[a]
- Fistula – Sinus – Wound breakdown
- Purulent drainage or the presence of pus

Suggestive criteria
- Clinical signs: local – systemic
  (eg, redness and fever)
- Radiological and/or nuclear imaging signs
- New-onset joint effusion
- Elevated serum inflammatory markers
  (ESR – WBC – CRP)
- Persistent, increasing or new-onset wound
  drainage

Consider the presence of FRI
(eg, observation or surgery). Low
threshold to look for confirmatory signs.

Surgical exploration

Confirmatory criteria
- Phenotypically indistinguishable pathogens
  identified by culture from at least two
  separate deep tissue/implant specimens.
- Presence of microorganisms in deep tissue
  specimens, confirmed by histopathological
  examination.[c]
- Presence of more than five PMNs/
  HPF, confirmed by histopathological
  examination.[d]

Suggestive criteria
- Pathogenic organism identified by
  culture from a single deep tissue/
  implant specimen.

In combination with other suggestive
criteria there should be a high suspicion
of the presence of FRI.[b]

Diagnosis of FRI

[a] In cases of purulent drainage or fistula/sinus/wound breakdown, the presence of pathogens identified by
  culture is not an absolute requirement (eg, in the case of chronic antibiotic suppression).
[b] If the positive culture is from sonication fluid, it is highly likely that FRI is present. This is especially true when
  virulent bacteria (ie, *Staphylococcus aureus*) are present.
[c] The presence of microorganisms is confirmed by using specific staining techniques for bacteria and fungi.
[d] The presence of an average of more than five PMNs/HPF on histopathological examination should only be
  considered diagnostic of FRI in chronic/late-onset cases (eg, fracture nonunion).
ESR: erythrocyte sedimentation rate, WBC: white blood cell count, CRP: C-reactive protein,
PMN(s): polymorphonuclear neutrophil(s), HPF: high-power field.

B

The diagnosis of FRI should always be considered in case of impaired fracture healing.
The presence of confirmatory signs of FRI should prompt the treating, multidisciplinary, medical team to proceed with developing a treatment strategy.
The presence of suggestive signs of FRI should prompt the treating, multidisciplinary, medical team to further investigate the probability of an FRI.
The only confirmatory clinical signs of FRI are the presence of a fistula, sinus, or wound breakdown and/or purulent drainage from the wound or presence of pus
  during surgery.
Caution when interpreting the results of serum inflammatory markers in FRI is warranted, as their predictive value is low.
The imaging modality of choice depends on the local availability of the technique and the questions to be answered.
Nuclear imaging (FDG-PET/CT or WBC scintigraphy + SPECT/CT) is more accurate than MRI for detecting FRI, but MRI is better in visualizing surgical
  relevant details. Therefore, apart from radiological signs, nuclear medicine signs should be included in the diagnostic pathway (definition) of FRI.
As evidence on histopathology is accumulating, it seems appropriate to include it in the diagnostic pathway (definition) of FRI for chronic/late-onset cases (eg,
  nonunion).

Fig. 4. (*A*) Descriptive flow chart of diagnostic criteria of fracture-related infection (FRI) and (*B*) recommendations. CRP, C-reactive protein; ESR, erythrocyte sedimentation rate; HPF, high-power field; PMN, polymorphonuclear neutrophil; WBC, white blood cell. (*From [A]* Metsemakers WJ, Morgenstern M, McNally MA, et al. Fracture-related infection: A consensus on definition from an international expert group. Injury. 2018;49(3):505-510; with permission; and [*B*] Govaert GAM, Kuehl R, Atkins BL, et al. Diagnosing Fracture-Related Infection: Current Concepts and Recommendations. Journal of Orthopaedic Trauma34(1):8-17, January 2020; with permission.)

28 days), 6.6% (11 of 166) of the 7-day group, and 5.5% (9 of 163) of the 14-day group. CRP-guided and fixed 7-day treatment were noninferior to 14-day treatment for gram-negative bacteremia. Study limitations include the large noninferiority margin and low event rate.

These study results are consistent with another trial of 7-day treatment for gram-negative bacteremia.[44] A multicenter open-label trial performed in Israel and Italy randomized inpatients (n = 604) with gram-negative bacteremia who were afebrile and hemodynamically stable for 48 hours to receive 7 or 14 days of antibiotic therapy. Patient with an uncontrolled focus of infection were excluded. The source of the infection was urinary in 69% of patients. No differences were noted in the 90-day composite outcome of all-cause mortality; relapse, suppurative, or distant complications; and readmission or extended hospitalization (>14 days) (45.8%, 7-day treatment, vs 48.3%, 14-day treatment). Ninety-day mortality was not different (11.8%, 7-day treatment, vs 10.7%, 14-day treatment). No significant differences were noted in all other outcomes/adverse events, but the 7-day group had a shorter time to return to baseline functional status.

It is important to review the inclusion criteria for these 2 studies. In the vonDach study, patients were afebrile for 24 hours without evidence for complicated infection (eg, abscess) or severe immunosuppression. In the Yahav study, patients were afebrile and hemodynamically stable for at least 48 hours.

Based on the results of these 2 recent trials, 7 days is emerging as the optimal duration of antimicrobial therapy for gram-negative bacteremia rather than a duration of 14 days. A systematic review and meta-analysis also confirmed that short-course was noninferior to long-course antibiotic treatment for patients with uncomplicated gram-negative bacteremia.[45]

An ongoing randomized controlled trial in ICU patients (planned enrollment 3622, February 2017–March 2022) with bacteremia (BALANCE, Bacteremia Antibiotic Length Actually Needed for Clinical Effectiveness, http://balance.ccctg.ca/; https://clinicaltrials.gov/ct2/show/NCT03005145) is comparing 7 with 14 days of antibiotic treatment and includes most bacterial pathogens except S aureus.[46] The BALANCE study has recently been expanded to include non-ICU patient enrollment based on a pilot randomized trial.[47,48]

Skin and soft tissue infections

Skin and soft tissue infections (SSTIs) have a wide range from cellulitis and superficial SSI to organ/space SSI and rapidly progressive necrotizing soft tissue infections (NSTI). Complicated SSTIs can present with toxic shock syndrome, septic shock, and associated organ failure and require SICU admission.[23] SSI is the most common reason for unplanned hospital readmission following surgery in the United States.[49] A recent report found that of 414,851 noncardiac surgery patients, 35.9% did not receive appropriate perioperative antimicrobial prophylaxis (19.7% for antibiotic choice, 17.1% for weight-adjusted dosing, 0.6% for timing of first dose, and 26.8% for redosing), and nonadherence was especially common in emergency surgery.[50]

Complicated SSTIs include deep soft tissue infections, such as infected ulcers, infected burns, and abscesses that require significant surgical intervention. These infections arise in patients with significant comorbidities that complicate and often delay response to treatment and put patients at high risk for life- and limb-threatening conditions.

NSTIs are identified easily when there is the presence of bullae, crepitus, radiologic evidence of gas, hypotension, or visible skin necrosis. However, less than half of patients with NSTIs have these obvious "hard clinical signs" on examination.[51] Laboratory values (LRINEC score) can be helpful, but cannot rule out NSTI. With any suspicion for NSTI, surgical intervention with dissection down to the fascial and muscle level should promptly occur.[52]

After prompt NSTI diagnosis is established, early appropriate broad-spectrum IV antibiotics, including methicillin-resistant *S aureus* (MRSA) coverage, should be initiated. Prompt surgical debridement is the major determinant of outcome in NSTIs, to obtain adequate source control. If NSTI suspicion is present, surgical intervention should not be delayed for radiologic imaging. Although CT and MRI imaging may reveal deeper abscesses, soft tissue gas, or fascial thickening, they should not delay surgical intervention. Multiple cultures should be sent during the initial surgical debridement procedure for pathogen identification to ensure appropriate antimicrobial therapy. NSTIs can be polymicrobial (most common) or monomicrobial (group A streptococcus or MRSA). In immunocompromised patients or those with contact with seawater or raw seafood, uncommon microbiologic causes such as *Vibrio* and *Aeromonas* should be considered.

Posttransplant infections

Postoperative infection is associated with significant morbidity and mortality in solid organ transplant recipients.[53–55] Prevention of rejection with posttransplant immunosuppression is a significant risk factor for postoperative infections, particularly opportunistic infections. These patients are at risk for all of the usual postoperative SICU infections described previously, including SSIs and non-SSIs, but the infection may be more severe or progress more rapidly than in immunocompetent hosts. The possible causative pathogens are broad, but they are associated with the timing of infection in relation to the transplantation. It is important to determine whether immunosuppression should be significantly reduced in the treatment of patients with posttransplant infections.

Orthopedic and Prosthetic Material-Related Infections

Fracture-related infection

Fracture-related infection (FRI) is a severe complication that occurs after bony trauma. New consensus guidelines[56] have been established for FRI management (**Figs. 4** and **5**) and are summarized:

1. Important considerations such as biofilm presence, fracture consolidations, and stability of the fracture must be taken into account in decision making.
2. If FRI is suspected or confirmed, empirical IV antibiotics should be started immediately after operative sampling. Empirical therapy should include agents with gram-negative bacilli coverage and lipo/glycopeptide coverage; it should then be narrowed based on operative sample results.

When an FRI of an implant is suspected and it is within 6 weeks of index surgery, there is some evidence that hardware can be left in place as long as surgical debridement and sampling is obtained, hardware stability is confirmed, and local antibiotic use (in addition to IV antibiotics) should be considered.[57] A recent report confirmed a 71% fracture union success rate in patients with acute FRI who underwent irrigation, debridement, hardware retention, and antibiotic therapy.[58] However, in the setting of critically ill patients with FRI, all hardware may need to be removed and operative cultures collected to ensure appropriate definitive antimicrobial management.

Osteomyelitis

Patients with polytrauma can often develop bone and joint infections that can be difficult to diagnose and treat. The key to successful management is early diagnosis and

Procedure/strategy	Antimicrobial therapy	Total duration
Removal & osteomyelitis treatment		6 wk
Retention & eradication		12 wk
One-stage exchange & eradication		12 wk
Two-stage exchange & eradication (short interval)		12 wk
Two-stage exchange & eradication (long interval) without antibiotic-free interval		12 wk
Two-stage exchange & eradication (long interval) with antibiotic-free interval		1–2 weeks after implantation[a]
Debridement & suppression until fracture healing	individual	1–2 weeks after removal of implant

○   Debridement, irrigation, and acquisition of multiple tissue samples.

▬►   IV-antibiotics are continued until culture and sensitivity results are available and then, if there are appropriate oral agents available, the patient can be switched to oral antibiotic therapy (in general IV 1–2 wk).

▬►   Oral antibiotics without biofilm activity (approx. 4 weeks, to complete 6 weeks of total antibiotic course).

▬►   Oral antibiotics with biofilm activity.

▬►   Antibiotic free interval (≥2 wk).

   Ex- and implantation of fixation device.

   One stage exchange of the fixation device.

[a] When the cultures are negative, the antibiotic therapy can be stopped.
When positive continue to the guidelines for the one stage exchange (ie, 12 weeks of antibiotics).

Fig. 5. Recommendations for systemic antimicrobial therapy in fracture-related infection (FRI): a consensus from an international expert group. FDG, fludeoxyglucose; SPECT, single-photon emission computed tomography. (*From* Depypere M, Kuehl R, Metsemakers WJ, et al. Recommendations for Systemic Antimicrobial Therapy in Fracture-Related Infection: A Consensus From an International Expert Group. J Orthop Trauma. 2020;34(1):30-41. https://doi.org/10.1097/BOT.0000000000001626; with permission.)

treatment with appropriate antibiotics and surgical debridement. According to the landmark LEAP study, osteomyelitis rate was 9.4% following severe limb-threatening trauma to the lower extremity in a cohort of 330 patients.[59] Intervention must include debridement of all necrotic tissue, removal of foreign material, and abscess/infection drainage. The most common pathogenic organism is *S aureus,* which adheres to host tissues and biomaterials leading to a biofilm that is difficult to eradicate. Surgical treatment often requires a staged approach with multiple debridements, removal of nonessential hardware, and wound vacuum-assisted Closure (VAC) placement. Once all infection is eradicated with appropriate antibiotic treatment, bony stabilization and reconstruction of soft tissue can be performed, preferably with vascularized soft tissue flaps.[60]

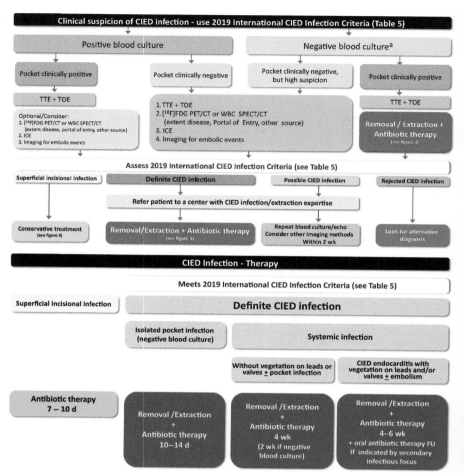

Fig. 6. Guideline recommendations for diagnosis and treatment of CIED infections. (*From* Blomström-Lundqvist C, Traykov V, Erba PA, et al. European Heart Rhythm Association (EHRA) international consensus document on how to prevent, diagnose, and treat cardiac implantable electronic device infections-endorsed by the Heart Rhythm Society (HRS), the Asia Pacific Heart Rhythm Society (APHRS), the Latin American Heart Rhythm Society (LAHRS), International Society for Cardiovascular Infectious Diseases (ISCVID) and the European Society of Clinical Microbiology and Infectious Diseases (ESCMID) in collaboration with the European Association for Cardio-Thoracic Surgery (EACTS). Europace. 2020;22(4):515-549; with permission.)

Mesh infections

Prosthetic mesh has demonstrated a clear benefit in reducing hernia recurrence. However, mesh placement can be associated with postoperative complications including seroma, mesh infection, or mesh fistula.[61] Mesh infections are the third leading cause for reoperation following ventral hernia repairs[62] and can present at varying times from immediately postoperatively to more than a year after surgery. In patients who are critically ill, broad-spectrum antibiotics and wound debridement with explantation of the mesh is frequently necessary for optimal source control. With this, there is an obvious expectation for hernia recurrence that follows the debridement of infected tissue and it is often a larger defect that results. In patients who are not critically ill, there is some evidence that mesh salvage can be successful; this includes medical management with antibiotics and local wound care. This strategy typically involves percutaneous drainage procedures or local debridement, prolonged antibiotic therapy, and negative pressure wound therapy.

Cardiac implantable electrophysiological device infections

Infections involving cardiac implantable electrophysiological devices (CIEDs) have been notoriously difficult to diagnose and manage. Any and all of the components can be infected, including the device leads and the generator pocket. When the endocardial structures are involved, there is associated high mortality. However, extracting the devices also carries a high risk of complications and mortality.[63] There are guidelines (**Fig. 6**) for the management of infected CIED that are helpful in the treatment of this challenging infection.[64,65]

SUMMARY

SICU patients are at risk for a wide range of postoperative infections. When postoperative ICU patients manifest signs and symptoms of infection, a meticulous diagnostic workup is required to determine the cause of the infection. Examination of the surgical site is the first priority given the risk for SSI. Then a careful assessment of all other potential causes based on the patient's signs and symptoms of infection is warranted.

CLINICS CARE POINTS

- Initial management of all surgical infections should include early empirical antibiotic therapy guided by the known common pathogens at the specific site of infection.

- Source control, or the physical intervention to remove or eliminate infection through drainage, debridement, or removal of hardware or device, is necessary to treat postoperative infections.

- Ideal principles for management of IAIs include early diagnosis, early addition of empirical antibiotics, fluid resuscitation, early source control, and deescalation of antibiotic therapy after the causative pathogen is identified.

- Optimal diverticulitis treatment is based on Hinchey stage and patient clinical condition, because the mortality rate for patients with diverticulitis with Hinchey III is 6% but increases greatly to 35% for fecal peritonitis (Hinchey IV).

- Infected pancreatic necrosis is treated by percutaneous catheter or endoscopic drainage and systemic antibiotics as the initial management strategy.

- Empyema is initially managed with tube drainage, antibiotics, and then intrapleural therapy with TPA/dornase and video-assisted thoracic surgery for source control.

- Optimal therapy for SSTIs includes:
  - Prompt identification of necrotizing versus nonnecrotizing infection.
  - Early empirical antibiotic coverage with consideration for MDRO risk factors
  - Early aggressive surgical debridement NSTI is required for source control
  - Cultures and pathogen identification are required for appropriate antibiotic therapy

- FRI is a severe complication that occurs after bony trauma, and new consensus guidelines have been established for FRI management

DISCLOSURE

The authors have no commercial or financial conflicts of interest and no funding sources.

REFERENCES

1. Vincent J-L, Sakr Y, Sprung CL, et al. Sepsis in European intensive care units: results of the SOAP study. Crit Care Med 2006;34(2):344–53.
2. Cheng B, Xie G, Yao S, et al. Epidemiology of severe sepsis in critically ill surgical patients in ten university hospitals in China. Crit Care Med 2007;35(11):2538–46.
3. Vincent J-L, Rello J, Marshall J, et al. International study of the prevalence and outcomes of infection in intensive care units. JAMA 2009;302(21):2323–9.
4. Vincent J-L, Sakr Y, Singer M, et al. Prevalence and Outcomes of Infection Among Patients in Intensive Care Units in 2017. JAMA 2020;323(15):1478–87.
5. Subramanian M, Hirschkorn C, Eyerly-Webb SA, et al. Clinical diagnosis of infection in Surgical Intensive Care Unit: You're not as good as you think! Surg Infections 2020;21(2):122–9.
6. De Waele J, De Bus L. How to treat infections in a surgical intensive care unit. BMC Infect Dis 2014;14:193.
7. Duncan RA. Antimicrobial Use in Surgical Intensive Care. Surg Intensive Care Med 2015;449–59. https://doi.org/10.1007/978-3-319-19668-8_33.
8. Evans LE, Rhodes A, Alhazzani W, et al. Surviving sepsis campaign: international guidelines for management of sepsis and septic shock 2021. Crit Care Med 2021;49(11):e1063–143.
9. Mazuski JE, Tessier JM, May AK. The surgical infection society revised guidelines on the management of intra-abdominal infection. Surg Infect (Larchmt) 2017; 18:1–76.
10. Solomkin JS, Mazuski JE, Bradley JS, et al. Diagnosis and management of complicated intra-abdominal infection in adults and children: Guidelines by the Surgical Infection Society and the Infectious Diseases Society of America. Clin Infect Dis 2010;50(2):133–64.
11. van de Groep K, Verhoeff TL, Verboom DM, et al. MARS consortium. Epidemiology and outcomes of source control procedures in critically ill patients with intra-abdominal infection. J Crit Care 2019;52:258–64.
12. Johnson S, Lavergne V, Skinner AM, et al. Clinical Practice Guideline by the Infectious Diseases Society of America (IDSA) and Society for Healthcare Epidemiology of America (SHEA): 2021 Focused Update Guidelines on Management of Clostridioides difficile Infection in Adults. Clin Infect Dis 2021;73(5):e1029–44.
13. Kalil A, Metersky ML, Klompas M, et al. Management of Adults with Hospital-acquired and Ventilator-associated Pneumonia: 2016 Clinical Practice Guidelines by the Infectious Diseases Society of America and the American Thoracic Society. Clin Infect Dis 2016;63(5):e61–111.
14. Mermel LA, Allon M, Bouza Em, et al. Clinical Practice Guidelines for the Diagnosis and Management of Intravascular Catheter-Related Infection: 2009 Update by the Infectious Diseases Society of America. Clin Infect Dis 2009;49(1):1–45.
15. Gould CV, Umscheid CA, Agarwal RK, et al, The Healthcare Infection Control Practices Advisory Committee (HICPAC). Guideline for prevention of Catheter-Associated Urinary Tract Infections. 2019. Available at: https://www.cdc.gov/infectioncontrol/pdf/guidelines/cauti-guidelines-H.pdf.

16. van de Groep K, Verhoeff TL, Verboom DM, et al. Epidemiology and outcomes of source control procedures in critically ill patients with intra-abdominal infection. J Crit Care 2019;52:258–64.

17. Bass GA, Dzierba AL, Taylor B, et al. Tertiary peritonitis: considerations for complex team-based care. Eur J Trauma Emerg Surg Off Publ Eur Trauma Soc 2021;1–15. https://doi.org/10.1007/s00068-021-01750-9.

18. Sartelli M, Catena F, Abu-Zidan FM, et al. Management of intra-abdominal infections: recommendations by the WSES 2016 consensus conference. World J Emerg Surg 2017;12:22.

19. Sartelli M, Catena F, Di Saverio S, et al. Current concept of abdominal sepsis: WSES position paper. World J Emerg Surg 2014;9(1):22.

20. Sartelli M, Catena F, Ansaloni L, et al. Complicated intra-abdominal infections in Europe: a comprehensive review of the CIAO study. World J Emerg Surg 2012; 7(1):36. https://doi.org/10.1186/1749-7922-7-36.

21. Sawyer RG, Claridge JA, Nathens AB, et al. Trial of short-course antimicrobial therapy for intraabdominal infection. N Engl J Med 2015;372(21):1996–2005.

22. Hassinger TE, Guidry CA, Rotstein OD, et al. Longer-Duration Antimicrobial Therapy Does Not Prevent Treatment Failure in High-Risk Patients with Complicated Intra-Abdominal Infections. Surg Infect (Larchmt) 2017;18(6):659–63.

23. Montravers P, Tubach F, Lescot T, et al. Short-course antibiotic therapy for critically ill patients treated for postoperative intra-abdominal infection: the DURA-POP randomised clinical trial. Intensive Care Med 2018;44:300–10.

24. Abidi HH, Sawyer RG. More evidence for shortening antibiotic therapy in peritonitis: the DURAPOP trial. J Thorac Dis 2018;10(Suppl 26):S3160–1.

25. Peery AF, Shaukat A, Strate LL. AGA Clinical Practice Update on medical management of colonic diverticulitis: Expert Review. Gastroenterology 2021;160: 906–11.

26. Wexner SD, Talamini MA. EAES/SAGES consensus conference on acute diverticulitis: a paradigm shift in the management of acute diverticulitis. Surg Endosc 2019;33(9):2724–5.

27. Lambrichts DP, Edomskis PP, van der Bogt RD, et al. Sigmoid resection with primary anastomosis versus the Hartmann's procedure for perforated diverticulitis with purulent or fecal peritonitis: a systematic review and meta-analysis. Int J Colorectal Dis 2020;35(8):1371–86.

28. Francis NK, Sylla P, Abou-Khalil M, et al. EAES and SAGES 2018 consensus conference on acute diverticulitis management: evidence-based recommendations for clinical practice. Surg Endosc 2019;33(9):2726–41.

29. Cirocchi R, Sapienza P, Anania G, et al. State-of-the-art surgery for sigmoid diverticulitis. Langenbecks Arch Surg 2022;407(1):1–14.

30. Nascimbeni R, Amato A, Cirocchi R, et al. Management of perforated diverticulitis with generalized peritonitis. A multidisciplinary review and position paper. Tech Coloproctol 2021;25(2):153–65.

31. Leppäniemi A, Tolonen M, Tarasconi A, et al. 2019 WSES guidelines for the management of severe acute pancreatitis. World J Emerg Surg 2019;14:27.

32. De Waele JJ, Rello J, Anzueto A, et al. Infections and use of antibiotics in patients admitted for severe acute pancreatitis: data from the EPIC II study. Surg Infect (Larchmt) 2014;15(4):394–8.

33. Garret C, Canet E, Corvec S, et al. Impact of prior antibiotics on infected pancreatic necrosis microbiology in ICU patients: a retrospective cohort study. Ann Intensive Care 2020;10(1):82.

34. van Santvoort HC, Besselink MG, Bakker OJ, et al. A step-up approach or open necrosectomy for necrotizing pancreatitis. N Engl J Med 2010;362(16):1491–502.

35. Warshaw AL. Improving the treatment of necrotizing pancreatitis–a step up. N Engl J Med 2010;362(16):1535–7.

36. Hollemans RA, Bakker OJ, Boermeester MA, et al. Superiority of Step-up Approach vs Open Necrosectomy in Long-term Follow-up of Patients With Necrotizing Pancreatitis. Gastroenterology 2019;156(4):1016–26.

37. Boxhoorn L, van Dijk SM, van Grinsven J, et al. Immediate versus postponed intervention for infected necrotizing pancreatitis. N Engl J Med 2021;385(15):1372–81.

38. Baron TH. Drainage for infected pancreatic necrosis – is the waiting the hardest part? October 7, 2021. N Engl J Med 2021;385:1433–5.

39. Baron TH, DiMaio CJ, Wang AY, et al. American Gastroenterological Association Clinical Practice Update: Management of Pancreatic Necrosis. Gastroenterology 2020;158(1):67–75.e1.

40. Hu K, Chopra A, Kurman J, et al. Management of complex pleural disease in the critically ill patient. J Thorac Dis 2021;13(8):5205–22. https://doi.org/10.21037/jtd-2021-31.

41. Egyud M, Suzuki K. Post-resection complications: abscesses, empyemas, bronchopleural fistulas. J Thorac Dis 2018;10(Suppl 28):S3408–18. Available at: https://jtd.amegroups.com/article/view/23821/18554.

42. von Dach E, Albrich WC, Brunel A-S, et al. Effect of C-reactive protein–guided antibiotic treatment duration, 7-day treatment, or 14-day treatment on 30-day clinical failure rate in patients with uncomplicated gram-negative bacteremia: A randomized clinical trial. JAMA 2020;323:2160–9. PMCID: PMC7267846. Available at: https://jamanetwork.com/journals/jama/fullarticle/2766635.

43. Daneman N, Fowler RA. Shortening Antibiotic Treatment Durations for Bacteremia. Editorial Clin Infect Dis 2019;69(7):1099–100.

44. Yahav D, Franceschini E, Koppel F, et al. Bacteremia Duration Study Group. Seven Versus 14 Days of Antibiotic Therapy for Uncomplicated Gram-negative Bacteremia: A Noninferiority Randomized Controlled Trial. Clin Infect Dis 2019;69(7):1091–8.

45. Li X, Liu C, Mao Z, et al. Short-course versus long-course antibiotic treatment in patients with uncomplicated gram-negative bacteremia: A systematic review and meta-analysis. J Clin Pharm Ther 2021;46:173–80.

46. Daneman N, Rishu AH, Xiong W, et al. Canadian Critical Care Trials Group. Bacteremia antibiotic length actually needed for clinical effectiveness (BALANCE): study protocol for a pilot randomized controlled trial. Trials 2015;16:173.

47. Daneman N, Rishu AH, Pinto R, et al. Canadian Critical Care Trials Group. 7 versus 14 days of antibiotic treatment for critically ill patients with bloodstream infection: a pilot randomized clinical trial. Trials 2018;19:111.

48. Daneman N, Rishu AH, Pinto R, et al. A pilot randomized controlled trial of 7 versus 14 days of antibiotic treatment for bloodstream infection on non-intensive care versus intensive care wards. Trials 2020;21:92.

49. Merkow RP, Ju MH, Chung JW, et al. Underlying reasons associated with hospital readmission following surgery in the United States. JAMA 2015;313(5):483–95.

50. Bardia A, Treggiari MM, Michel G, et al. Adherence to Guidelines for the Administration of Intraoperative Antibiotics in a Nationwide US Sample. JAMA Netw Open 2021;4(12):e2137296.

51. Chan T, Yaghoubian A, Rosing D, et al. Low sensitivity of physical examination findings in necrotizing soft tissue infection is improved with laboratory values: a prospective study. Am J Surg 2008;196(6):926–30 ; discussion 930.
52. Pelletier J, Gottlieb M, Long B, et al. Necrotizing soft tissue infection (NSTI): Pearls and Pitfalls for the emergency clinician. J Emerg Med 2022;62(4):480–91.
53. Kalil AC, Sandkovsky U, Florescu DF. Severe infections in critically ill solid organ transplant recipients. Clin Microbiol Infect 2018;24(12):1257–63. https://doi.org/10.1016/j.cmi.2018.04.022. Epub 2018 Apr 30. PMID: 29715551.
54. Kumar R, Ison MG. Opportunistic Infections in Transplant Patients. Infect Dis Clin North Am 2019;33(4):1143–57. https://doi.org/10.1016/j.idc.2019.05.008. PMID: 31668195.
55. Winterbottom F, Jenkins M. Infections in the Intensive Care Unit: Posttransplant Infections. Crit Care Nurs Clin North Am 2017;29(1):97–110. https://doi.org/10.1016/j.cnc.2016.09.002. Epub 2016 Nov 24. PMID: 28160960; PMCID: PMC7135544.
56. Depypere M, Kuehl R, Metsemakers W-J, et al. Recommendations for Systemic Antimicrobial Therapy in Fracture-Related Infection: A Consensus From an International Expert Group. J Orthop Trauma 2020;34(1):30–41. https://doi.org/10.1097/BOT.0000000000001626.
57. Hoit G, Bonyun M, Nauth A. Hardware considerations in infection and nonunion management: When and how to revise the fixation. OTA Int Open Access J Orthop Trauma 2020;3(1):e055. https://doi.org/10.1097/OI9.0000000000000055.
58. Berkes M, Obremskey WT, Scannell B, et al. Maintenance of hardware after early postoperative infection following fracture internal fixation. J Bone Joint Surg Am 2010;92(4):823–8. https://doi.org/10.2106/JBJS.I.00470.
59. Bosse MJ, MacKenzie EJ, Kellam JF, et al. An analysis of outcomes of reconstruction or amputation after leg-threatening injuries. N Engl J Med 2002;347(24):1924–31. https://doi.org/10.1056/NEJMoa012604.
60. Chan JKK, Ferguson JY, Scarborough M, et al. Management of Post-Traumatic Osteomyelitis in the Lower Limb: Current State of the Art. Indian J Plast Surg 2019;52(1):62–72. https://doi.org/10.1055/s-0039-1687920.
61. Mavros MN, Athanasiou S, Alexiou VG, et al. Risk factors for mesh-related infections after hernia repair surgery: a meta-analysis of cohort studies. World J Surg 2011;35(11):2389–98. https://doi.org/10.1007/s00268-011-1266-5.
62. Sanchez VM, Abi-Haidar YE, Itani KMF. Mesh infection in ventral incisional hernia repair: incidence, contributing factors, and treatment. Surg Infect (Larchmt) 2011;12(3):205–10. https://doi.org/10.1089/sur.2011.033.
63. Athan E, Chu VH, Tattevin P, et al. Clinical characteristics and outcome of infective endocarditis involving implantable cardiac devices. JAMA 2012;307(16):1727–35. https://doi.org/10.1001/jama.2012.497.
64. Blomström-Lundqvist C, Traykov V, Erba PA, et al. European Heart Rhythm Association (EHRA) international consensus document on how to prevent, diagnose, and treat cardiac implantable electronic device infections—endorsed by the Heart Rhythm Society (HRS), the Asia Pacific Heart Rhythm Society (APHRS), the Latin American Heart Rhythm Society (LAHRS), International Society for Cardiovascular Infectious Diseases (ISCVID), and the European Society of Clinical Microbiology and Infectious Diseases (ESCMID) in collaboration with the European Association for Cardio-Thoracic Surgery (EACTS). Eur Heart J 2020; 41(21):2012–32.
65. Wang A, Gaca JG, Chu VH. Management considerations in infective endocarditis: A review. JAMA 2018;320(1):72–83.

ICU Management of Invasive β-Hemolytic Streptococcal Infections

Ahmed Babiker, MBBS[a,b], Sameer S. Kadri, MD, MS, FIDSA[c,*]

KEYWORDS

- Invasive streptococcal infection • Streptococcal toxic shock syndrome • STSS
- Necrotizing fasciitis • Necrotizing soft tissue infection

KEY POINTS

- *Microbiology:* β-hemolytic *Streptococci* (BHS) exhibit complete (β) hemolysis on blood-containing agars and can further be subtyped based on the presence of the surface C-polysaccharide antigens. They include Group A Streptococcus (GAS; *Streptococcus pyogenes*), Group B Streptococcus (GBS; *Streptococcus agalactiae*), and non-group A or B *Streptococci* (NABS).
- *Epidemiology: Streptococci* are a leading cause of invasive bacterial disease worldwide. Common risk factors for developing invasive BHS infection include advanced age, diabetes mellitus, cardiovascular disease, malignancy, immunosuppression, and postpartum states.
- *Clinical syndrome:* Invasive BHS disease is defined as the isolation of BHS from the normally sterile site in patients with a compatible clinical syndrome. Compatible clinical syndromes include streptococcal toxic shock syndrome (STSS), necrotizing soft tissue infection (NSTI), bacteremia (with or without a primary source), lower respiratory tract infections, musculoskeletal infections, meningitis, skin and soft tissue infection with bacteremia and puerperal/postpartum infections. STSS and NSTI carry a significant degree of mortality and require early recognition and prompt intervention.
- *Diagnosis:* Diagnosis of invasive BHS streptococcal infection relies on the identification of the organism in a culture from a normally sterile site, such as blood, synovial fluid, or cerebrospinal fluid (CSF) in the setting of a compatible clinical syndrome.

Continued

[a] Department of Medicine, Division of Infectious Diseases, Emory University School of Medicine, Atlanta, GA, USA; [b] Department of Laboratory Medicine and Pathology, Emory University School of Medicine; [c] Critical Care Medicine Department, Clinical Epidemiology Section, National Institutes of Health Clinical Center, Bethesda, MA, USA
* Corresponding author.
E-mail address: sameer.kadri@nih.gov

Infect Dis Clin N Am 36 (2022) 861–887
https://doi.org/10.1016/j.idc.2022.07.007
0891-5520/22/© 2022 Elsevier Inc. All rights reserved.

id.theclinics.com

Continued

- *Treatment:* Management is multi-disciplinary and should include intensivists, infectious diseases specialists, surgeons, and clinical microbiologists. Resuscitation, source control and prompt antibiotic administration are the cornerstone of managements. Patients with suspected NSTI require early and aggressive surgical intervention. β-lactam agents remain the drugs of choice as isolates are uniformly susceptible. For GAS, adjunctive clindamycin (in clindamycin susceptible strains) is recommended. In β-lactam allergic patients, vancomycin and linezolid should be considered due to varying resistance to other non–β-lactam agents. Intravenous immunoglobulin administration could be considered when available for STSS.

INTRODUCTION

Streptococci sp. are a large heterogeneous genus of Gram-positive bacteria that are widely distributed across the normal flora of human and animals that have a propensity to cause invasive disease.

General Microbiology

Streptococci sp. are a diverse group of Gram-positive nonspore forming, catalase negative (distinguishing them from *Staphylococci sp.*) cocci arranged in pairs and chains. Traditionally the classification of *Streptococci sp* was primarily by patterns of hemolysis on blood agar. Using this methodology streptococci can be classified into 3 distinctive patterns; α (partial hemolysis), β (complete hemolysis), and γ (no hemolysis).[1,2] β-hemolytic *Streptococci* (BHS) are *Streptococci sp.* that exhibit β-hemolysis on blood agar. Dr. Rebecca Craighill Lancefield systematized the classification of *Streptococci sp.* based on the presence of the surface C-polysaccharide antigens.[3] BHS generally exhibit A, B, C, G, F, or L antigens. Over the past decades, we have witnessed changes in taxonomy and nomenclature of the *Streptococcus* genus as a result of the application of advanced molecular techniques (such as 16S rDNA gene sequencing) that help delineate differences in bacterial genera and species with higher precision.[2] However, the Lancefield system of serogrouping and the hemolysis reactions of bacteria on blood agar plates remains a useful clinical classification system of *Streptococci* sp. for patient management.[2,4] This despite its limitations as captured wittily in the poem (parody on the famous T. S. Eliot poem, "The Naming of Cats") by Dr. Musher.[5] (**Table 1**).

Group A Streptococcus Microbiology

Streptococcus pyogenes, Group A *Streptococcus* (GAS), is the sole member of Lancefield group A. On blood agar they form small 1 to 2 mm, grey–white colonies with a zone of β-hemolysis.[1] (see **Table 1**).

Group B Streptococcus Microbiology

Streptococcus agalactiae, Group B *Streptococcus* (GBS), is the sole member of Lancefield group B. They form small 3 to 4 mm, grey–white colonies that have a narrow zone of β-hemolysis (compared with other BHS) on blood agar.[3] Although up to 11% of GBS colonies can be nonhemolytic.[6] (see **Table 1**).

Non-Group A or B β-hemolytic Streptocci Microbiology

Unlike GAS and GBS, no single *Streptococcal* species is uniquely identifiable via the expression of non-A and B antigens. These can include groups C, G, F, and L, of which

Table 1
Classification and microbiologic features of β-hemolytic *streptococci*

Species	Lancefield Antigen(s)[a]	Hemolytic Reaction[b]	Unique Biochemical Properties
S. pyogenes	A	β	+ve PYR, -ve bile esculin hydrolysis, bacitracin susceptible
S. agalactiae	B	β	+ve CAMP test, -ve bile esculin hydrolysis, -ve PYR test, +ve hippurate hydrolysis, +ve granadaene, bacitracin resistant
S. dysgalactiae subsp. (includes subsp. equismilis, dysgalactiae, equi, and zooepidemicus)	C, G and rarely A	β	+ve LAP, -ve PYR, -ve hippurate hydrolysis, SXT susceptible

Abbreviations: CAMP, Christie–Atkins–Munch-Peterson; LAP, leucine aminopeptidase; PYR, pyrrolidonylarylamidase; trimethoprim-sulfamethoxazole.
[a] Lancefield antigen based on the presence of the surface C-polysaccharide antigens.[3]
[b] Hemolytic reaction classification based on activity on blood-containing agars.[4]
Data from G. W. Procop et al., in Koneman's Color Atlas and Textbook of Diagnostic Microbiology; and Bennett JE, Dolin R, Blaser MJ. Mandell, Douglas, and Bennett's Principles and Practice of Infectious Diseases. Elsevier Inc., 2015, pp 2283-2284.

the most common are groups C and G.[7] The vast majority of non-group A or B β-hemolytic Streptococci (NABS) clinical isolates associated with human infection that are identified as group C or G streptococci belong to *Streptococcus dysgalactiae* and in particular the subspecies *S. dysgalactiae subsp equisimilis*[7,8] (see **Table 1**). A population-based survey of invasive NABS found that 212 (80%) were caused by SDSE.[7] Rarely, *Streptococci* of animal origin which also express the group C or G antigen are implicated in human infection. These include *Streptococcus equi subsp equi* and *Streptococcus equi subsp zooepidemicus* which are associated primarily with horses and *Streptococcus canis* is associated with several animal species, including dogs, cats, and cattle.[7]

NABS form large colonies, typically surrounded by a large zone of β-hemolysis. Some group G strains may have a golden cast on close inspection.[1] *Streptococci* in the *S. anginosus* or *S. milleri* group, which also have the propensity to cause invasive infection,[9,10] may also react with C or G typing sera, but these organisms are distinguished by the fact that they form small (<0.5 mm) non B-hemolytic colonies[2] (see **Table 1**).

PATHOGENESIS
Group A Streptococcus Pathogenesis

The virulence factors of GAS are the most well defined, which involve a host of adhesion molecules and immunomodulator factors such as the hyaluronic capsule, M protein, streptolysin O, streptolysin S, streptococcal pyrogenic exotoxins A and B, and NAD glycohydrolase NADase.[11,12] Some of these exotoxin act as superantingens, which trigger excessive stimulation of T lymphocytes by binding to class II major histocompatibility complex molecules, leading to a massive release of T cell mediators, proinflammatory cytokines and subsequent shock.[13] The major virulence and adhesion factor of GAS is the M protein which is encoded by the *emm* gene. Sequencing of the hypervariable 5' end of the *emm* gene is used in molecular typing. The M protein disrupts and inhibits complement activation by binding to complement factors which inhibits phagocytosis.[14] For a full review of pathogenicity factors readers are directed toward reference.[11]

Group B Streptococcus Pathogenesis

The best-characterized GBS virulence factors are the capsular polysaccharide and the secreted hemolysin.[15] The polysaccharide capsule, which confers serotype specificity to GBS, is made of complex carbohydrates composed of approximately 150 repeating oligosaccharide subunits. The 10 capsular serotypes (Ia, Ib, II, III, IV, V, VI, VII, VIII, and IX) currently recognized differ in their arrangements of monosaccharides within the oligosaccharide repeating units. The capsule confers virulence to the organism, at least in part, by inhibiting the deposition of complement components and inhibition of phagocytosis.[13]

Non–group A or B β-Hemolytic Streptococci Pathogenesis

Molecular studies have described virulence determinants of NABS (in particular *S. dysgalactiae subsp equisimilis*) that are similar to known alleles in GAS.[16] Evidence of horizontal transfer and recombination events between GAS and NABS has been demonstrated and may play a role in the acquisition of these virulence factors and its pathogenicity.[17] Sequencing has revealed that they share up to 72% sequence homology,[18] including the antiphagocytic M protein, streptolysin O, streptolysin S, streptokinase, streptococcal phospholipase A2 and one or more pyrogenic exotoxins.[17] Species-specific streptococcal superantigen gene *sepG* and the occasional recombinant event from GAS leading to the acquisition of GAS superantigen genes *sepA/B* has been documented among NABS.[14,19] However, the presence of these genes were not by themselves associated with invasive disease.[17] The occurrence of streptococcal toxic shock syndrome (STSS) and necrotizing soft tissue infection (NSTI) and other severe forms of infection is considerably less in NABS compared with GAS, even in the presence of such genes.[18,19] For a review of the full pathogenicity factors in NABS, readers are directed toward reference.[20]

INVASIVE β-HEMOLYTIC STREPTOCOCCI EPIDEMIOLOGY

Invasive BHS disease, defined as the presence of BHS in a normally sterile site, causes a large burden of disease worldwide. Common risk factors for the development of invasive diseases include, increasing age, cardiovascular disease (CVD), diabetes mellites (DM), malignancy and immunosuppressed or postpartum states.[21] Organisms-specific risk factors are listed later in discussion and in **Table 2**.

Invasive Group A Streptococcus Epidemiology

Within the US, the Centers for Diseases Control and Prevention (CDC) estimates that approximately 11,000 to 24,000 cases of invasive GAS disease occur with between 1,200 and 1,900 people dying each year.[22] In the year 2019, 7.6 cases per 100,000 population were estimated, with a mortality rate of 0.7% per 100,000 population across all syndromes.[23]

Several risk actors have been identified as predisposing to invasive GAS infection. The skin is the most frequent portal of entry and skin lesions such as minor trauma, chronic skin conditions, burns, surgical procedures, peripheral vascular diseases, and the use of intravenous drugs can predispose to the development of invasive

Table 2
Invasive β-hemolytic Streptococcal clinical syndromes and risk factors

BHS Species	Common Risk Factors for Invasive Disease	Invasive Clinical Syndrome(s)
GAS	Skin lesions	SSTI with bacteremia
	Trauma	NSTI
	Chronic skin conditions (eczema, and so forth)	STSS
		Bacteremia (with/without primary source)
	Burns	Lower respiratory tract infections
	PVD	(Pneumonia/Empyema)
	IVDU	Musculoskeletal infections (Septic arthritis/
	CVD	Osteomyelitis)
	DM	Meningitis
	Homelessness	Puerperal/postpartum infection
	Alcohol abuse	Deep-seated abscesses
	Malignancy	Peritonitis
	Immunosuppression	
	Preceding varicella or influenza infection	
	NSAID use	
GBS	Age	SSTI with bacteremia
	Smoking	Endocarditis
	CVD	Arthritis
	DM	Pneumonia
	Obesity	Osteomyelitis
	Malignancy	Meningitis
	Neurological disease	Pyelonephritis
	Immunosuppression	Neonatal sepsis
	ESLD	
	ESRD	
	Postpartum state	
NABS	Age	SSTI with bacteremia
	DM	NSTI
	CVD	STSS
	Malignancy	Bacteremia (with/without primary source)
	Immunosuppression	Lower respiratory tract infections
	ESLD	(Pneumonia/Empyema)
	Alcohol use	Endocarditis
	IVDU	Septic arthritis
		Osteomyelitis
		Meningitis
		Puerperal/postpartum infection
		Deep-seated abscesses
		Peritonitis

Abbreviations: CKD, chronic kidney disease; CVD, cardiovascular disease; DM, diabetes mellitus; ESLD, end-stage liver disease; ESRD, end-stage renal diseases; GAS, Group A streptococcus; GBS, Group B streptococcus; IVDU, intravenous drug use; NABS, non-group A or B Streptococcus; NSAID, non-steroidal anti-inflammatory drugs; NSTI, necrotizing soft tissue infection; PVD, peripheral vascular disease; SSTI, skin and soft tissue infection; STSS, streptococcal toxic shock syndrome.

GAS. This in addition to comorbid conditions such as CVD, DM, postpartum states, homelessness, alcohol abuse, malignancy and immunosuppression.[24–27] Preceding infections with varicella (particularly in children) and influenza[26–28] and use of nonsteroidal anti-inflammatory drugs have also been linked to increased risk of subsequent invasive GAS.[26,29]

Close contacts of patients with invsive GAS infection have a high likelihood of becoming colonized with a virulent strain.[30] The risk of subsequent invasive GAS disease among household contacts of persons with invasive GAS is increased when compared with the general population.[31-35] The most common relationships among confirmed household clusters of invasive GAS transmission are spouses and parent/child pairs.[31,33] Clinicians should be aware that GAS can be associated with transmission and outbreaks within health care settings.[36-39]

Invasive Group B Streptococcus Epidemiology

Within the US, the CDC estimates approximately 30,800 cases of invasive GBS disease occur annually in all age groups.[40] Invasive GBS incidence among nonpregnant adults is rising and has increased from 8.1 cases per 100,000 population in 2008 to 10.9 cases per 100,000 population in 2017.[41] In 2019 across all invasive GBS syndromes, 9.9 cases per 100,000 population with a mortality rate of 0.6 deaths per 100,00 population was observed.[42]

Several risk actors have been identified as predisposing to invasive GBS infection. These include advanced age, smoking, DM, CVD, obesity, malignancy, neurological disease (such as cerebrovascular accidents), end-stage liver diseases (ESLD), end-stage renal disease (ESRD) and immunosuppression.[6,43,44]

Invasive Non-group A or B Streptococci Epidemiology

NABS have become increasingly recognized to cause invasive disease with increased rates reported worldwide.[18,45] Due to the microbiological heterogeneity of NABS and different definitions in previous studies, the true burden of disease is not clearly known. However, it is thought to be similar to that attributable to GAS.[7] Among NABS, S dysgalactiae subsp equisimilis is responsible for most cases of invasive infections in humans, and has surpassed GAS as a leading cause of invasive Streptococcal infections in some centers globally.[5,12,15] A US population-based surveillance study of invasive NABS performed over a 2-year period estimated an incidence of 3.2 cases per 100,000 population.

Risk factors associated with invasive NABS infection include advanced age, DM, CVD, malignancies, immunosuppression, ESLD, alcohol, and IV drug use.[7,18,24,46,47] Rarely members of the NABS group such as S. equi subsp equi, S. equi subsp zooepidemicus, and S. canis can be acquired by direct contact with animals such as dogs, cats and cattle.[7,48]

INVASIVE β-HEMOLYTIC STREPTOCOCCI CLINICAL SYNDROMES

BHS are more commonly associated with noninvasive diseases such as pharyngitis or mild skin and soft tissue (nonnecrotizing) infections. However, these species have the potential to cause invasive infection, defined as the presence of bacteria in a normally sterile site.[49] These frequently include skin and soft tissue infections (SSTI) with bacteremia, NSTIs, STSS, musculoskeletal infections, (septic arthritis and osteomyelitis), lower respiratory tract infections (pneumonia and empyema), bacteremia without a focus of infection and postpartum infections of the female genital tract.[21]

Invasive Group A Streptococcus Clinical Syndromes

The nasopharyngeal mucosa and skin are the principal sites of GAS asymptomatic colonization.[11] GAS is commonly associated with noninvasive infections such as pharyngitis and SSTIs. Less commonly, GAS causes invasive infection which encompass several clinical syndromes which include SSTI (necrotizing or nonnecrotizing with bacteremia), musculoskeletal infections (septic arthritis and osteomyelitis), lower respiratory tract infections (pneumonia and empyema), bacteremia without a focus of infection, STSS, endocarditis, myositis, peritonitis, postpartum/puerperal infections and deep-seated abscesses such as pelvic or retropharyngeal abscesses.[50] (see **Table 2**). The case fatality rate within the US across different clinical syndromes of invasive GAS has been estimated to be 11.7% but can be as high as 70%[50–52] when associated with NSTI in the presence of STSS.[50] Among all the invasive GAS clinical syndromes, two manifestations are of particular importance to intensive care unit providers due to the high degree of mortality they carry: NSTI (aka necrotizing fasciitis) and STSS. These manifestations while typically associated with GAS, can occur with NABS and to a lesser extent GBS.[8,53,54]

Necrotizing soft tissue infection (necrotizing fasciitis)

The term necrotizing fasciitis was first coined in the 1950s and refers to an aggressive subcutaneous tissue infection that tracks along the superficial fascia and compromises all the tissues between the skin and underlaying muscle.[55,56] Toxin-induced inflammatory responses are believed to be involved in both tissue pathology and systemic toxicity.[57] The incidence of NSTI due to invasive group A streptococcal (GAS) infections is estimated to be 0.4 per 100,000 in the US.[50]

It most commonly involves the extremities (lower extremities more commonly than upper extremities), particularly in patients with diabetes and/or peripheral vascular disease. NSTI usually presents acutely (over hours); rarely, it may present subacutely (over days).[12] Extension from a skin lesion is seen in most cases, which can be trivial, such as a minor abrasion, insect bite, injection site, varicella lesion or boil, and a small minority of patients have no visible skin lesion.[12] Examination of the local site typically reveals cutaneous inflammation, edema, and discoloration or gangrene and anesthesia. A distinguishing clinical feature is the wooden-hard induration of the subcutaneous tissues and pain that is out of proportion to exam findings.[58,59] Rapid progression to extensive destruction can occur, leading to systemic toxicity, limb loss, and death.[55] Case fatality rates, even in the presence of appropriate therapy can be as high 30–40%.[60,61] Successful management of necrotizing fasciitis is dependent on early recognition, prompt administration of antimicrobials and debridement.

Streptococcal toxic shock syndrome

STSS is a complication of invasive BHS characterized by shock and multiorgan failure.[29] Bacterial exotoxins act as superantigens to trigger polyclonal T-cell activation, cytokine cascade, and refractory shock.[29] While it has been reported among other BHS, in particular NABS, it most frequently occurs with invasive GAS.[8,18,19] Most recent CDC surveillance reporting shows STSS occurring at a rate of 3–4% among invasive GAS cases[50,62] although prior reports show it can be associated with NSTI in up to 50% of cases caused by certain emm types.[60]

STSS is characterized by an acute, progressive illness associated with fever, rapid-onset hypotension, and accelerated multi-system failure in the presence of a positive GAS culture (**Table 3**).[29] Initial symptoms include an influenza-like illness prodrome, characterized by fever, chills, confusion, myalgia, nausea, vomiting, and diarrhea. A diffuse, scarlatina-like erythema may occur in a small percentage of cases.[63] Subsequently symptoms of the underlaying invasive GAS syndrome can be seen. If the skin is the portal of entry, this is followed by early and visible signs of inflammation, such localized swelling and erythema, followed by ecchymoses and sloughing of skin. In the absence of a defined portal of entry, clinical evidence of a deep infection becomes more obvious as the illness progresses.[29,51,60] Ultimately end-organ failure rapidly

Table 3
Centers for diseases prevention and control streptococcal toxic shock diagnostic criteria

Criteria	Definition
Clinical Criteria	
Hypotension	Systolic blood pressure less than or equal to 90 mm Hg for adults
Multi-organ involvement	Characterized by 2 or more of the below
Renal Impairment	Creatinine greater than or equal to 2 mg/dL for adults or greater than or equal to twice the upper limit of normal for age. In patients with preexisting renal disease, a greater than twofold elevation over the baseline level.
Coagulopathy	Platelets less than or equal to 100,000/mm³ or disseminated intravascular coagulation, defined by prolonged clotting times, low fibrinogen level, and the presence of fibrin degradation products.
Liver Involvement	Alanine aminotransferase, aspartate aminotransferase, or total bilirubin levels greater than or equal to twice the upper limit of normal for the patient's age. In patients with preexisting liver disease, a greater than twofold increase over the baseline level.
Acute respiratory distress syndrome	Acute onset of diffuse pulmonary infiltrates and hypoxemia in the absence of cardiac failure or by evidence of diffuse capillary leak manifested by acute onset of generalized edema, or pleural or peritoneal effusions with hypoalbuminemia.
A generalized erythematous macular rash	Rash may desquamate
Soft-tissue necrosis	Necrotizing fasciitis , myositis, or gangrene.
Laboratory Criteria	
Confirmed	Isolation of from sterile site
Probable	Isolation of a nonsterile site

Adapted from Streptococcal Toxic Shock Syndrome: For Clinicians. Centers for Disease Control and Prevention. Available at https://www.cdc.gov/groupastrep/diseases-hcp/Streptococcal-Toxic-Shock-Syndrome.html.

ensues which includes renal failure, hepatic failure, acute respiratory distress syndrome, and disseminated intravascular coagulation[64] The diagnosis of STSS is established based on the presence of clinical criteria and a positive culture as outlined in **Table 3**. Mortality can be as high as 30%-70%.[50–52]

Invasive Group B Streptococcus Clinical Syndromes

GBS frequently colonizes the human genital and gastrointestinal tracts.[65] It is an important cause of infection in 3 populations: pregnant adults, nonpregnant adults, and neonates where GBS has long been a leading cause of neonatal infection.[21] Invasive clinical syndromes in nonpregnant adults commonly include SSTI with bacteremia, musculoskeletal infections, lower respiratory tract infections, pyelonephritis, endocarditis and bacteremia without focus of infection[43] (see **Table 2, Fig. 1**). In a US national surveillance network conducted between 2008 and 2016 case fatality rate averaged 6.5% across clinical syndromes in nonpregnant adults.[41]

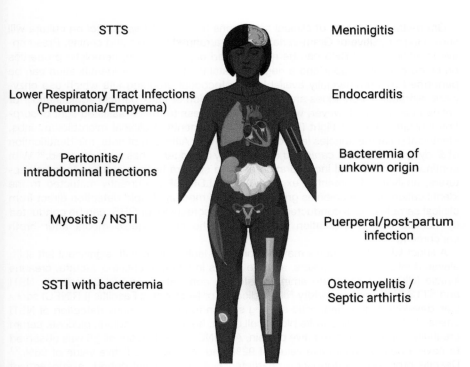

Fig. 1. Common invasive β-hemolytic Streptococcal clinical syndromes *(Created with Bio-Render).* NSTI, necrotizing soft tissue infection; SSTI, skin and soft tissue infectionl; STSS, Streptococcal Toxic Shock Syndrome. (Created with BioRender.com.)

Non–group A or B β-Hemolytic Streptococcal Clinical Syndromes

NABS are frequent commensals of the skin, oropharynx, gastrointestinal and genitourinary tracts and were historically considered normal commensal flora.[3] NABS have a wide spectrum of clinical syndrome which mirrors that of GAS. It most commonly presents as SSTI (NSTI or SSTI with bacteremia)[7] with a high rate of associated bacteremia, especially *S. dysgalactiae subsp equisimilis* with rates of bacteriemia as high as 94%.[7] Other invasive clinical syndromes include musculoskeletal infections (septic arthritis and osteomyelitis), lower respiratory tract infections (pneumonia and empyema), peritonitis, meningitis, endocarditis, postpartum/puerperal infections, myositis, and STSS[7,15,16,22] Mortality rates ranging between 2% and 21% have been reported globally.[7,66,67]

DIAGNOSIS

Diagnosis of invasive BHS infection relies on the identification of the organism in a culture from a normally sterile site, such as blood, synovial fluid, or cerebrospinal fluid and can be considered definitive evidence of infection in the setting of a compatible clinical syndrome. Bacterial cultures should be obtained from the clinically relevant infection sites. Blood cultures (at least 2 sets) should be drawn (ideally prior to antibiotic administration), as a high proportion of patients with invasive BHS syndromes may have positive blood cultures.[21,47,63] Patients who undergo debridement should have surgical specimens (not swabs) sent to the microbiology lab for Gram-stain and cultures. Specimens should be inoculated into a suitable blood-containing medium that has a peptone base.

Gram-stained smears of clinical specimens that yield *Streptococci* on culture will show Gram-positive or Gram-variable cocci arranged in pairs and chains. Presumptive identification of BHS can be made based on, Gram-stain, hemolytic properties on blood containing agar and a negative catalase test. Further identification can be performed by commercially available streptococcal grouping kits which use enzymatic extraction techniques and either coagulation or latex particle agglutination for antigen detection. However, with increasing access to matrix-assisted light desorption ionization time of flight (MALDI-TOF) instruments in clinical microbiology labs, identification at the species level can be achieved. Although of note, misidentification of *S. dysgalactiae* as *S. canis* and occasionally *S pyogenes* has been reported.[68] With continued updates and incorporation of more spectra to the database by manufacturers, analytic refinement is expected.[68] MALDI-TOF is currently restricted to the identification of pure colonies grown on a solid medium. Rapid detection direct from clinical samples, as is conducted for antenatal screening for GBS, can be conducted by nucleic acid amplification or plating to the chromogenic media after broth enrichment.[69]

Adjunct laboratory studies may demonstrate leukocytosis with significant left shift, elevated inflammatory markers, and elevations in serum creatinine, lactate, creatine kinase (CK), and aspartate aminotransferase concentrations can be seen in NSTI and STTS.[63,70] The Laboratory Risk Indicator for Necrotizing Fasciitis (LRINEC) score was developed as a diagnostic scoring system to aid in the early detection of NSTI cases.[71] The score uses white blood cell count, hemoglobin, sodium, glucose, serum creatinine, and serum c-reactive protein. A LRINEC cut-off score of ≥ 6 was observed to have a positive predictive value of 92% and negative predictive value of 96%.[71] Despite promising performance characteristics in the initial cohort, a subsequent multicenter prospective evaluation of the LRINEC score has lessened the excitement around this predictive tool. In the study, a cut-off of ≥ 6 in patients with NSTI failed to discriminate between those with and without high cytokine levels, septic shock, and death.[72]

Imaging such as computed tomography (CT) or magnetic resonance imaging (MRI) may be helpful in the confirmation of NSTI to assess the source of invasive BHS infections. In NSTI cases it may show edema extending along the fascial plane, although the sensitivity and specificity of these imaging studies are ill-defined and thus not definitive. Clinical judgment is the most important element in the diagnosis of NSTI, STSS, and severe invasive BHS syndromes and imaging should not delay preemptive supportive, antibiotic, and surgical management of these cases.[73] For NSTI cases the diagnosis is confirmed by the appearance of the subcutaneous tissues or fascial planes at the time of debridement and positive Gram-stains, cultures and/or histopathology from tissue.[58]

GAS and GBS are included as targets on FDA-approved commercial panel-based molecular diagnostics for the rapid detection of pathogens in positive blood culture bottles (Biofire FilmArray Blood Culture Identification panel [BioFire Diagnostics, LLC]), respiratory specimens (BioFire FilmArray Pneumonia Panel [[BioFire Diagnostics, LLC]), cerebrospinal fluid (BioFire FilmArray Meningitis/Encephalitis [[BioFire Diagnostics, LLC]), and synovial fluid (BioFire Bone and Joint Infection (BJI) Panel (BioFire Diagnostics, Salt Lake City, UT). These panels have the added advantage of rapid turnaround time and the detection of many microorganisms simultaneously, even in the setting of antibiotic therapy.[74,75] However, a clear understanding of the specific performance characteristics for each panel/target and limitations when implementing multiplex assays is important for result interpretation.[74,75]

TREATMENT

General Principles and Supportive Management

The management of invasive BHS admitted to the intensive care unit requires a multidisciplinary approach involving input from infectious diseases specialists, surgeons, and clinical microbiologists when appropriate.[73] Early recognition of invasive BHS clinical syndromes and rapid resuscitation, antibiotic therapy, and source control are crucial to the management of such cases. In the early stages of illness, the causative organism will be unknown, and the same basic strategy should be applied to any case of bacterial sepsis and managed as per surviving sepsis guidelines.[76] This includes resuscitation with large quantities of intravenous fluids to maintain perfusion, prompt the administration of empiric antibiotic therapy and supportive management with mechanical ventilation, vasopressors and renal replacement therapy as needed.

Antibacterial Therapy

As patients with invasive BHS may not be readily distinguished from bacterial sepsis syndromes due to other pathogens empiric therapy should initially consist of broad-spectrum antibiotic treatment which can be subsequently tailored, as receiving discordant or delayed empirical antibiotic therapy is associated with a significantly increased odds of mortality.[77–79] The most common etiological agents of culture-positive sepsis include Gram-negative lactose fermenters (Escherichia coli and Klebsiella species), Gram-negative nonfermenters (Pseudomonas species and Acinetobacter species), Gram-positive organisms such as Staphylococcal species and Enterococcus species and Candida species, which underlies the need for broad empiric antimicrobial therapy initially.[80,81]

The final duration of treatment with consideration for step-down oral therapy should be tailored to clinical response and site of infection and guided by antimicrobial susceptibility testing. After the confirmation of invasive BHS, targeted therapy with penicillin and other β-lactams are the treatment of choice given high rates of susceptibility[42,55] (**Fig. 2**).

β-Lactam Hypersensitivity

For patients with confirmed severe hypersensitivity reactions to β-lactams that preclude their use vancomycin may be used. Linezolid and daptomycin are active in vitro, but clinical experience in treating invasive BHS infections is limited.[82] The prevalence of resistance to clindamycin, macrolides, tetracyclines, and fluoroquinolones varies based on geography and type of BHS and the use of these agents should be guided by local resistance patterns and susceptibility testing as there is a significant and rising resistance among BHS isolates to these agents and thus they should be avoided for empiric therapy (**Table 4**, see **Fig. 2**).[41,83]

Surgical Management

For patients with a suspected diagnosis of NSTI, prompt and aggressive surgical exploration to perform the debridement of necrotic tissue and/or to confirm the diagnosis is the single most important treatment intervention.[55,58] Delays in surgical treatment (mostly defined > 24h in the literature) has been found to correlate with higher mortality, increased length of stay, morbidity and number of subsequent operations needed among survivors.[23,71,84–86] Debridement should be aggressive and consists of removal of all nonviable tissue including muscle, fascial layers, subcutaneous tissue, and skin. The incision should be extended until healthy viable tissue is

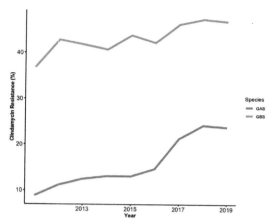

Fig. 2. Proportion of clindamycim resistant isolates through CDC Active Bacterial Core surveillance between 2011 and 2019. Both figures are adapted from the Active Bacterial Core surveillance ABCs 2019 interactive dashboard. Active Bacterial Core surveillance is laboratory- and population-based surveillance program that monitors invasive bacterial infections. GAS, Group A streptococcus; GBS, Group B streptococcus.

seen.[73,87] Scheduled reexplorations should be conducted at least every 12–24 h after the initial operation or sooner if any local or systemic signs of clinical worsening become evident.[73] Delay in reexploration, similar to primary exploration has been associated with decreased survival and increased morbidity.[88] Reexplorations should be repeated until no further need for debridement, patients typically require 3–4 debridements.[55,87] Patients with an invasive BHS infection and an ongoing deep-seated source (e.g., intra-abdominal abscess) should also be evaluated for intervention and source control either by general surgery or interventional radiology.

Table 4
Reported antimicrobial resistance in the US

BHS Species	Agent	Resistance Rates	Time Period, Methodology, Sample Size	Reference
GAS[a]	Penicillin	0%	2019,	42
	Clindamycin	24.7%	Active population surveillance, n = 2,235	
GBS[a]	Penicillin	0%	2019,	42
	Clindamycin	46.8%	Active population surveillance, n = 2318	
NABS[b]	Penicillin	0%	2002–2004,	
	Clindamycin	5.7%	Active population surveillance, n = 212	7

Abbreviations: GAS, Group A streptococcus; GBS, Group B streptococcus; NABS, non-group A; non-group B Streptococcus.
[a] Data from Active Bacterial Core Surveillance 2019 Interactive Dashboard. Active Bacterial Core surveillance is the laboratory- and population-based surveillance program that monitors invasive bacterial infections.
[b] Unlike GAS and GBS, NABS data from 2 (vs full) Active Bacterial Core surveillance sites from 2002 to 2004 (vs. 2019).

Adjunctive Therapies

Adjunctive clindamycin

Clindamycin, a protein synthesis inhibitor with activity during the stationary phase of bacterial growth has been shown to decrease the expression and production of GAS virulence factors and exotoxins.[89] The addition of adjunctive clindamycin therapy to β-lactams is recommended by multiple professional societies for the management of severe invasive GAS and associated NSTI.[55,73] These recommendations were initially made based on in vitro, animal models and observational studies which demonstrated that penicillin had reduced efficacy with a high inoculum size. This was hypothesized to be due to a physiological stationary growth phase and associated down-regulation of penicillin-binding proteins that the bacteria exhibited with a large inoculum size, later termed the inoculum effect.[90] In a streptococcus myositis mouse model the efficacy of clindamycin was not altered by the inoculum size and was found to be superior to penicillin at the inoculum size studied.[91]

The preponderance of observational studies has shown a benefit or trend towards benefit with the use of adjunctive clindamycin in invasive GAS.[8,32,53,54,92,93] The largest of these was propensity-matched retrospective study of 1956 invasive patients with BHS (1079 with GAS) admitted to 118 US hospitals over a 15-year period. In-hospital mortality in propensity-matched patients with GAS who received adjunctive clindamycin was significantly lower than in those who did not (6.5%, (18/277) vs 11.0% (55/500); aOR 0.44 [95% CI 0.23–0.81]). This survival benefit was observed even in patients without shock or NSTI; however, the number of patients within the NSTI subgroup was too small for any conclusions to be made.[8] These findings suggest there is room for wider utilization of clindamycin, as adjunctive clindamycin might be beneficial in patients with invasive GAS infections outside of STSS and NSTI, a population in whom clindamycin utilization is currently low.[8,53] In contrast to prior studies, a recent observational study of NSTI due to GAS which utilized propensity overlap weighting methods found that patients receiving clindamycin did not have a statistically significant reduced in-hospital mortality (19.2% vs. 17.5%; aOR, 1.11 [95% 0.59–2.09]).[94] Similar findings were reported from a prospectively enrolled cohort of streptococcal NSTI where clindamycin therapy prior to ICU admission was not associated with improved mortality.[95] These findings among NSTI cases may reflect improvements in recognition and prompt antibiotic therapy, surgical intervention and IVIG use.[95]

Observational studies of non-GAS (specifically NABS) have failed to show a similar mortality benefit.[8,53,96] One contributing factor to the differential impact of clindamycin could be different clindamycin resistance rates in GAS, NABS, and GBS,[97] with resistance rates typically highest for GBS.[98] As species information may not be readily available early on in the course of infection the risk-benefit balance of early clindamycin administration on the basis of clinical presentation seems reasonable, at least in high mortality conditions such as NSTI and suspected STSS. Given that these severe presentations are more likely to be due to GAS vs. NABS, in aggregate, more patients with GAS (than NABS) are likely to appropriately receive prompt clindamycin.[8] Moreover, the impact of clindamycin resistance remains unclear, as myositis animal models have shown a reduction in lesions and virulence factors with clindamycin use in clindamycin-resistant GAS strains.[89.8,53] However, clinical data examining impact of clindamycin resistance remains scant. In a reterospective cohort of 118 patients with culture confirmed BHS NSTI, clindamycin resistance was associated with increased risk of amputation in adjusted MV analysis, but not with increased mortality or STSS risk. Importantly, the study was not limited to GAS and included those with polymicrobial infection (28% had cocultured *Staphylococcus aureus*) thus adding potential confounding. Ultimately clindamycin use should be guided by local and patient-specific susceptibility as clindamycin resistance rates across BHS species can show considerable geographic variation[99] and are rising over time (see **Fig. 2**).[100] Although recent US population-based estimates of clindamycin resistance among NABS are not available[42]

The optimal duration of adjunctive clindamycin is uncertain as data are limited. Contemporary real-world data reveal the median duration of *adjunctive* clindamycin *administration* ranges between 4 and 5 days. We recommend a minimum of 72 hours with the patient's clinical course to be taken into consideration, until further prospective data are available.

Alternatively, linezolid has become more widely used in clinical practice as an adjunctive agent[8,101] in lieu of clindamycin. This is primarily due to its toxin inhibiting properties,[102] broad-spectrum status, and concern for rising clindamycin resistance. However, experience to date is limited to *in vitro* data and case reports.[82,102,103]

Antimicrobial Resistance Considerations for Management

The CDC conducts active, laboratory- and population-based surveillance for invasive GAS and GBS in 10 geographically diverse sites in the US.[100] Through this surveillance program, called Active Bacterial Core surveillance, no β-lactam resistant isolates have been identified to date (see **Table 4**). However, a 2017 GAS hospital outbreak lead to the identification of GAS strains with elevated minimum inhibitory concentrations (MICs) to ampicillin, amoxicillin, and cefotaxime (despite the increase MICs remained within the range of what is considered susceptible) consistent with a first step in developing β-lactam resistance.[39] Identified strains contained a mutation that altered the amino acid composition of the key peptidoglycan synthetic enzyme (PBP2x) at a site previously associated with reduced susceptibility to β-lactams in other streptococci through the remodeling of the transpeptidase domain that results in reduced affinity.[104] A recent genomic interrogation of 7,025 global genome sequences of GAS clinical isolates collected as part of population-based studies conducted in the United States, Finland, and Iceland revealed 137 (2%) strains with similar mutations in PBP2X, some of which correlated with increased MICs to β-lactam antibiotics.[105] Importantly none of the mutations identified resulted in frank resistance. Similarly, elevated MICs to β-lactams antibiotics conferred by PBP2x point mutations have also been described in GBS and NABS (*Streptococcus dysgalactiae subspecies* equisimilis).[106,107] These reports provide evidence that BHS have the potential to adapt to β-lactam antibiotic selective pressure and the importance of continued phenotypic surveillance.

Within the US, clindamycin resistance among invasive BHS is monitored through the Active Bacterial Core surveillance. In contrast to the continued susceptibility of BHS to β-lactams, clindamycin resistance has been increasing over time for both GAS and GBS (see **Fig. 2**, see **Table 4**). However, continued active surveillance of invasive NABS disease is currently not performed by the CDC, and no recent population-based estimates of clindamycin resistance among NABS are available with the last systematic estimates from 2002 to 2004[7] (see **Table 4**). In the above-mentioned propensity-matched retrospective study of invasive patients with BHS (GAS and NABS) admitted to 118 US hospitals between 2000 and 2015, patients with clindamycin-resistant isolates were removed from the final cohort. Initial data exploration revealed a significantly higher proportion of patients with invasive NABS infections had clindamycin-resistant cultures (80 [16.2%] of 492) compared with those who had invasive GAS infections (76 [11.4%] of 669, p = 0.02) which suggest higher clindamycin resistance among NABS in the US.[8] Outside the US, studies which have examined clindamycin resistance among NABS, compared with GAS and/or GBS have found higher rates of clindamycin among NABS compared with GAS.[97,108,109]

Intravenous Immunoglobulin

Polyspecific intravenous immunoglobulin (IVIG) has widely been used as adjunctive treatment of STSS to aid in the neutralization of superantigens and enhanced bacterial clearance by including the opsonization of GAS for phagocytosis.[110] Additional proposed mechanisms of actions include inhibition of T cell proliferation, and inhibition of inflammatory cytokines such as TNF-alpha and interleukin 6.[111]

Prior data from observational and statistically underpowered prospective trials have been inconclusive and mixed on the efficacy of IVIG for streptococcal TSS. A prospective study of patients with invasive GAS infection (with or without STSS) who were admitted to the intensive care units at 4 tertiary hospitals (n = 62) in Canada concluded that IVIG had no effect on mortality.[112] While a small (n = 21) observational study in Canada, a comparative observational studies of prospectively identified cases of GAS STTS from Sweden (N = 67; 27% with NF)[54] and invasive GAS disease from Australia (N = 84; 79% with shock and 35% with NF)[32] found the administration of IVIG in the clindamycin-treated subgroup was associated with lower mortality rates. However, these studies were likely underpowered and mortality associations did not reach statistical significance in any of the studies.[113] Moreover, as IVIG is often coadministered with clindamycin, this has complicated studying the impact of IVIG independent of clindamycin.[32,54,114] The only randomized trial of IVIG in STSS was prematurely terminated due to low enrollment, but a favorable, nonsignificant effect was observed.[115] These studies were included in a 2018 meta-analysis of IVIG administration in clindamycin-treated patients which found a significant mortality reduction on pooled analysis (risk ratio: 0.46; 95% confidence interval, 0.26–0.83; p = 0.01).[113] A large (n = 322) propensity-matched analysis of administrative data from 121 US centers evaluating the role of adjunctive IVIG in NSTI with shock[116] observed no clinical benefit to IVIG therapy, regardless of timing of treatment and specific subgroup analysis for GAS, and/or clindamycin recipients and did not identify a subgroup for which IVIG significantly improved outcomes.[116] The study also found that IVIG use in NSTI associated shock was infrequent (4%) and highly variable across centers in the US, highlighting potential barriers to usage and access. Addition of the 49 patients with specific coding for GAS and clindamycin from this study to the abovementioned meta-analysis had negligible effects on the overall results of the meta-analysis.[113] In a more recent prospectively enrolled cohort of GAS and NABS NSTI (n = 192), lack of IVIG administration was found to be independently associated with mortality.[95] A randomized trial assessing the effect of IVIG compared with placebo on self-reported physical function and mortality (as a secondary outcome) among ICU admitted patients with NSTI of all microbiological etiologies found no difference in mortality between IVIG and placebo groups.[117] Possibly, the lack of effect in the latter study, as well as in the study by Kadri and colleagues[116] was the consequence of not restricting these studies to BHS NSTIs.

While the results remain mixed, given the high rate of mortality and the potential benefit of IVIG, it should be considered as adjunctive therapy for STSS cases in centers where it is available. We recommend an initial dose of 1 g/kg intravenously on day 1 followed by 0.5 g/kg intravenously on days 2 and 3.[115] However, providers should be aware there are considerable batch-to-batch variations or variations between manufacturers of IVIG in terms of the quantity of neutralizing antibodies, further complicating the interpretation of the literature.[114]

Hyperbaric Oxygen

Hyperbaric oxygen has been proposed as adjunctive therapy to surgical debridement for NSTI.[58] Hyperbaric oxygen therapy uses delivery of 100% oxygen at a pressure of 2–3 absolute atmospheric pressure. Its use is motivated by the fact that oxygen delivery at these parameters achieves a much higher concentration of dissolved oxygen in the blood. By increasing plasma dissolved oxygen concentration, hyperbaric oxygen is believed to potentially enhance oxygen delivery to hypoxic tissues surrounding areas of necrosis, directly killing anaerobic bacteria and improving leukocyte activity.[118]

However, despite theoretical benefits, no prospective literature exists to support its use as adjuvant therapy. Given mixed results from a series of observational studies society guidelines do not recommend its routine use.[55,58] Moreover, access to hyperbaric oxygen might be limited depending on the area of practice and patients might be too unstable to tolerate transfer. While it may be beneficial, we believe that administration (or transfer for administration) should not interfere with the standard treatment and in particular ICU level supportive care and prompt surgical evaluation and intervention[73]

AB103 (Reltecimod)

AB103 (previously p2TA) is a novel synthetic CD28 mimetic octapeptide that selectively inhibits the direct binding of superantigen exotoxins to the CD28 costimulatory receptor on T-helper 1 lymphocytes.[119] Preclinical studies demonstrated that AB103 and related superantigen mimetic peptides are associated with improved survival, attenuation of plasma cytokine levels and decreased necrosis. In a GAS murine model of NSTI (thigh infection with *S pyogenes*), 100% survival was observed with decreased bacterial burden at the site of infection.[120,121]

A phase 2a multicenter, randomized, double-blinded, placebo-controlled trial of adjuvant AB103 vs placebo established safety of the drug. While positive trends across several important clinical endpoints were seen it was not adequately powered to assess efficacy.[119] A subsequent phase 3 trial assessed the efficacy and safety of Reltecimod (0.5 mg/kg) versus placebo in patients with NSTI. A previously validated composite endpoint was used which included 28-day mortality, number of debridements, amputations after the first operation, and the resolution of organ dysfunction within the first two weeks based on the change in the modified Sequential Organ Failure Assessment Score (which excluded the hepatic component) was utilized.[122] Whereas it did not reach statistical significance for the primary composite endpoint in the modified intention to treat population, the per-protocol population did show evidence of significant benefit, which was driven by the definitive improvement in the resolution of organ dysfunction.[123] Larger trials that can examine both the timing and dose of AB103 with clinically relevant endpoints will determine whether this agent will enter the mainstream armamentarium for NSTI.[124]

Prevention of Invasive β-hemolytic Streptococcal Disease

Chemoprophylaxis

The optimal approach and effectiveness of postexposure prophylaxis for the prevention of secondary invasive GAS infections remains uncertain. Current CDC guidance does not recommend routine prophylaxis for household contacts but provides a permissive recommendation to offer chemoprophylaxis to household members aged ≥65 years or with other risk factors for invasive GAS infection.[33,34] The CDC recommended regimen is intramuscular benzathine penicillin and rifampin.[34] Oral penicillin or an oral cephalosporin likely represents an adequate oral option and is recommended by Canadian and United Kingdom health authorities.[33,34,125,126] For those with a β-lactam allergy which precludes the use of β-lactams, alternatives include clindamycin or azithromycin after the confirmation of susceptibility of the index patient isolate.[34] The CDC does not recommend routine use of culture to identify household contacts who are colonized.[34] They recommend that health care providers routinely inform household contacts of persons with invasive GAS disease about risk of developing GAS diseases and emphasize the importance of seeking medical attention if contacts develop compatible symptoms.[34]

Both the World Health Organization and CDC recommend intrapartum antibiotic prophylaxis administered intravenously for women with GBS colonization or other select risk factors for the prevention of neonatal GBS sepsis.[65,127] Drug of choice for prophylaxis is penicillin G or ampicillin. For patients with allergies that preclude the use of penicillin or ampicillin, alternative options include cefazolin (if the patient is low risk for anaphylaxis), clindamycin if susceptibility results are available, or vancomycin. The effectiveness of alternative agents in the prevention of early-onset GBS has not been evaluated. In particular, vancomycin's pharmacokinetic profile is not favorable for achieving bactericidal concentrations in the amniotic fluid.[128]

Vaccines

GAS vaccine development has been ongoing since the 1940's.[129] Candidates for a GAS vaccine have mainly focused on the M protein as it is highly immunogenic and responsible for eliciting strain-specific immunity to GAS.[11] Current candidates include N-terminal M protein peptides configured in recombinant multivalent proteins, conserved M epitopes from the central region of the M protein, cell wall carbohydrate, and multiple secreted and cell surface proteins,[129] However, lack of relevant animal models, high genetic diversity of antigen targets,[130] safety concerns due to cross-reactive immune responses to human tissues and lack of consensus on clinical endpoints for the establishment of proof of concept have created major impediments to progress in GAS vaccine development to date.[129,131] Most current vaccine candidates remain in the preclinical investigation phase, with only 2 candidates actively under evaluation in human trials.[132,133] Previously, a 26-valent vaccine candidate was shown to be safe, well tolerated and immunogenic in phase I and II trials; however, the development of this candidate was halted for commercial reasons.[134]

Similarly, to GAS, there are no commercially available GBS vaccines. Given the low uptake globally of intrapartum antibiotic prophylaxis, immunization of pregnant women with a GBS vaccine represents a promising strategy to protect newborns through transplacental antibody transfer and reducing vaginal GBS colonization.[135] The GBS capsular polysaccharide represents the main vaccine candidate target, in addition to proteins such as alpha-C-protein (bca), C alpha-like proteins 2 and 3 (alp2 and alp3), epsilon/Alp1, Rib (rib), and beta-C-protein (bac) which are embedded in the GBS bacterial surface.[136] Currently, capsular polysaccharide conjugate vaccines and protein-based GBS vaccines are under development. The most advanced vaccine candidates are hexavalent vaccines (targeting serotypes Ia, Ib, II, III, IV, and V) which are now in phase II trials and a recombinant protein vaccine has been shown to be immunogenic and well tolerated in healthy nonpregnant women and is being further evaluated in a phase 2 trials.[137,138]

Future Directions

Given the large global disease burden by BHS continued efforts to update and improve global estimates of disease burden globally are required.[139] With improvements in accessibility, turnaround time, cost, and bioinformatic tools integration of whole genome sequencing as part of routine surveillance has the ability to allow for more in-depth characterization of invasive strains and allow for the identification of putative antimicrobial resistance determinants and virulence factors.[42,105,107,140] This is in particular needed for NABS which have been neglected in comparison to other BHS species. Continued broad efforts toward vaccine development to increase the number of pipeline vaccine candidates, these include antigen discovery efforts, determination of immunological surrogates/correlates of protection, and support of preclinical and clinical vaccine trials[131] Pathogen-specific comparative therapeutic trials have been hampered by the ability to enroll adequate numbers.[115] Global consortiums which can perform novel adaptive platform trial methodologies at large scale (such as Staphylococcus aureus Network Adaptive Platform Trial[141]) have the ability to overcome such issues and address lingering questions regarding adjunctive therapies such as clindamycin, linezolid, and IVIG. Finally continued investigation and development of novel agents, such as microbial therapeutics or novel immunomodulatory agents which will aid in bypassing potential emerging bacterial resistance is required.

SUMMARY

Invasive BHS streptococcal disease results in diverse clinical manifestations and can carry a high degree of morbidity and mortality. Overall, these infections are becoming more frequent because of an aging population and the increasing burden of chronic illness. Management is multi-disciplinary and should include intensivists, infectious diseases specialists, surgeons, and clinical microbiologists. Resuscitation, source control, and prompt antibiotic administration are the cornerstone of management. Patients with suspected NSTI require early and aggressive surgical intervention. β-lactam agents remain the drugs of choice as isolates are uniformly susceptible. Among adjunctive therapies, clindamycin (in clindamycin susceptible GAS strains) is recommended and IVIG could be considered.

CLINICS CARE POINTS

- Invasive b-hemolytic streptococci (BHS) are a leading cause of invasive bacterial disease worldwide and can present with a wide array of clinical syndromes.

- Among all the invasive BHS clinical syndromes, two manifestations are of particular importance to intensive care unit providers due to the high degree of mortality they carry: Necrotizing skin and tissue infection (NSTI) and streptococcal toxic shock syndrome (STSS).

- NSTI refers to an aggressive subcutaneous tissue infection which tracks along the superficial fascia and compromises all the tissues between the skin and under laying muscle. STSS is characterized by an acute, progressive illness associated with fever, rapid-onset hypotension, and accelerated multi-system failure in the presence of a positive BHS culture.

- Diagnosis of invasive BHS streptococcal infection relies on identification of the organism in a culture from a normally sterile site in the setting of a compatible clinical syndrome. While, culture data and imaging such as computed tomography or magnetic resonance imaging may be helpful in confirmation of NSTI to assess the source of invasive BHS infections clinical judgment is the most important element in diagnosis and imaging should not delay preemptive supportive, antibiotic and surgical management of these cases.

- Early recognition of invasive BHS clinical syndromes and rapid resuscitation, antibiotic therapy and source control are crucial to the management IBHS. In the early stages of illness, the causative organism will be unknown, and the same basic strategy should be applied as to any case of bacterial sepsis and managed as per surviving sepsis guidelines.

- Patients with a suspected diagnosis of NSTI require prompt and aggressive surgical exploration and will likely need multiple scheduled explorations and repeat debridement. Delays in primary and repeat debridement has been associated with poor outcomes.
- β-lactam agents remain the drugs of choice as isolates are uniformly susceptible. Among adjunctive therapies, clindamycin is recommended in clindamycin susceptible GAS strains. Clinicians should be aware that clindamycin resistance is rising among BHS strains. IVIG could be considered for STSS when available.

DISCLOSURE

The authors have no disclosures.

REFERENCES

1. Procop GW, Church DL, Hall GS, et al. Gram-Positive Cocci Part II: Streptococci, Enterococci, and the "Streptococcus-Like" Bacteria. Koneman's Color Atlas and Textbook of Diagnostic Microbiology. Seventh ed: Wolters Kluwer.
2. Facklam R. What happened to the streptococci: overview of taxonomic and nomenclature changes. Clin Microbiol Rev 2002;15(4):613–30.
3. Lancefield RC. A SEROLOGICAL DIFFERENTIATION OF HUMAN AND OTHER GROUPS OF HEMOLYTIC STREPTOCOCCI. J Exp Med 1933;57(4):571–95.
4. Brown JH. The use of blood agar for the study of streptococci. New York, N.Y.: The Rockefeller Institute for Medical Research; 1919.
5. Musher DM. The Naming of Strep, with Apologies to T. S. Eliot. Clinical Infectious Diseases 2009;49(12):1959–60.
6. Edwards MS, Baker CJ. Streptococcus agalactiae. In: Bennet John E, Dolin Raphael, Blaser MJ, editors. Mandell, Douglas, and Bennett's Principle and Practice of Infectious Diseases. 2020.
7. Broyles LN, Van Beneden C, Beall B, et al. Population-Based Study of Invasive Disease Due to β-Hemolytic Streptococci of Groups Other than A and B. Clinical Infectious Diseases 2009;48(6):706–12.
8. Babiker A, Li X, Lai YL, et al. Effectiveness of adjunctive clindamycin in β-lactam antibiotic-treated patients with invasive β-haemolytic streptococcal infections in US hospitals: a retrospective multicentre cohort study. The Lancet Infectious diseases 2020.
9. Ruoff KL. Streptococcus anginosus ("Streptococcus milleri"): the unrecognized pathogen. Clin Microbiol Rev 1988;1(1):102–8.
10. Decker John P, Ruoff Kathryn L. Classification of Streptocci. In: Mandell D, Bennetts, editors. Principles and Practice of Infectious Diseases. Elsevier; 2020.
11. Walker MJ, Barnett TC, McArthur JD, et al. Disease manifestations and pathogenic mechanisms of Group A Streptococcus. Clin Microbiol Rev 2014;27(2): 264–301.
12. Bryant AE, Stevens DL. Streptococcus pyogenes. In: Bennet JE, Dolin R, Blaser MJ, editors. Mandell, Douglas, and Bennett's Principle and Practice of Infectious Diseases. 2020.
13. Lindahl G, Stålhammar-Carlemalm M, Areschoug T. Surface proteins of Streptococcus agalactiae and related proteins in other bacterial pathogens. Clin Microbiol Rev 2005;18(1):102–27.
14. Koskiniemi S, Sellin M, Norgren M. Identification of two genes, cpsX and cpsY, with putative regulatory function on capsule expression in group B streptococci. FEMS Immunol Med Microbiol 1998;21(2):159–68.

15. Brandt CM, Spellerberg B. Human infections due to Streptococcus dysgalactiae subspecies equisimilis. Clinical infectious diseases : an official publication of the Infectious Diseases Society of America 2009;49(5):766–72.

16. Davies MR, McMillan DJ, Beiko RG, et al. Virulence Profiling of Streptococcus dysgalactiae Subspecies equisimilis Isolated from Infected Humans Reveals 2 Distinct Genetic Lineages That Do Not Segregate with Their Phenotypes or Propensity to Cause Diseases. Clinical Infectious Diseases 2007;44(11):1442–54.

17. Hashikawa S, Iinuma Y, Furushita M, et al. Characterization of group C and G streptococcal strains that cause streptococcal toxic shock syndrome. Journal of clinical microbiology 2004;42(1):186–92.

18. Lother SA, Demczuk W, Martin I, et al. Clonal Clusters and Virulence Factors of Group C and G Streptococcus Causing Severe Infections, Manitoba, Canada, 2012-2014. Emerging infectious diseases 2017;23(7):1079–88.

19. Ekelund K, Skinhøj P, Madsen J, Konradsen HB. Invasive group A, B, C and G streptococcal infections in Denmark 1999–2002: epidemiological and clinical aspects. Clinical Microbiology and Infection 2005;11(7):569–76.

20. Turner CE, Bubba L, Efstratiou A. Pathogenicity Factors in Group C and G Streptococci. Microbiol Spectr 2019;7(3).

21. Parks T, Barrett L, Jones N. Invasive streptococcal disease: a review for clinicians. Br Med Bull 2015;115(1):77–89.

22. Centers for Disease Control and Prevention. Group A Streptococcal (GAS) Disease. 2018. https://www.cdc.gov/groupastrep/surveillance.html (accessed Feb 7th 2022).

23. Kobayashi L, Konstantinidis A, Shackelford S, et al. Necrotizing soft tissue infections: delayed surgical treatment is associated with increased number of surgical debridements and morbidity. J Trauma 2011;71(5):1400–5.

24. Rantala S, Vuopio-Varkila J, Vuento R, Huhtala H, Syrjänen J. Clinical presentations and epidemiology of beta-haemolytic streptococcal bacteraemia: a population-based study. Clin Microbiol Infect 2009;15(3):286–8.

25. Lamagni TL, Neal S, Keshishian C, et al. Severe Streptococcus pyogenes infections, United Kingdom, 2003-2004. Emerging infectious diseases 2008;14(2): 202–9.

26. Stevens DL. Invasive group A streptococcus infections. Clinical infectious diseases : an official publication of the Infectious Diseases Society of America 1992;14(1):2–11.

27. Steer AC, Lamagni T, Curtis N, Carapetis JR. Invasive group a streptococcal disease: epidemiology, pathogenesis and management. Drugs 2012;72(9): 1213–27.

28. Tasher D, Stein M, Simões EA, Shohat T, Bromberg M, Somekh E. Invasive bacterial infections in relation to influenza outbreaks, 2006-2010. Clinical infectious diseases : an official publication of the Infectious Diseases Society of America 2011;53(12):1199–207.

29. Lappin E, Ferguson AJ. Gram-positive toxic shock syndromes. The Lancet Infectious Diseases 2009;9(5):281–90.

30. Sablier F, Slaouti T, Drèze PA, et al. Nosocomial transmission of necrotising fasciitis. Lancet (London, England) 2010;375(9719):1052.

31. Lamagni TL, Oliver I, Stuart JM. Global Assessment of Invasive Group A Streptococcus Infection Risk in Household Contacts. Clinical Infectious Diseases 2014;60(1):166–7.

32. Carapetis JR, Jacoby P, Carville K, Ang SJ, Curtis N, Andrews R. Effectiveness of clindamycin and intravenous immunoglobulin, and risk of disease in contacts,

in invasive group a streptococcal infections. Clinical infectious diseases : an official publication of the Infectious Diseases Society of America 2014;59(3): 358–65.

33. Adebanjo T, Apostol M, Alden N, et al. Evaluating Household Transmission of Invasive Group A Streptococcus Disease in the United States Using Population-based Surveillance Data. Clinical infectious diseases : an official publication of the Infectious Diseases Society of America 2020;70(7):1478–81, 2013-2016.

34. Prevention of Invasive Group A Streptococcal Infections Workshop Partcipants. Prevention of invasive group a streptococcal disease among household contacts of case patients and among postpartum and postsurgical patients: recommendations from the Centers for Disease Control and Prevention. Clinical infectious diseases : an official publication of the Infectious Diseases Society of America 2002;35(8):950–9.

35. Robinson KA, Rothrock G, Phan Q, et al. Risk for severe group A streptococcal disease among patients' household contacts. Emerging infectious diseases 2003;9(4):443–7.

36. Raymond J, Schlegel L, Garnier F, Bouvet A. Molecular characterization of Streptococcus pyogenes isolates to investigate an outbreak of puerperal sepsis. Infection control and hospital epidemiology 2005;26(5):455–61.

37. Turner CE, Dryden M, Holden MT, et al. Molecular analysis of an outbreak of lethal postpartum sepsis caused by Streptococcus pyogenes. Journal of clinical microbiology 2013;51(7):2089–95.

38. Daneman N, McGeer A, Low DE, et al. Hospital-Acquired Invasive Group A Streptococcal Infections in Ontario, Canada, 1992–2000. Clinical Infectious Diseases 2005;41(3):334–42.

39. Vannice K, Ricaldi J, Nanduri S, et al. Streptococcus pyogenes pbp2x Mutation Confers Reduced Susceptibility to β-lactam antibiotics. Clinical Infectious Diseases 2019.

40. Centers for Disease Control and Prevention. Group B Strep (GBS) 2020. https://www.cdc.gov/groupbstrep/clinicians/index.html (accessed Feb 7th 2022).

41. Francois Watkins LK, McGee L, Schrag SJ, et al. Epidemiology of Invasive Group B Streptococcal Infections Among Nonpregnant Adults in the United States, 2008-2016. JAMA Intern Med 2019;179(4):479–88.

42. Centers for Disease Control and Prevention. ABCs Bact Facts interactive data dashboard: group B Streptococcus (2019). 2021. https://www-cdc-gov/abcs/bact-facts-interactive-dashboard.html (accessed April 6th 2022).

43. Jump RLP, Wilson BM, Baechle D, et al. Risk Factors and Mortality Rates Associated With Invasive Group B Streptococcus Infections Among Patients in the US Veterans Health Administration. JAMA Netw Open 2019;2(12):e1918324.

44. Jackson LA, Hilsdon R, Farley MM, et al. Risk factors for group B streptococcal disease in adults. Ann Intern Med 1995;123(6):415–20.

45. Harris P, Siew DA, Proud M, Buettner P, Norton R. Bacteraemia caused by beta-haemolytic streptococci in North Queensland: changing trends over a 14-year period. Clin Microbiol Infect 2011;17(8):1216–22.

46. Cohen-Poradosu R, Jaffe J, Lavi D, et al. Group G streptococcal bacteremia in Jerusalem. Emerging infectious diseases 2004;10(8):1455–60.

47. Rantala S. Streptococcus dysgalactiae subsp. equisimilis bacteremia: an emerging infection. European journal of clinical microbiology & infectious diseases : official publication of the European Society of Clinical Microbiology 2014;33(8):1303–10.

48. Cunha CB. Viridans Streptococci, Nutrionally Variant Streptococci, and Group C and G Streptococci. In: Bennet JE, Dolin R, Blaser MJ, editors. Mandell, Douglas, and Bennett's Principle and Practice of Infectious Diseases. 2020.

49. Centers for Disease Control and Prevention. Case definitions for infectious conditions under public health surveillance. Centers for Disease Control and Prevention. MMWR Recomm Rep 1997;46(Rr-10):1–55.

50. Nelson GE, Pondo T, Toews KA, et al. Epidemiology of Invasive Group A Streptococcal Infections in the United States, 2005-2012. Clinical infectious diseases : an official publication of the Infectious Diseases Society of America 2016;63(4):478–86.

51. Stevens DL, Tanner MH, Winship J, et al. Severe Group A Streptococcal Infections Associated with a Toxic Shock-like Syndrome and Scarlet Fever Toxin A. New England Journal of Medicine 1989;321(1):1–7.

52. Centers for Disease Control and Prevention. Streptococcal Toxic Shock Syndrome. 2020. https://www.cdc.gov/groupastrep/diseases-hcp/Streptococcal-Toxic-Shock-Syndrome.html (accessed April 6th 2022)

53. Couture-Cossette A, Carignan A, Mercier A, Desruisseaux C, Valiquette L, Pépin J. Secular trends in incidence of invasive beta-hemolytic streptococci and efficacy of adjunctive therapy in Quebec, Canada, 1996-2016. PloS one 2018;13(10):e0206289–.

54. Linner A, Darenberg J, Sjolin J, Henriques-Normark B, Norrby-Teglund A. Clinical efficacy of polyspecific intravenous immunoglobulin therapy in patients with streptococcal toxic shock syndrome: a comparative observational study. Clinical infectious diseases : an official publication of the Infectious Diseases Society of America 2014;59(6):851–7.

55. Stevens DL, Bisno AL, Chambers HF, et al. Executive Summary: Practice Guidelines for the Diagnosis and Management of Skin and Soft Tissue Infections: 2014 Update by the Infectious Diseases Society of America. Clinical Infectious Diseases 2014;59(2):147–59.

56. Wilson B. Necrotizing fasciitis. Am Surg 1952;18(4):416–31.

57. Johansson L, Thulin P, Low DE, Norrby-Teglund A. Getting under the skin: the immunopathogenesis of Streptococcus pyogenes deep tissue infections. Clinical infectious diseases : an official publication of the Infectious Diseases Society of America 2010;51(1):58–65.

58. Bonne SL, Kadri SS. Evaluation and Management of Necrotizing Soft Tissue Infections. Infect Dis Clin North Am 2017;31(3):497–511.

59. Alayed KA, Tan C, Daneman N. Red Flags for Necrotizing Fasciitis: A Case Control Study. Int J Infect Dis 2015;36:15–20.

60. Kaul R, McGeer A, Low DE, Green K, Schwartz B. Population-based surveillance for group A streptococcal necrotizing fasciitis: Clinical features, prognostic indicators, and microbiologic analysis of seventy-seven cases. Ontario Group A Streptococcal Study. Am J Med 1997;103(1):18–24.

61. Ward RG, Walsh MS. Necrotizing fasciitis: 10 years' experience in a district general hospital. Br J Surg 1991;78(4):488–9.

62. Centers for Disease Control and Prevention. Group A Streptococcal (GAS) Surveillance Report. 2019. https://www.cdc.gov/abcs/downloads/GAS_Surveillance_Report_2019.pdf (accessed Feb 7th 2022).

63. Stevens DL. Streptococcal toxic-shock syndrome: spectrum of disease, pathogenesis, and new concepts in treatment. Emerging infectious diseases 1995;1(3):69–78.

64. Breiman RF, Davis JP, Facklam RR, et al. Defining the Group A Streptococcal Toxic Shock Syndrome: Rationale and Consensus Definition. Jama 1993; 269(3):390–1.
65. Verani JR, McGee L, Schrag SJ. Prevention of perinatal group B streptococcal disease–revised guidelines from CDC, 2010. MMWR Recomm Rep 2010; 59(Rr-10):1–36.
66. Kittang BR, Bruun T, Langeland N, Mylvaganam H, Glambek M, Skrede S. Invasive group A, C and G streptococcal disease in western Norway: virulence gene profiles, clinical features and outcomes. Clin Microbiol Infect 2011;17(3): 358–64.
67. Woo PC, Fung AM, Lau SK, Wong SS, Yuen KY. Group G beta-hemolytic streptococcal bacteremia characterized by 16S ribosomal RNA gene sequencing. Journal of clinical microbiology 2001;39(9):3147–55.
68. Nybakken EJ, Oppegaard O, Gilhuus M, Jensen CS, Mylvaganam H. Identification of Streptococcus dysgalactiae using matrix-assisted laser desorption/ionization-time of flight mass spectrometry; refining the database for improved identification. Diagnostic Microbiology and Infectious Disease 2021;99(1): 115207.
69. Rosa-Fraile M, Spellerberg B. Reliable Detection of Group B Streptococcus in the Clinical Laboratory. Journal of clinical microbiology 2017;55(9):2590–8.
70. Stevens DL, Bryant AE. Necrotizing Soft-Tissue Infections. N Engl J Med 2017; 377(23):2253–65.
71. Wong CH, Khin LW, Heng KS, Tan KC, Low CO. The LRINEC (Laboratory Risk Indicator for Necrotizing Fasciitis) score: a tool for distinguishing necrotizing fasciitis from other soft tissue infections. Critical care medicine 2004;32(7): 1535–41.
72. Hansen MB, Rasmussen LS, Svensson M, et al. Association between cytokine response, the LRINEC score and outcome in patients with necrotising soft tissue infection: a multicentre, prospective study. Sci Rep 2017;7:42179.
73. Sartelli M, Guirao X, Hardcastle TC, et al. 2018 WSES/SIS-E consensus conference: recommendations for the management of skin and soft-tissue infections. World Journal of Emergency Surgery 2018;13(1):58.
74. Ramanan P, Bryson AL, Binnicker MJ, Pritt BS, Patel R. Syndromic Panel-Based Testing in Clinical Microbiology. Clin Microbiol Rev 2017;31(1). e00024–17.
75. Hanson KE, Couturier MR. Multiplexed Molecular Diagnostics for Respiratory, Gastrointestinal, and Central Nervous System Infections. Clinical infectious diseases : an official publication of the Infectious Diseases Society of America 2016;63(10):1361–7.
76. Rhodes A, Evans LE, Alhazzani W, et al. Surviving Sepsis Campaign: International Guidelines for Management of Sepsis and Septic Shock: 2016. Intensive care medicine 2017;43(3):304–77.
77. Kadri SS, Lai YL, Warner S, et al. Inappropriate empirical antibiotic therapy for bloodstream infections based on discordant in-vitro susceptibilities: a retrospective cohort analysis of prevalence, predictors, and mortality risk in US hospitals. The Lancet Infectious diseases 2021;21(2):241–51.
78. Kumar A, Roberts D, Wood KE, et al. Duration of hypotension before initiation of effective antimicrobial therapy is the critical determinant of survival in human septic shock. Critical care medicine 2006;34(6):1589–96.
79. Nawijn F, DPJ Smeeing, Houwert RM, Leenen LPH, Hietbrink F. Time is of the essence when treating necrotizing soft tissue infections: a systematic review and meta-analysis. World Journal of Emergency Surgery 2020;15(1):4.

80. Vincent JL, Rello J, Marshall J, et al. International study of the prevalence and outcomes of infection in intensive care units. Jama 2009;302(21):2323–9.

81. Mayr FB, Yende S, Angus DC. Epidemiology of severe sepsis. Virulence 2014; 5(1):4–11.

82. Bryant AE, Bayer CR, Aldape MJ, McIndoo E, Stevens DL. Emerging erythromycin and clindamycin resistance in group A streptococci: Efficacy of linezolid and tedizolid in experimental necrotizing infection. J Glob Antimicrob Resist 2020;22:601–7.

83. Oppegaard O, Skrede S, Mylvaganam H, Kittang BR. Emerging Threat of Antimicrobial Resistance in β-Hemolytic Streptococci. Front Microbiol 2020;11:797.

84. Hadeed GJ, Smith J, O'Keeffe T, et al. Early surgical intervention and its impact on patients presenting with necrotizing soft tissue infections: A single academic center experience. J Emerg Trauma Shock 2016;9(1):22–7.

85. V K, Hiremath BV, V A I. Necrotising soft tissue infection-risk factors for mortality. J Clin Diagn Res 2013; 7(8): 1662-1665.

86. Boyer A, Vargas F, Coste F, et al. Influence of surgical treatment timing on mortality from necrotizing soft tissue infections requiring intensive care management. Intensive care medicine 2009;35(5):847–53.

87. Hakkarainen TW, Kopari NM, Pham TN, Evans HL. Necrotizing soft tissue infections: review and current concepts in treatment, systems of care, and outcomes. Curr Probl Surg 2014;51(8):344–62.

88. Okoye O, Talving P, Lam L, et al. Timing of Redébridement after Initial Source Control Impacts Survival in Necrotizing Soft Tissue Infection. The American Surgeon 2013;79(10):1081–5.

89. Andreoni F, Zurcher C, Tarnutzer A, et al. Clindamycin Affects Group A Streptococcus Virulence Factors and Improves Clinical Outcome. The Journal of infectious diseases 2017;215(2):269–77.

90. Eagle H. Experimental approach to the problem of treatment failure with penicillin. I. Group A streptococcal infection in mice. Am J Med 1952;13(4):389–99.

91. Stevens DL, Gibbons AE, Bergstrom R, Winn V. The Eagle effect revisited: efficacy of clindamycin, erythromycin, and penicillin in the treatment of streptococcal myositis. The Journal of infectious diseases 1988;158(1):23–8.

92. Zimbelman J, Palmer A, Todd J. Improved outcome of clindamycin compared with beta-lactam antibiotic treatment for invasive Streptococcus pyogenes infection. The Pediatric infectious disease journal 1999;18(12):1096–100.

93. Mulla ZD, Leaverton PE, Wiersma ST. Invasive group A streptococcal infections in Florida. Southern medical journal 2003;96(10):968–73.

94. Hamada S, Nakajima M, Kaszynski RH, et al. Association between adjunct clindamycin and in-hospital mortality in patients with necrotizing soft tissue infection due to group A Streptococcus: a nationwide cohort study. European Journal of Clinical Microbiology & Infectious Diseases 2022;41(2):263–70.

95. Bruun T, Rath E, Madsen MB, et al. Risk Factors and Predictors of Mortality in Streptococcal Necrotizing Soft-tissue Infections: A Multicenter Prospective Study. Clinical infectious diseases : an official publication of the Infectious Diseases Society of America 2021;72(2):293–300.

96. Hamada S, Nakajima M, Kaszynski RH, et al. In-hospital mortality among patients with invasive non-group A β-hemolytic Streptococcus treated with clindamycin combination therapy: a nationwide cohort study. Acute medicine & surgery 2021;8(1):e634–.

97. Merino Díaz L, Torres Sánchez MJ, Aznar Martín J. Prevalence and mechanisms of erythromycin and clindamycin resistance in clinical isolates of β-haemolytic

streptococci of Lancefield groups A, B, C and G in Seville, Spain. Clinical Microbiology and Infection 2008;14(1):85–7.

98. Compain F, Hays C, Touak G, et al. Molecular characterization of Streptococcus agalactiae isolates harboring small erm(T)-carrying plasmids. Antimicrobial agents and chemotherapy 2014;58(11):6928–30.

99. Haenni M, Lupo A, Madec JY. Antimicrobial Resistance in Streptococcus spp. Microbiol Spectr 2018;6(2).

100. Fay K, Onukwube J, Chochua S, et al. Patterns of Antibiotic Nonsusceptibility Among Invasive Group A Streptococcus Infections—United States, 2006–2017. Clinical Infectious Diseases 2021;73(11):1957–64.

101. Nori P, Nadeem N, Saraiya N, Szymczak W, Boland-Reardon C, Kahn M. Beta-hemolytic group a streptococcal orthopaedic infections: Our institutional experience and review of the literature. J Orthop 2020;21:150–4.

102. Coyle EA, Cha R, Rybak MJ. Influences of linezolid, penicillin, and clindamycin, alone and in combination, on streptococcal pyrogenic exotoxin a release. Antimicrobial agents and chemotherapy 2003;47(5):1752–5.

103. Rac H, Bojikian KD, Lucar J, Barber KE. Successful Treatment of Necrotizing Fasciitis and Streptococcal Toxic Shock Syndrome with the Addition of Linezolid. Case Rep Infect Dis 2017;2017:5720708.

104. Grebe T, Hakenbeck R. Penicillin-binding proteins 2b and 2x of Streptococcus pneumoniae are primary resistance determinants for different classes of beta-lactam antibiotics. Antimicrobial agents and chemotherapy 1996;40(4):829–34.

105. Musser JM, Beres SB, Zhu L, et al. Reduced In Vitro Susceptibility of Streptococcus pyogenes to β-Lactam Antibiotics Associated with Mutations in the pbp2x Gene Is Geographically Widespread. Journal of clinical microbiology 2020;58(4).

106. Fuursted K, Stegger M, Hoffmann S, et al. Description and characterization of a penicillin-resistant Streptococcus dysgalactiae subsp. equisimilis clone isolated from blood in three epidemiologically linked patients. The Journal of antimicrobial chemotherapy 2016;71(12):3376–80.

107. Metcalf BJ, Chochua S, Gertz RE Jr, et al. Short-read whole genome sequencing for determination of antimicrobial resistance mechanisms and capsular serotypes of current invasive Streptococcus agalactiae recovered in the USA. Clin Microbiol Infect 2017;23(8):574, e7-.e14.

108. Buter CC, Mouton JW, Klaassen CH, et al. Prevalence and molecular mechanism of macrolide resistance in beta-haemolytic streptococci in The Netherlands. Int J Antimicrob Agents 2010;35(6):590–2.

109. Gajdács M, Ábrók M, Lázár A, Burián K. Beta-Haemolytic Group A, C and G Streptococcal Infections in Southern Hungary: A 10-Year Population-Based Retrospective Survey (2008-2017) and a Review of the Literature. Infect Drug Resist 2020;13:4739–49.

110. Sriskandan S, Ferguson M, Elliot V, Faulkner L, Cohen J. Human intravenous immunoglobulin for experimental streptococcal toxic shock: bacterial clearance and modulation of inflammation. The Journal of antimicrobial chemotherapy 2006;58(1):117–24.

111. Norrby-teglund A, Ihendyane N, Darenberg J. Intravenous Immunoglobulin Adjunctive Therapy in Sepsis, with Special Emphasis on Severe Invasive Group A Streptococcal Infections. Scandinavian Journal of Infectious Diseases 2003;35(9):683–9.

112. Mehta S, McGeer A, Low DE, et al. Morbidity and mortality of patients with invasive group A streptococcal infections admitted to the ICU. Chest 2006;130(6): 1679–86.

113. Parks T, Wilson C, Sriskandan S, Curtis N, Norrby-Teglund A. Polyspecific Intravenous Immunoglobulin in Clindamycin-treated Patients With Streptococcal Toxic Shock Syndrome: A Systematic Review and Meta-analysis. Clinical Infectious Diseases 2018;67(9):1434–6.

114. Kaul R, McGeer A, Norrby-Teglund A, et al. Intravenous immunoglobulin therapy for streptococcal toxic shock syndrome–a comparative observational study. The Canadian Streptococcal Study Group. Clinical infectious diseases : an official publication of the Infectious Diseases Society of America 1999;28(4):800–7.

115. Darenberg J, Ihendyane N, Sjölin J, et al. Intravenous immunoglobulin G therapy in streptococcal toxic shock syndrome: a European randomized, double-blind, placebo-controlled trial. Clinical infectious diseases : an official publication of the Infectious Diseases Society of America 2003;37(3):333–40.

116. Kadri SS, Swihart BJ, Bonne SL, et al. Impact of Intravenous Immunoglobulin on Survival in Necrotizing Fasciitis With Vasopressor-Dependent Shock: A Propensity Score-Matched Analysis From 130 US Hospitals. Clinical infectious diseases : an official publication of the Infectious Diseases Society of America 2017;64(7):877–85.

117. Madsen MB, Hjortrup PB, Hansen MB, et al. Immunoglobulin G for patients with necrotising soft tissue infection (INSTINCT): a randomised, blinded, placebo-controlled trial. Intensive care medicine 2017;43(11):1585–93.

118. Jallali N, Withey S, Butler PE. Hyperbaric oxygen as adjuvant therapy in the management of necrotizing fasciitis. Am J Surg 2005;189(4):462–6.

119. Bulger EM, Maier RV, Sperry J, et al. A Novel Drug for Treatment of Necrotizing Soft-Tissue Infections: A Randomized Clinical Trial. JAMA Surgery 2014;149(6): 528–36.

120. Arad G, Levy R, Nasie I, et al. Binding of superantigen toxins into the CD28 homodimer interface is essential for induction of cytokine genes that mediate lethal shock. PLoS Biol 2011;9(9):e1001149.

121. Ramachandran G, Tulapurkar ME, Harris KM, et al. A peptide antagonist of CD28 signaling attenuates toxic shock and necrotizing soft-tissue infection induced by Streptococcus pyogenes. The Journal of infectious diseases 2013;207(12):1869–77.

122. Bulger EM, May A, Dankner W, Maislin G, Robinson B, Shirvan A. Validation of a clinical trial composite endpoint for patients with necrotizing soft tissue infections. J Trauma Acute Care Surg 2017;83(4):622–7.

123. Bulger EM, May AK, Robinson BRH, et al. A Novel Immune Modulator for Patients With Necrotizing Soft Tissue Infections (NSTI): Results of a Multicenter, Phase 3 Randomized Controlled Trial of Reltecimod (AB 103). Ann Surg 2020; 272(3):469–78.

124. Nathens AB. Commentary on "Results of a Multicenter, Phase 3 Randomized Controlled Trial of Reltecimod. Ann Surg 2020;272(3):479–80.

125. Health Protection Agency; Group A Streptococcus Working Group. Interim UK guidelines for management of close community contacts of invasive group A streptococcal disease. Commun Dis Public Health 2004;7(4):354–61.

126. Allen U, Moore D. Invasive group A streptococcal disease: Management and chemoprophylaxis. Paediatr Child Health 2010;15(5):295–302.

127. World Health Organization. WHO recommendations for prevention and treatment of maternal peripartum infections 2015. Geneva, Switzerland.

128. Onwuchuruba CN, Towers CV, Howard BC, Hennessy MD, Wolfe L, Brown MS. Transplacental passage of vancomycin from mother to neonate. Am J Obstet Gynecol 2014;210(4):352, e1-.e4.

129. Dale JB, Walker MJ. Update on group A streptococcal vaccine development. Current opinion in infectious diseases 2020;33(3):244–50.

130. Davies MR, McIntyre L, Mutreja A, et al. Atlas of group A streptococcal vaccine candidates compiled using large-scale comparative genomics. Nat Genet 2019;51(6):1035–43.

131. Vekemans J, Gouvea-Reis F, Kim JH, et al. The Path to Group A Streptococcus Vaccines: World Health Organization Research and Development Technology Roadmap and Preferred Product Characteristics. Clinical Infectious Diseases 2019;69(5):877–83.

132. Sekuloski S, Batzloff MR, Griffin P, et al. Evaluation of safety and immunogenicity of a group A streptococcus vaccine candidate (MJ8VAX) in a randomized clinical trial. PLoS One 2018;13(7):e0198658.

133. Pastural É, McNeil SA, MacKinnon-Cameron D, et al. Safety and immunogenicity of a 30-valent M protein-based group a streptococcal vaccine in healthy adult volunteers: A randomized, controlled phase I study. Vaccine 2020;38(6): 1384–92.

134. McNeil SA, Halperin SA, Langley JM, et al. A double-blind, randomized phase II trial of the safety and immunogenicity of 26-valent group A streptococcus vaccine in healthy adults. International Congress Series 2006;1289:303–6.

135. Kobayashi M, Schrag SJ, Alderson MR, et al. WHO consultation on group B Streptococcus vaccine development: Report from a meeting held on 27-28 April 2016. Vaccine 2019;37(50):7307–14.

136. Carreras-Abad C, Ramkhelawon L, Heath PT, Le Doare K. A Vaccine Against Group B Streptococcus: Recent Advances. Infect Drug Resist 2020;13: 1263–72.

137. Buurman ET, Timofeyeva Y, Gu J, et al. A Novel Hexavalent Capsular Polysaccharide Conjugate Vaccine (GBS6) for the Prevention of Neonatal Group B Streptococcal Infections by Maternal Immunization. The Journal of infectious diseases 2019;220(1):105–15.

138. Fischer P, Pawlowski A, Cao D, et al. Safety and immunogenicity of a prototype recombinant alpha-like protein subunit vaccine (GBS-NN) against Group B Streptococcus in a randomised placebo-controlled double-blind phase 1 trial in healthy adult women. Vaccine 2021;39(32):4489–99.

139. Carapetis JR, Steer AC, Mulholland EK, Weber M. The global burden of group A streptococcal diseases. The Lancet Infectious diseases 2005;5(11):685–94.

140. Babiker A. mSphere of Influence: Whole-Genome Sequencing, a Vital Tool for the Interruption of Nosocomial Transmission. mSphere 2021;6(2). e00230–21.

141. Campbell AJ, Dotel R, Braddick M, et al. Clindamycin adjunctive therapy for severe Staphylococcus aureus treatment evaluation (CASSETTE)-an open-labelled pilot randomized controlled trial. JAC Antimicrob Resist 2022;4(1): dlac014.

Severe *Clostridioides difficile* Infection in the Intensive Care Unit—Medical and Surgical Management

Ramzy Husam Rimawi, MD[a],*, Stephanie Busby, MD[b],
Wendy Ricketts Greene, MD, FCCM[c]

KEYWORDS

- *Clostridioides difficile* • Colitis • Intensive care unit • Sepsis

KEY POINTS

- *Clostridioides difficile* guidelines have recently been updated with new medical and surgical management recommendations.
- Fidaxomicin is now the suggested treatment of initial and recurrent *C difficile* infections.
- *C difficile* colitis remains a major cause of morbidity and mortality in the intensive care unit.
- Patients with *C difficile* infections refractory to medical management should have urgent surgical evaluations.

MEDICAL MANAGEMENT

Clostridioides difficile infection (CDI) occurs in approximately 4% of intensive care unit (ICU) patients and causes fulminant colitis, prolonged hospitalization, significant morbidity, and death in nearly 60% of infected patients.[1,2] The Infectious Diseases Society of America (IDSA) and Society for Healthcare Epidemiology of America (SHEA) have recently changed their treatment recommendations. In this article, the authors review the latest CDI medical and surgical recommendations in the adult patients in the ICU.[3]

Whether CDI is confirmed or suspected, appropriate precautions should be initiated to prevent the transmission of bacterial spores. No single infection precaution method

[a] Department of Medicine, Division of Pulmonary, Sleep, Allergy, and Critical Care Medicine, Emory University School of Medicine, 550 Peachtree Street NorthWest, Atlanta, GA 30308, USA;
[b] Department of Surgery, Emory University School of Medicine; [c] Emory University, Emory University Hospital, American College of Surgeons Board of Governors, SESC DEI Committee, ECCC IDEA Committee, Surgical Section of the NMA and Surgical Leaders Foundation, Emory School of Medicine African American Women's Collaborative
* Corresponding author.
E-mail address: RamzyRimawi@emory.edu

Infect Dis Clin N Am 36 (2022) 889–895
https://doi.org/10.1016/j.idc.2022.07.006
0891-5520/22/© 2022 Elsevier Inc. All rights reserved.

can fully eliminate *C difficile* spores. Because of the discrepancy in hand-washing products and institutional preventative measures globally, some articles have demonstrated that intensification in hand hygiene practices is not an effective measure for preventing CDI. Nonetheless, the use of gloves, disposable gowns, and washing hands with soap and water rather than alcohol-based sanitizers can help reduce the bacterial burden and is the current Center for Disease Control and Prevention recommendation.

Whenever possible, patients with confirmed or suspected CDI should be placed into private rooms and/or cohorted separately. Although visitor contact precautions are commonly used, the association between visitor contact precautions and hospital-onset CDI is minimal.[4,5] CDI precautions should be continued either until the diarrhea resolves or a predetermined (by institutional policy) duration after hospital discharge is reached. Any shared medical equipment, environmental surface, or reusable device should be properly cleaned and disinfected with Environmental Protection Agency (EPA)-registered disinfectant having a sporicidal claim.

After the diagnosis of CDI is established, antibiotic therapy is critical. International society antibiotic recommendations are frequently changed not only because of the robust data regarding CDI antibiotic treatment efficacy but also because of the increasing risk of recurrence. Furthermore, antibiotic recommendations can differ based on first or recurrent exposures. Because of the high encumbrance CDI causes to critically ill patients, ICU providers must remain cognizant of the latest CDI recommendations.

There are several antibiotics with activity against *C difficile*, including oral vancomycin, metronidazole, fidaxomicin, fusidic acid, nitazoxanide, teicoplanin, rifampin, rifaximin, bacitracin, cadazolid, LFF517, and surotomycin. However, it is still unknown whether the in vitro activity of some of these antibiotics against *C difficile* can disrupt the microbial flora enough to prevent, treat, or delay CDI. Clinical data on the effectiveness of these agents are often lacking, controversial, or inconsistent.

Metronidazole is 100% bioavailable, therefore reducing colonic concentrations and increasing the risk of resistance and recurrence. Consequently, it is no longer the recommended therapy for CDI unless the infection is mild and vancomycin or fidaxomicin is unavailable. Oral vancomycin inhibits cell wall synthesis, has minimal systemic absorption, and has high colonic concentrations. Although oral vancomycin is an accepted therapy for CDI, the risk of recurrence after primary therapy is approximately 25%.[6] The risk is even higher if other systemic antibiotics are given concomitantly. Consequently, the latest IDSA/SHEA guidelines now suggest using fidaxomicin, 200 mg, twice daily for 10 days as the first-line agent for initial and recurrent CDI. Because of its narrow spectrum of activity selective for *C difficile* over other gastrointestinal microbes and inhibition of spore production, fidaxomicin has 52% fewer second occurrences and 40% reduction in persistent diarrhea and death when compared with vancomycin.[7,8]

Rifaximin is commonly used to treat CDI as a ducktail agent following the initial dose of oral vancomycin. Nitazoxanide is an analogue of the nitrothiazole drug principally investigated for its' effects against *Helicobacter pylori* and has been shown to have activity against *C difficile*; however, clinical data are needed.[9] Actoxumab and bezlotoxumab are human monoclonal antibodies with activity against *C difficile* toxins A and B, respectively. In the MODIFY I and II trials, bezlotoxumab, 10 mg/kg, given once intravenously, but not actoxumab, was associated with a substantially lower rate of recurrent infection than placebo.[10]

Although encapsulated mixtures of *Lactobacillus* probiotics have been shown to reduce the risk of developing CDI by 64%, the role of probiotics in curtailing primary or recurrent CDI remains inconsistent.[11] When systemic antibiotics are needed in patients at risk of CDI, primary or secondary prophylactic strategies become appealing. Data on the use of antibiotic prophylaxis however are controversial. Oral vancomycin prophylaxis only decreases risk of CDI in patients with prior CDI actively receiving systemic antimicrobial therapy but lacks benefit as a primary prophylaxis.[12]

SURGICAL MANAGEMENT

Fulminant *Clostridioides difficile* colitis (FCDC) results in clinical deterioration due to multiorgan failure, peritonitis, abdominal compartment syndrome, and sepsis. Although 1% to 3% of CDI progresses to fulminant colitis, only 36% go onto surgery and had a 19% to 80% mortality.[13,14] The World Society of Emergency Surgery (WSES) and The Eastern Association Surgery for Trauma (EAST) provide guidelines for surgically treating patients with CDI and FCDC.[14–16]

Although surgery is a known risk factor for CDI development, it is also a treatment option in severe cases. Kim and colleagues found the CDI rate was 0.4 during a retrospective review of 4720 surgical ward patients.[17] The factors that disrupt the microbiome include nasogastric tubes and the specific type of surgery performed.[18] Emergency surgeries, in general, have a higher risk of CDI than elective surgery.[19–21] Cholecystectomy and appendectomy carry the lowest risk of CDI. However, colectomy, small-bowel resection, and gastric resection, especially with a hospital length of stay more than 10 days are associated with a high risk of CDI. A retrospective colectomy database review of the 2015 American College of Surgeons National Surgical Quality Improvement Project demonstrated that stoma reversal, smoking, steroids, and disseminated cancer were all associated with CDI in the 30-day postoperative period.

Although diarrhea is the hallmark symptom of CDI, it may not be present in surgical patients initially, possibly due to colonic dysmotility either from previous underlying conditions or possibly from the disease process itself[22]; this is especially important in surgical patients who may have a concomitant ileus. Therefore, it is essential that providers caring for surgical patients routinely have a high index of suspicion for CDI development. For those unable to produce stool specimens, polymerase chain reaction testing of perirectal swabs provides an acceptable alternative to stool specimen analysis. Colonoscopy should be avoided when FCDC is present. Because of the high risk of perforation when FCDC is present, alternative diagnostic strategies include point-of-care ultrasound and flexible endoscopy.[23] Point-of-care ultrasound may especially be beneficial in patients too unstable for transport. Ultrasonographic findings of pseudomembranous colitis in severe cases include a thickened colonic wall with heterogeneous echogenicity as well as narrowing of the colonic lumen.[24] Pseudomembranes can also be visualized as hyperechoic lines covering the mucosa.

In 2013, Miller and colleagues published an analysis of 2 clinical trials aimed to validate a categorization system that stratify CDI patients into severe or mild-to-moderate groups. A combination of 5 simple and commonly available clinical and laboratory variables (ATLAS) (Age, Treatment with systemic antibiotics, Leukocyte count, Albumin, and Serum creatinine), measured at the time of CDI diagnosis, was able to accurately predict treatment response to CDI therapy.[25] Later, a different risk scoring system for daily clinical practice included the following[25,26]:

- Age greater than 70 years—2 points
- White blood cell counts greater than 20,000/μL or less than 2000/μL – 1 point
- Cardiorespiratory failure—7 points
- Diffuse abdominal tenderness—6 points

Patients with a value of 6 points were deemed low risk, whereas patients with a score greater than or equal to 6 were considered high risk. Unfortunately, no clinical or laboratory finding can predict which patient will not respond to medical therapy and eventually need surgical intervention. Therefore, some common indications for consulting surgery include, but are not limited to, the following:

- Hypotension with or without vasopressor requirements
- Temperature greater than or equal to 38.5°C
- Ileus or significant abdominal distention
- Megacolon (>7 cm diameter in the colon)
- Peritonitis or significant abdominal tenderness
- Free abdominal air on imaging
- Altered mental status
- White blood cell count greater than 2000 cells/mL
- Serum lactate levels greater than 2.2 mmol/L
- Intensive care admission due to clinical deterioration or end-organ failure
- Transplant recipient
- Failure to improve after 3 to 5 days of medical therapy

Patients with FCDC who progress to systemic toxicity should initiate antibiotics while awaiting surgical consultation. Delaying surgery increases the likelihood of adverse outcomes.[14] Therefore, adult patients infected with *C difficile* should undergo surgery early, before developing shock and requiring vasopressors. Although optimal timing remains controversial, the practice management guidelines recommend surgical intervention 3 to 5 days after failure to improve with medical efforts.[27] Although a total abdominal colectomy (TAC) or subtotal colectomy can be done in adult patients with CDI undergoing surgery, the guidelines also recommend a TAC in patients with FCDC. This recommendation is based on low-quality evidence but highly values patient preferences for a definitive surgical intervention that may reduce mortality rates.

A multiinstitutional randomized controlled trial (ClinicalTrials.gov identifier NCT01441271) entitled "Optimal surgical treatment of fulminant Clostridium difficile colitis" was initiated to determine the best operative procedure for patients with CDI.[16] In this study, patients were randomized to ileostomy with colonic lavage versus TAC. Unfortunately, the study was closed due to a lack of adequate enrollment. Neal and colleagues described an innovative procedure in which an ileostomy is created to allow colonic washing and direct topical treatment with vancomycin enemas.[28] This article found a 19% mortality rate in these patients compared with a 50% mortality rate in historical controls who had undergone a TAC. Although the article showed encouraging results, there was a high recurrence rate after ileostomy reversal.

In summary, fidaxomicin, as a standard or extended-pulsed regimen, is the suggested treatment of initial and recurrent CDI. Vancomycin (in a tapered or pulsed regimen) is an acceptable alternative, followed by rifaximin and fecal microbiota transplantation. Bezlotoxumab, in combination with standard-of-care antibiotics, is suggested for patients with recurrent CDI within 6 months. Several antimicrobial agents in the pipeline are being developed to increase the CDI armamentarium, neutralize the disease-causing toxins, and reduce spore formation.[29] Unfortunately, there are several technical and physiologic barriers that make it challenging to assess the clinical impact of the newly discovered CDI drugs. Moreover, some of the compound concentrations dramatically alter the other bacterial gut flora and can increase the risk of recurrence. To date, the combination of selective antibiotic and microbial restorative therapy is proving to be the winning formula. If the patients fail to improve after 3 to 5 days, a possible consequence, FCDC, continues to carry a high rate of adverse outcomes and mortality. Patients with FCDC should have early surgical consultation and be considered for total colectomy. Major risk factors specific to the surgical population include nasogastric tubes and the need for emergency surgery. Alternative methods for diagnosing FCDC in a postoperative patient with an ileus include perform perirectal swab, point-of-care ultrasound, and flexible sigmoidoscopy.

CLINICS CARE POINTS

- When a patient is infected with *C difficile*, fidaxomicin should be considered. If unavailable, oral vancomycin is an acceptable alternative.
- Even if a postsurgical patient does not have diarrhea, they could still be infected with *C difficile*.
- If patients fail to improve within 3 to 5 days of therapy, get a surgical consultation for possible total colectomy.

REFERENCES

1. Kyne L, Hamel MB, Polavaram R, et al. Health care costs and mortality associated with nosocomial diarrhea due to Clostridium difficile. Clin Infect Dis 2002; 34:346–53.
2. Lawrence SJ, Puzniak LA, Shadel BN, et al. Clostridium difficile in the intensive care unit: epidemiology, costs, and colonization pressure. Infect Control Hosp Epidemiol 2007;28(2):123–30.
3. Johnson S, Lavergne V, Skinner AM, et al. Clinical practice guideline by the Infectious Diseases Society of America (IDSA) and Society for Healthcare Epidemiology of America (SHEA): 2021 focused update guidelines on management of Clostridioides difficile infection in adults. Clin Infect Dis 2021;ciab549.
4. Scaria E, Barker AK, Alagoz O, et al. Association of Visitor Contact Precautions with Estimated Hospital-Onset Clostridioides difficile Infection Rates in Acute Care Hospitals. JAMA Netw Open 2021;4(2):e210361.
5. Louh IK, Greendyke WG, Hermann EA, et al. Clostridium difficile infection in acute care hospitals: Systematic review and best practices for prevention. Infect Control Hosp Epidemiol 2017;38:476–82. https://doi.org/10.1017/ice.2016.324.
6. Kelly CP, LaMont JT. Clostridium difficile – more difficult than ever. N Engl J Med 2008;359:1932–40.
7. Cornely OA, Miller MA, Louie TJ, et al. Treatment of First Recurrence of Clostridium difficile Infection: Fidaxomicin Versus Vancomycin. Clin Infect Dis 2012; 55(Suppl. 2S154–S161).
8. Crook DW, Walker AS, Kean Y, et al. Fidaxomicin Versus Vancomycin for Clostridium difficile Infection: Meta-Analysis of Pivotal Randomized Controlled Trials. Clin Infect Dis 2012;55:S93–103.
9. Ballard TE, Wang X, Olekhnovich I, et al. Biological Activity of Modified and Exchanged 2-Amino-5-Nitrothiazole Amide Analogues of Nitazoxanide. Bioorg Med Chem Lett 2010;20:3537–9.
10. Wilcox MH, Gerding DN, Poxton IR, et al. Bezlotoxumab for Prevention of Recurrent Clostridium difficile Infection. N Engl J Med 2017;376:305–17.

11. Goldenberg JZ, Ma SS, Saxton JD, et al. Probiotics for the prevention of Clostridium difficile-associated diarrhea in adults and children. Cochrane Database Syst Rev 2013;CD006095. PMID:23728658.

12. Tariq R, Laguio-Vila M, Tahir MW, et al. Efficacy of oral vancomycin prophylaxis for prevention of Clostridioides difficile infection: a systematic review and meta-analysis. Therap Adv Gastroenterol 2021;14. 1756284821994046.

13. Seder CW, et al. Early colectomy may be associated with improved survival in fulminant Clostridium difficile colitis: an 8-year experience. The Am J Surg 2009;197(3):302–7.

14. Dallal Ramsey M, Harbrecht Brian G, Boujoukas Arthur J, et al. Fulminant Clostridium difficile: an underappreciated and increasing cause of death and complications. Ann Surg 2002;235(3):363–72.

15. Sartelli Massimo, Di Bella Stefano, McFarland Lynne V, et al. 2019 update of the WSES guidelines for management of Clostridioides (Clostridium) difficile infection in surgical patients. World J Emerg Surg 2019;14(1):1–29.

16. Ferrada Paula, Velopulos Catherine G, Sultan Shahnaz, et al. Timing and type of surgical treatment of Clostridium difficile–associated disease: a practice management guideline from the Eastern Association for the Surgery of Trauma. J Trauma Acute Care Surg 2014;76(6):1484–93.

17. Kim Min Jeong, Kim Byung Seup, Kwon Jae Woo, et al. Risk factors for the development of Clostridium difficile colitis in a surgical ward. J Korean Surg Soc 2012; 83(1):14–20.

18. Wijarnpreecha Karn, Sornprom Suthanya, Thongprayoon Charat, et al. Nasogastric tube and outcomes of Clostridium difficile infection: A systematic review and meta-analysis. J Evidence-Based Med 2018;11(1):40–5.

19. Zerey Marc, Paton Lauren B, Lincourt Amy E, et al. The burden of Clostridium difficile in surgical patients in the United States. Surg infections 2007;8(6):557–66.

20. Skancke Matthew, Vaziri Khashayar, Umapathi Bindu, et al. Elective stoma reversal has a higher incidence of postoperative Clostridium difficile infection compared with elective colectomy: an analysis using the American College of Surgeons National Surgical Quality Improvement Program and targeted colectomy databases. Dis Colon Rectum 2018;61(5):593–8.

21. Khanna Sahil, Baddour Larry M, Dibaise John K, et al. Appendectomy Is Not Associated with Adverse Outcomes inClostridium difficile Infection: A Population-Based Study. Official J Am Coll Gastroenterol ACG 2013;108(4):626–7.

22. Jaber Raffat M, Olafsson Snorri, Fung Wesley L, et al. Clinical review of the management of fulminant Clostridium difficile infection. Official J Am Coll Gastroenterol ACG 2008;103(12):3195–203.

23. Revzin Margarita V, Moshiri Mariam, Bokhari Jamal, et al. Sonographic assessment of infectious diseases of the gastrointestinal tract: from scanning to diagnosis. Abdom Radiol 2020;45(2):261–92.

24. Abu-Zidan Fikri M, Arif Alper Cevik. Diagnostic point-of-care ultrasound (POCUS) for gastrointestinal pathology: state of the art from basics to advanced. World J Emerg Surg 2018;13(1):1–14.

25. Miller Mark A, Louie Thomas, Mullane Kathleen, et al. Derivation and validation of a simple clinical bedside score (ATLAS) for Clostridium difficile infection which predicts response to therapy. BMC Infect Dis 2013;13(1):1–7.

26. Van Der Wilden Gwendolyn M, Chang Yuchiao, Cropano Catrina, et al. Fulminant Clostridium difficile colitis: prospective development of a risk scoring system. J Trauma Acute Care Surg 2014;76(2):424–30.

27. Halabi Wissam J, Nguyen Vinh Q, Carmichael Joseph C, et al. Clostridium difficile colitis in the United States: a decade of trends, outcomes, risk factors for colectomy, and mortality after colectomy. J Am Coll Surg 2013;217(5):802–12.
28. Neal Matthew D, Alverdy John C, Hall Daniel E, et al. Diverting loop ileostomy and colonic lavage: an alternative to total abdominal colectomy for the treatment of severe, complicated Clostridium difficile associated disease. Ann Surg 2011; 254(3):423–9.
29. Jarrad AM, Karoli T, Blaskovich MA, et al. Clostridium difficile Drug Pipeline: Challenges in Discovery and Development of New Agents. J Med Chem 2015;58(13): 5164–85.

Uses of Procalcitonin as a Biomarker in Critical Care Medicine

Ryan C. Maves, MD[a,b],*, Chukwunyelu H. Enwezor, MD[a]

KEYWORDS

- Procalcitonin • Biomarkers • Sepsis • Antimicrobial stewardship

KEY POINTS

- Procalcitonin (PCT) is a polypeptide produced by multiple tissues in the body and is up-regulated in response to pro-inflammatory cytokines, including interleukin-1, interleukin-6, and tumor necrosis factor alpha.
- Although serum PCT levels tend to be higher in patients with bacterial as opposed to viral pneumonia, this difference is not sufficiently significant in critically ill patients to withhold antibacterial drugs empirically at the time of presentation.
- Elevated PCT levels are independently correlated with the risk of critical illness and death in patients with lower respiratory tract infections and sepsis, like that seen with other traditional illness severity scores such as Acute Physiology and Chronic Health Evaluation II (APACHE-II) and Acute Physiology and Chronic Health Evaluation IV (APACHE-IV).
- Serum PCT levels should decline with effective antibacterial therapy. Algorithms to permit the safe discontinuation of antibiotics have been validated, using PCT cutoffs of 0.25 to 0.50 ng/mL or a decline in PCT of greater than 80% above the maximum. These algorithms require clinician teaching and support from institutional antimicrobial stewardship programs to be effective.
- While promising, PCT-guided antibiotic algorithms have not yet been compared with newer, evidence-based shorter courses of antibiotics in many common infections. The benefit of PCT in those settings remains to be proven.

INTRODUCTION AND BACKGROUND

Distinguishing between bacterial and nonbacterial sources of fever and sepsis is challenging in the acute setting. Rapid administration of effective antimicrobial drugs is one of the few modifiable risk factors for mortality in the septic patient,[1] although the precise timing varies depending on illness severity.[2] As such, there is a strong

[a] Department of Internal Medicine, Section of Infectious Diseases, Wake Forest University School of Medicine, Winston-Salem, NC, USA; [b] Department of Anesthesiology, Section of Critical Care Medicine, Wake Forest University School of Medicine, Winston-Salem, NC, USA
* Corresponding author. Section on Infectious Diseases, Atrium Health Wake Forest Baptist Medical Center, Medical Center Boulevard, Winston-Salem, NC 27157.
E-mail address: rmaves@wakehealth.edu

Infect Dis Clin N Am 36 (2022) 897–909
https://doi.org/10.1016/j.idc.2022.07.004
0891-5520/22/© 2022 Elsevier Inc. All rights reserved.

id.theclinics.com

impetus for emergency departments (EDs) and inpatient units to identify sepsis and initiate therapy quickly.

We lack rapid, reliable techniques to establish (or exclude) bacterial infection quickly in the potentially septic host. Prior studies have shown limited accuracy in physicians' abilities to diagnose sepsis reliably. Approximately 40% of hospitalized patients with features of the systemic inflammatory response syndrome may have noninfectious causes of disease,[3] whereas 35% of patients who receive empiric broad-spectrum intravenous antibacterial drugs in ED settings for suspected sepsis do not have bacterial infections.[4] Culture-based methods for diagnosis require a minimum of 48 h, and usually longer, for pathogen identification and drug susceptibility testing results. Although newer molecular methods for rapid pathogen detection are promising, systems such as whole-blood multiplex PCR are limited in their sensitivity,[5] and emerging technologies such as cell-free DNA detection from plasma remain investigational.[6]

Given this gap between diagnostic uncertainty and management, clinicians have looked to biomarkers as an approach to improve care. As a concept, this is not new; leukocytosis is a biomarker, after all. Procalcitonin (PCT) is a 116-amino-acid residue, a precursor of the hormone calcitonin that is produced by parafollicular cells of the thyroid and by neuroendocrine cells in the lungs and intestine, described initially in 1984 by Le Moullec and colleagues.[7] PCT was subsequently found to increase in cases of bacterial infection and decline with effective antibiotic treatment.[8]

The role that PCT plays in the pathogenesis of bacterial infections is unclear. Rapid synthesis and release of cytokines such as tumor necrosis factor alpha (TNF-α), interleukin (IL)-1 and IL-6 occur with *in vitro* bacterial stimulation of macrophages; upregulation of these cytokines *in vivo* is followed by synthesis of PCT within hours. Viral infections often lead to upregulation of interferon gamma (IFN-γ), which has the opposite effect of downregulating PCT expression.[9] These observations have led investigators and clinicians to evaluate PCT as a biomarker for three main purposes: as a marker of disease severity, to distinguish viral from bacterial infections, and to guide the duration of antibiotic treatment for bacterial infections.

PROCALCITONIN AS A BIOMARKER FOR DISEASE SEVERITY

Increased PCT levels are linked to increased disease severity in infected patients. In observational studies of PCT incorporated into previously-validated risk scores for pneumonia severity (including the pneumonia severity index, the American Thoracic Society [ATS] minor criteria for severe community-acquired pneumonia [CAP], and SMART-COP), the addition of PCT improved the performance of these scores for prediction of need for invasive mechanical ventilation, vasopressor support, or both,[10–12] albeit with reported areas under the receiver-operator curve (AUROC) scores of only 0.63 to 0.70. When analyzed in a population of patients with pneumonia requiring mechanical ventilation in the intensive care unit (ICU), PCT levels were predictive of the risk of 28-day mortality, with AUROC for initial PCT of 0.70 and maximum PCT of 0.74, although this was not meaningfully different from the risk derived from calculated Acute Physiology and Chronic Health Evaluation II (APACHE-II) scores (AUROC 0.69).[13]

In general populations of patients with sepsis and septic shock, PCT levels are similarly predictive of adverse outcomes. Schuetz and colleagues[14] evaluated PCT levels at baseline and at 72 h in derivation ($n = 154$) and validation ($n = 102$) cohorts in two US ICUs in patients with sepsis. In this study, those patients with PCT decreases of 80% or more from baseline had reduced risks of in-hospital mortality (positive predictive value [PPV] for death, 34%; negative predictive value [NPV] 79% in the validation cohort.) As with the prior study, PCT trends were similar in their predictive performance to Acute Physiology and Chronic Health Evaluation IV (APACHE-IV) in assessing risk of in-hospital death (AUROC 0.70 for PCT vs 0.68 for APACHE-IV), although a model that integrated both PCT and APACHE-IV had some improved performance (AUROC 0.75).

Similar results and predictive trends were observed in the Multicenter Procalcitonin Monitoring Sepsis (MOSES) study, a randomized trial of PCT-guided antimicrobial management conducted in 13 US hospitals. In this trial, ICU patients with decreases in PCT levels ≤80% from baseline at 4 days had an increased risk of death compared with those patients whose PCT levels declined greater than 80% (PPV for death, 29.5%; NPV 81.1%).[15]

PROCALCITONIN IN COMMUNITY-ACQUIRED PNEUMONIA

Empiric antibacterial drugs are routinely recommended for the care of patients with CAP. Bacterial pathogens are identified only in a minority of patients with CAP when cultures of blood and sputum are combined with urine antigen testing,[16] although molecular testing of lower respiratory tract specimens may identify bacteria in up to 78% of hospitalized patients, including many with bacterial and viral coinfections.[17] Given that a considerable proportion of CAP is of purely viral origin, antimicrobial stewardship efforts could be improved by distinguishing those patients with viral CAP versus those with bacterial infections.

Elevated PCT levels are associated with a greater likelihood of bacterial versus viral pneumonia. The question for the clinician at the bedside becomes: at what threshold of PCT is it safe to withhold empiric antibiotics? A prospective trial of 210 patients evaluated a diagnostic bundle using a combination of rapid multiplex polymerase chain reaction (PCR) testing, including viruses and Streptococcus pneumoniae, in combination with PCT. Although those patients with serum PCT levels ≤0.1 ng/mL and only viral pathogens detected received fewer antibiotics and had shorter lengths of stay, relatively few patients in that group had their antibiotics discontinued (8/25, 32%) despite the low likelihood of a bacterial infection.[18]

The optimum cutoff point for serum PCT and viral versus bacterial pneumonia is uncertain. In a multicenter, prospective cohort of 1735 hospitalized adult patients with CAP, participants with confirmed typical bacterial pneumonia (eg, due to S pneumoniae or Haemophilus) had higher median PCT levels (2.5 ng/mL; interquartile range (IQR) 0.29, 12.2) when compared with those with viral (median PCT 0.09 ng/mL; IQR <0.05, 0.54) or atypical bacterial (median PCT 0.20 ng/mL; IQR <0.05, 0.87) infections. Importantly, these data could not identify a PCT cutoff level that precluded the use of empiric antibacterial therapy at the time of presentation. At a cutoff of less than 0.1 ng/mL, the NPV of PCT to exclude bacterial pneumonia was only 82.4%. Although this risk is relatively low, many intensivists would be uncomfortable withholding antibiotics to critically ill patients with a greater than 1-in-6 odds of a life-threatening infection.[19]

Confoundingly, severe viral pneumonia may present with elevated PCT, suggesting that disease acuity may play a role in PCT expression in addition to pathogen type. In a cohort study of 2075 hospitalized adults with viral pneumonias, PCT levels were higher in patients with bacterial coinfections compared with isolated viral pneumonia (AUROC 0.666), but the predictive power of PCT decreased significantly (AUROC 0.584) when normalized for disease severity. This was further evaluated in a murine lethal influenza model, with marked elevations in PCT seen in mice with bacteriologically sterile experimental influenza in addition to increased IL-6 expression. These elevations persisted despite similarly elevated IFN-γ levels in infected mice, suggesting that IFN-mediated inhibition of PCT expression may be overcome by high levels of competing cytokines.[20] Comparable findings were described in a cohort of 1608 adult patients admitted with severe influenza to ICUs in Spain; PCT elevations were associated with increased mortality on univariate analysis but were insufficient in distinguishing between pure viral pneumonia and bacterial coinfections (AUROC 0.32–0.67, depending on coinfecting pathogen).[21]

Overall, the evidence for PCT in CAP is strongest as a prognostic marker than a diagnostic marker, at least at the time of initial presentation. The 2019 CAP guidelines from the Infectious Diseases Society of America (IDSA) and ATS do not recommend PCT for determining the need for empiric antibacterial drugs in CAP.[22] It may have a role in ambiguous cases, where clinical and radiographic data alone are inadequate to guide management.[23]

PROCALCITONIN AS A GUIDE FOR ANTIMICROBIAL TREATMENT DURATION

Once bacterial infection has been established, the duration of antibacterial therapy can be unclear. Typical durations of therapy are often 7 to 14 days (or some other multiple of seven, based presumably upon the days of the week, the number of visible planets in the sky, or both[24]). Multiple trials have established the efficacy of shorter antibiotic courses, for syndromes ranging from gram-negative bacteremia[25,26] to ventilator-associated pneumonia.[27,28] Despite this, extended courses of antibiotics are frequently prescribed in hospitals, with increased lengths of stay,[29] antibiotic toxicity[30] and risks for *Clostridioides difficile* infection.[31] Conversely, shorter courses of therapy can reduce lengths of stay and hospital costs,[32,33] often with improved outcomes.[34]

Given that PCT tends to decrease in bacterial infections with adequate treatment, PCT-based algorithms have been to personalize durations of therapy. The PRORATA trial randomized 621 medical and surgical ICU patients in France to PCT-guided therapy versus usual care, with antibiotics recommended to be stopped in the intervention arm when PCT levels decreased to 0.5 ng/mL or less. PCT-guided therapy led to fewer days of antibiotics (14.3 vs 11.6 days), with no change in mortality at 28 or 60 days and with similar lengths of stay.[35] Subsequently, the Simplified Acute Physiology Score (SAPS) II trial evaluated mortality differences in 1546 ICU patients in the Netherlands managed using PCT-guided antimicrobial therapy. SAPS II identified a similar reduction in days of antimicrobial exposure (9.3 vs 7.5 d), with noninferior results in both 28-day and 1-year mortality.[36]

A comparable trial by Shehabi and colleagues,[37] conducted in 11 Australian ICUs, failed to show a significant reduction in time to antibiotic cessation (9 days with PCT guidance vs 11 days without, $P = .18$ days), although there was a reduction noted in total daily defined doses of antibiotics administered in the PCT guidance arm and no difference in overall mortality. This trial used a lower PCT cutoff for antibiotic cessation (0.1 ng/mL vs 0.5 ng/mL in the PRORATA trial), which may have attenuated its findings. Interestingly, an association with peak PCT levels, rate of decline, and mortality were noted in the Shehabi trial, consistent with the observational prognostic literature cited previously.

Although most trials show at least some reduction in antibiotic use with PCT monitoring, this has not been universal. A 2011 study by Jensen and colleagues,[38] conducted with 1200 ICU patients in Denmark, evaluated PCT-guided treatment versus usual care. Per the study protocol, increases in PCT during monitoring could be met with the broadening of antimicrobial therapy. As a result, the PCT arm received significantly greater amounts of meropenem, piperacillin-tazobactam, and ciprofloxacin and had more days receiving three or more antimicrobial drugs than the usual care arm. Patients in the PCT-guided arm had greater time requiring mechanical ventilation (65.5% of ICU patient-days, vs 60.7% of patient-days among controls, $P < .001$), although 60-day mortality between arms was similar (38.2% with PCT, vs 36.9% with usual care).

Retrospective series have shown comparable results. A 2017 industry-funded retrospective study compared 33,569 patients admitted to ICUs in the United States managed using PCT-guided therapy with 98,543 propensity-matched controls. Using registry data, the investigators found a reduction in antibiotic exposure from 17.3 days to 14.9 days with PCT monitoring without adjustment for illness severity; regression adjustment reduced the difference from 16.9 days without PCT monitoring to 16.2 days with PCT, a significant but comparatively small result.[39] Across all subjects, inpatient mortality was slightly higher with PCT monitoring (18.3% without PCT, vs 19.0% with PCT, $P = .001$), although the retrospective nature of the study makes it difficult to assign causality.

Despite these inconsistent findings, there is a trend supporting the use of PCT guidance for antibiotic cessation across multiple studies. A 2019 meta-analysis of patient-level data from 13 randomized trials of PCT-guided therapy for bacteremia confirmed a reduction in days of antimicrobial therapy without increased mortality, although the actual benefits may be small: patients with *Escherichia coli* bacteremia in the included trials received a mean 12.4 days of antimicrobial therapy with PCT guidance; those with pneumococcal bacteremia received 11.3 days.[40] Although these represent improvements, they are also significantly longer than the currently recommended durations of 7 days for *E coli* bacteremia and 5 to 7 days for pneumococci.

PROCALCITONIN AND CORONAVIRUS DISEASE-2019

Like so many aspects of medicine, efforts at antimicrobial stewardship have suffered during the coronavirus disease-2019 (COVID-19) pandemic. Bacterial coinfection is rare among patients with severe acute respiratory syndrome coronavirus-2 (SARS-CoV-2) infection and respiratory failure presenting from community settings, but empiric antibiotic prescription is common and likely occurs in the majority of cases. Early in the pandemic, a prospective cohort of 1705 hospitalized adults with severe COVID-19 in the United States reported that only 3.5% had a confirmed bacterial coinfection, but early empiric antibacterial drugs were administered to 56.6%,[41] with similar rates of bacterial coinfection and antibiotic use noted in observational studies conducted in the same time period in the United Kingdom.[42,43]

Rates of hospital-acquired infections, particularly ventilator-associated pneumonia (VAP), are conversely quite high in patients with COVID-19 requiring intubation and mechanical ventilation, due in part to the prolonged duration of invasive ventilation needed in these patients. The cumulative incidence of VAP in intubated patients with COVID-19 is estimated at 25% to 30% during hospitalization and is quantitatively greater than in other intubated patients in the ICU.[44-46] With these overlapping factors, a study of antibiotic use in 716 US hospitals showed that 49.2% of patients admitted to ICUs with COVID-19 in 2020 received antibiotics, including 95.9% of those requiring invasive mechanical ventilation, as compared with 31.2% of ICU patients without COVID-19.[47]

Biomarkers, including PCT, have been studied to better identify patients with COVID-19 likely to benefit from empiric antibiotics. Early in the pandemic, a single-center study in an Italian university hospital found serum PCT (with a cutoff of

0.5 ng/mL) to have inadequate sensitivity (43%) and specificity (72%) for non-COVID-19 pneumonia.[48] Similar to influenza, COVID-19 can cause increases in PCT independently of bacterial superinfection. An observational study of 332 patients in the Netherlands, for example, showed a markedly increased risk of critical illness in patients with COVID-19 presenting with a PCT greater than 1.0 ng/mL, with an adjusted odds ratio (OR) of 2.11 and an AUROC of 0.85 in a multivariate analysis that adjusted for C-reactive protein, age, sex, comorbidity, and known bacterial superinfections.[49]

In a meta-analysis of 10 studies, Shen and colleagues[50] reported an increased OR for death of 1.77 in patients with COVID-19 presenting with elevated baseline serum PCT levels, although this analysis is somewhat hampered by varying cutoffs for "elevated" in the included trials. Similarly, PCT-guided antibiotic de-escalation and discontinuation appear to be viable in COVID-19. In small studies, antibiotic discontinuation appeared to be safe using cutoffs of 0.25 ng/mL and 0.5 ng/mL.[51–54] Further studies will be necessary to understand better the interactions between SARS-CoV-2 and PCT kinetics.

CONFOUNDING FACTORS

Multiple factors can confound PCT measurement. In addition to the effects of severe viral pneumonia due to influenza and SARS-CoV-2 described above, other conditions can lead to false-positive results. Some of these disorders are infrequent in North American and European ICUs, such as malaria[55] and dengue,[56] but other are not: candidemia,[57] chronic kidney disease (CKD) and renal replacement therapy (RRT),[58] lung cancer,[59] and hematologic malignancies.[60]

CKD and end-stage renal disease (ESRD) are common among critically-ill patients. Uninfected control patients with ESRD on hemodialysis (HD) were compared with a cohort of ESRD patients with confirmed bacterial infection in Israel; although infected patients tended to have higher PCT levels than those without infection, the uninfected patients had a mean serum PCT of 1.0 ng/mL, markedly higher than that seen in patients with normal kidney function.[61] In a meta-analysis of seven studies with 1444 patients, Tao and colleagues[62] identified a serum PCT of 1.5 ng/mL as a potential cutoff for predicting bacterial infection in patients with ESRD requiring HD. Conversely, CRRT membranes can remove molecules as large as 35 kDa, larger than the 14.5 kDa PCT molecule, raising the possibility that CRRT could lead to artificially low PCT values.[63]

Invasive *Candida* infections account for approximately 10% of nosocomial bloodstream infections (BSIs) in the ICU and have a crude mortality of nearly 50%, despite the availability of effective antifungal therapy.[64] Blood cultures are negative in half of cases of invasive candidiasis, leading to delays in diagnosis and presumably contributing to the high mortality.[65] A 2019 systematic review by Cortegiani and colleagues[57] noted that, although PCT levels in patients with candidemia tended to be lower from patients with bacteremia, the wide ranges in both populations precluded the use of PCT to predict fungal versus bacterial BSI.

PROPOSED USES

Based on available data and existing guidelines, including the 2019 ATS/IDSA guidelines for CAP as well as the 2021 Surviving Sepsis Campaign guidelines, we do not recommend the routine use of PCT to distinguish between bacterial or viral pneumonia[22] or to determine whether to initiate antibacterial therapy in patients at high risk for critical illness.[66]

The best-validated use for PCT in critically-ill patients is to promote antibiotic de-escalation and reducing duration of total therapy. It is worth reflecting that early studies of intramuscular penicillin for the treatment of severe bacteremic pneumococcal pneumonia reported treatment durations of usually one and often no more than 4 days.[67] Our current durations of therapy evolved on a frequently *ad hoc* basis, based in part on concerns for preventing complications (eg, empyema from bacterial pneumonia) but on frequently flimsy scientific grounds. As such, PCT gives us a potential mechanism for individualizing therapy with a goal of both total antibiotic reduction and improved overall outcomes, both on the patient level and ecologically.

In implementing PCT-based algorithms for antibiotic guidance, it is important to remember that the outputs of any algorithm matter as much as the inputs. As noted in the Jensen trial, protocols that escalate therapy based on rising levels can lead to increased broad-spectrum drug usage.[38] Similarly, the lower cutoff of 0.1 ng/mL (compared with 0.25–0.50 ng/mL in other studies) used in the Shehabi trial may attenuate the benefits of PCT monitoring by requiring unnecessarily low serum levels to discontinue antibiotics.[37] With these in mind, PCT algorithms appear to be best supported by using:

- Serial monitoring at fixed intervals (eg, at presentation, 6–24 h later, and then every 24–28 h until antibiotic discontinuation).
- A cutoff of 0.25 to 0.50 ng/mL (or relative decline of >80% from peak levels) for antibiotic discontinuation.
- An avoidance of reflexive antibiotic escalation in the face of rising serum PCT levels but instead consideration of the patient's physiologic status and investigation of other potential causes for rising biomarker levels (eg, abscess) beyond inadequate antibiotic therapy alone.

A sample PCT algorithm for sepsis is provided in **Fig. 1**.

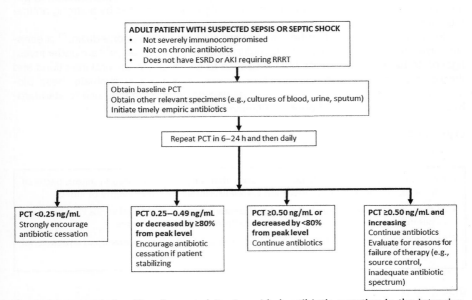

Fig. 1. A proposed algorithm for procalcitonin-guided antibiotic cessation in the intensive care unit. AKI, acute kidney injury; ESRD, end-stage renal disease; PCT, procalcitonin; RRT, renal replacement therapy.

Along with PCT cutoffs, close partnerships with antimicrobial stewardship programs are critical. Outcomes in the PRORATA trial may have been limited because of poor adherence to the study protocol.[35] In the Procalcitonin Antibiotic Consensus Trial (ProACT), 1656 patients with lower respiratory tract infections in 14 US hospital EDs were randomized to usual care versus PCT-guided antibiotic therapy; no difference was noted in antibiotic use between arms, in large part due to only 72.9% of patients receiving care that conformed to the treatment protocol.[68] Similarly, a retrospective review in a large academic health system in California showed that more than 80% of antibiotic regimens were continued despite low PCT levels and electronic health record-embedded decision support tools.[69] If algorithms are only as good as the outputs they generate, then clinicians must act on those outputs to make them useful. Regular clinician education, outreach, and active involvement of stewardship teams are necessary to make these outputs occur.

Furthermore, although the improvements in antimicrobial duration seen in some PCT trials are real, they are also insufficient; a decrease in treatment duration for *E coli* bacteremia to 12.4 days from 15.2 days may be an improvement, but it is no triumph when most cases of gram-negative bacteremia only need 7 days of antibiotics.[40] As such, PCT algorithms must also be interpreted in the context of shorter courses of optimally-dosed therapy.

SUMMARY AND FUTURE DIRECTIONS

PCT-based testing currently lacks sufficient sensitivity and specificity to withhold antibacterial therapy safely from patients with lower respiratory tract infections or suspected sepsis at the time of presentation. As a diagnostic marker, PCT elevation is associated with an increased risk of progression to critical illness and death, but its contribution to existing illness severity scores is mostly incremental. There is generally positive support for PCT-based algorithms to guide antibiotic discontinuation in patients in the ICU if adherence to algorithms is high and supported by a strong antimicrobial stewardship program.

Along with PCT, multiple other biomarkers such as proadrenomedullin,[70] presepsin,[71] pancreatic stone protein,[72] and multiplex host–protein assays[73] are under investigation to better delineate the host response to bacterial versus viral infections and the patient response to therapy. Future research will need to evaluate these biomarkers, both alone and in combination, as well as comparing their use to standardized, evidence-based short-course antimicrobial regimens.

CLINICS CARE POINTS

- Procalcitonin (PCT) is a widely-used biomarker that tends to be elevated in serious bacterial infections. The degree of PCT elevation correlates closely with the severity of illness.
- At the time of presentation, PCT is not sufficiently specific for bacterial versus viral infection to permit the safe withholding of antibiotics from seriously-ill patients.
- Serial measurement of PCT may be a useful tool to guide the discontinuation of antibacterial therapy in seriously-ill patient.

DISCLOSURE

No funding was obtained or used for this work. The authors report no financial conflicts of interest.

REFERENCES

1. Kumar A, Roberts D, Wood KE, et al. Duration of hypotension before initiation of effective antimicrobial therapy is the critical determinant of survival in human septic shock. Crit Care Med 2006;34(6):1589–96.
2. Taylor SP, Anderson WE, Beam K, et al. The Association Between Antibiotic Delay Intervals and Hospital Mortality Among Patients Treated in the Emergency Department for Suspected Sepsis. Crit Care Med 2021;49(5):741–7.
3. Comstedt P, Storgaard M, Lassen AT. The Systemic Inflammatory Response Syndrome (SIRS) in acutely hospitalised medical patients: a cohort study. Scand J Trauma Resusc Emerg Med 2009;17:67.
4. Shappell CN, Klompas M, Ochoa A, et al. Likelihood of Bacterial Infection in Patients Treated With Broad-Spectrum IV Antibiotics in the Emergency Department. Crit Care Med 2021;49(11):e1144–50.
5. Zboromyrska Y, Cilloniz C, Cobos-Trigueros N, et al. Evaluation of the Magicplex Sepsis Real-Time Test for the Rapid Diagnosis of Bloodstream Infections in Adults. Front Cell Infect Microbiol 2019;9:56.
6. Grumaz S, Grumaz C, Vainshtein Y, et al. Enhanced Performance of Next-Generation Sequencing Diagnostics Compared With Standard of Care Microbiological Diagnostics in Patients Suffering From Septic Shock. Crit Care Med 2019; 47(5):e394–402.
7. Le Moullec JM, Jullienne A, Chenais J, et al. The complete sequence of human preprocalcitonin. FEBS Lett 1984;167(1):93–7.
8. Assicot M, Gendrel D, Carsin H, et al. High serum procalcitonin concentrations in patients with sepsis and infection. Lancet 1993;341(8844):515–8.
9. Linscheid P, Seboek D, Nylen ES, et al. In vitro and in vivo calcitonin I gene expression in parenchymal cells: a novel product of human adipose tissue. Endocrinology 2003;144(12):5578–84.
10. Self WH, Grijalva CG, Williams DJ, et al. Procalcitonin as an Early Marker of the Need for Invasive Respiratory or Vasopressor Support in Adults With Community-Acquired Pneumonia. Chest 2016;150(4):819–28.
11. Huang DT, Weissfeld LA, Kellum JA, et al. Risk prediction with procalcitonin and clinical rules in community-acquired pneumonia. Ann Emerg Med 2008;52(1): 48–58 e2.
12. Ramirez P, Ferrer M, Marti V, et al. Inflammatory biomarkers and prediction for intensive care unit admission in severe community-acquired pneumonia. Crit Care Med 2011;39(10):2211–7.
13. Bloos F, Marshall JC, Dellinger RP, et al. Multinational, observational study of procalcitonin in ICU patients with pneumonia requiring mechanical ventilation: a multicenter observational study. Crit Care 2011;15(2):R88.
14. Schuetz P, Maurer P, Punjabi V, et al. Procalcitonin decrease over 72 hours in US critical care units predicts fatal outcome in sepsis patients. Crit Care 2013;17(3): R115.
15. Schuetz P, Birkhahn R, Sherwin R, et al. Serial Procalcitonin Predicts Mortality in Severe Sepsis Patients: Results From the Multicenter Procalcitonin MOnitoring SEpsis (MOSES) Study. Crit Care Med 2017;45(5):781–9.
16. Restrepo MI, Mortensen EM, Velez JA, et al. A comparative study of community-acquired pneumonia patients admitted to the ward and the ICU. Chest 2008; 133(3):610–7.

17. Gadsby NJ, Russell CD, McHugh MP, et al. Comprehensive Molecular Testing for Respiratory Pathogens in Community-Acquired Pneumonia. Clin Infect Dis 2016; 62(7):817–23.

18. Gilbert D, Gelfer G, Wang L, et al. The potential of molecular diagnostics and serum procalcitonin levels to change the antibiotic management of community-acquired pneumonia. Diagn Microbiol Infect Dis 2016;86(1):102–7.

19. Self WH, Balk RA, Grijalva CG, et al. Procalcitonin as a Marker of Etiology in Adults Hospitalized With Community-Acquired Pneumonia. Clin Infect Dis 2017; 65(2):183–90.

20. Gautam S, Cohen AJ, Stahl Y, et al. Severe respiratory viral infection induces procalcitonin in the absence of bacterial pneumonia. Thorax 2020;75(11):974–81.

21. Carbonell R, Moreno G, Martin-Loeches I, et al. Prognostic Value of Procalcitonin and C-Reactive Protein in 1608 Critically Ill Patients with Severe Influenza Pneumonia. Antibiotics (Basel) 2021;(4):10. https://doi.org/10.3390/antibiotics10040350.

22. Metlay JP, Waterer GW, Long AC, et al. Diagnosis and Treatment of Adults with Community-acquired Pneumonia. An Official Clinical Practice Guideline of the American Thoracic Society and Infectious Diseases Society of America. Am J Respir Crit Care Med 2019;200(7):e45–67.

23. Schuetz P. Procalcitonin Is Useful for Evaluating Patients with Ambiguous Presentation and for Early Discontinuation of Antibiotics in Community-acquired Pneumonia. Am J Respir Crit Care Med 2020;201(6):744–5.

24. Maves RC. Procalcitonin Is Not an Adequate Tool for Antimicrobial De-Escalation in Sepsis. Crit Care Med 2020;48(12):1848–50.

25. Yahav D, Franceschini E, Koppel F, et al. Seven Versus 14 Days of Antibiotic Therapy for Uncomplicated Gram-negative Bacteremia: A Noninferiority Randomized Controlled Trial. Clin Infect Dis 2019;69(7):1091–8.

26. Molina J, Cisneros JM. Seven-versus 14-day course of antibiotics for the treatment of bloodstream infections by enterobacterales: a randomized, controlled trial: authors' response. Clinical microbiology and infection : the official publication of the European Society of Clinical Microbiology and Infectious Diseases 2021. https://doi.org/10.1016/j.cmi.2021.12.008.

27. Chastre J, Wolff M, Fagon JY, et al. Comparison of 8 vs 15 days of antibiotic therapy for ventilator-associated pneumonia in adults: a randomized trial. JAMA 2003;290(19):2588–98.

28. Capellier G, Mockly H, Charpentier C, et al. Early-onset ventilator-associated pneumonia in adults randomized clinical trial: comparison of 8 versus 15 days of antibiotic treatment. PloS one 2012;7(8):e41290.

29. Yi SH, Hatfield KM, Baggs J, et al. Duration of Antibiotic Use Among Adults With Uncomplicated Community-Acquired Pneumonia Requiring Hospitalization in the United States. Clin Infect Dis 2018;66(9):1333–41.

30. Vaughn VM, Flanders SA, Snyder A, et al. Excess Antibiotic Treatment Duration and Adverse Events in Patients Hospitalized With Pneumonia: A Multihospital Cohort Study. Ann Intern Med 2019;171(3):153–63.

31. Feazel LM, Malhotra A, Perencevich EN, et al. Effect of antibiotic stewardship programmes on Clostridium difficile incidence: a systematic review and meta-analysis. J Antimicrob Chemother 2014;69(7):1748–54.

32. Ruttimann S, Keck B, Hartmeier C, et al. Long-term antibiotic cost savings from a comprehensive intervention program in a medical department of a university-affiliated teaching hospital. Clin Infect Dis 2004;38(3):348–56.

33. Niwa T, Shinoda Y, Suzuki A, et al. Outcome measurement of extensive implementation of antimicrobial stewardship in patients receiving intravenous antibiotics in a Japanese university hospital. Int J Clin Pract 2012;66(10):999–1008.
34. Hanretty AM, Gallagher JC. Shortened Courses of Antibiotics for Bacterial Infections: A Systematic Review of Randomized Controlled Trials. Pharmacotherapy 2018;38(6):674–87.
35. Bouadma L, Luyt CE, Tubach F, et al. Use of procalcitonin to reduce patients' exposure to antibiotics in intensive care units (PRORATA trial): a multicentre randomised controlled trial. Lancet 2010;375(9713):463–74.
36. de Jong E, van Oers JA, Beishuizen A, et al. Efficacy and safety of procalcitonin guidance in reducing the duration of antibiotic treatment in critically ill patients: a randomised, controlled, open-label trial. Lancet Infect Dis 2016;16(7):819–27.
37. Shehabi Y, Sterba M, Garrett PM, et al. Procalcitonin algorithm in critically ill adults with undifferentiated infection or suspected sepsis. A randomized controlled trial. Am J Respir Crit Care Med 2014;190(10):1102–10.
38. Jensen JU, Hein L, Lundgren B, et al. Procalcitonin-guided interventions against infections to increase early appropriate antibiotics and improve survival in the intensive care unit: a randomized trial. Crit Care Med 2011;39(9):2048–58.
39. Balk RA, Kadri SS, Cao Z, et al. Effect of Procalcitonin Testing on Health-care Utilization and Costs in Critically Ill Patients in the United States. Chest 2017;151(1):23–33.
40. Meier MA, Branche A, Neeser OL, et al. Procalcitonin-guided Antibiotic Treatment in Patients With Positive Blood Cultures: A Patient-level Meta-analysis of Randomized Trials. Clin Infect Dis 2019;69(3):388–96.
41. Vaughn VM, Gandhi TN, Petty LA, et al. Empiric Antibacterial Therapy and Community-onset Bacterial Coinfection in Patients Hospitalized With Coronavirus Disease 2019 (COVID-19): A Multi-hospital Cohort Study. Clin Infect Dis 2021; 72(10):e533–41.
42. Hughes S, Troise O, Donaldson H, et al. Bacterial and fungal coinfection among hospitalized patients with COVID-19: a retrospective cohort study in a UK secondary-care setting. Clin Microbiol Infect 2020;26(10):1395–9.
43. Wang L, Amin AK, Khanna P, et al. An observational cohort study of bacterial co-infection and implications for empirical antibiotic therapy in patients presenting with COVID-19 to hospitals in North West London. J Antimicrob Chemother 2021;76(3):796–803.
44. Vacheron CH, Lepape A, Savey A, et al. Increased Incidence of Ventilator-Acquired Pneumonia in Coronavirus Disease 2019 Patients: A Multicentric Cohort Study. Crit Care Med 2022;50(3):449–59.
45. Grasselli G, Scaravilli V, Mangioni D, et al. Hospital-Acquired Infections in Critically Ill Patients With COVID-19. Chest 2021;160(2):454–65.
46. Hedberg P, Ternhag A, Giske CG, et al. Ventilator-Associated Lower Respiratory Tract Bacterial Infections in COVID-19 Compared With Non-COVID-19 Patients. Crit Care Med 2022.
47. Rose AN, Baggs J, Wolford H, et al. Trends in Antibiotic Use in United States Hospitals During the Coronavirus Disease 2019 Pandemic. Open Forum Infect Dis 2021;8(6):ofab236.
48. Nazerian P, Gagliano M, Suardi LR, et al. Procalcitonin for the differential diagnosis of COVID-19 in the emergency department. Prospective monocentric study. Intern Emerg Med 2021;16(6):1733–5.
49. Tong-Minh K, van der Does Y, Engelen S, et al. High procalcitonin levels associated with increased intensive care unit admission and mortality in patients with a

COVID-19 infection in the emergency department. BMC Infect Dis 2022; 22(1):165.

50. Shen Y, Cheng C, Zheng X, et al. Elevated Procalcitonin Is Positively Associated with the Severity of COVID-19: A Meta-Analysis Based on 10 Cohort Studies. Medicina (Kaunas) 2021;(6):57.

51. Williams EJ, Mair L, de Silva TI, et al. Evaluation of procalcitonin as a contribution to antimicrobial stewardship in SARS-CoV-2 infection: a retrospective cohort study. The J Hosp Infect 2021;110:103–7.

52. Cortes MF, de Almeida BL, Espinoza EPS, et al. Procalcitonin as a biomarker for ventilator associated pneumonia in COVID-19 patients: Is it an useful stewardship tool? Diagn Microbiol Infect Dis 2021;101(2):115344.

53. Peters C, Williams K, Un EA, et al. Use of procalcitonin for antibiotic stewardship in patients with COVID-19: A quality improvement project in a district general hospital. Clin Med (Lond) 2021;21(1):e71–6.

54. Heesom L, Rehnberg L, Nasim-Mohi M, et al. Procalcitonin as an antibiotic stewardship tool in COVID-19 patients in the intensive care unit. J Glob Antimicrob Resist 2020;22:782–4.

55. Hesselink DA, Burgerhart JS, Bosmans-Timmerarends H, et al. Procalcitonin as a biomarker for severe Plasmodium falciparum disease: a critical appraisal of a semi-quantitative point-of-care test in a cohort of travellers with imported malaria. Malar J 2009;8:206.

56. Thanachartwet V, Desakorn V, Sahassananda D, et al. Serum Procalcitonin and Peripheral Venous Lactate for Predicting Dengue Shock and/or Organ Failure: A Prospective Observational Study. Plos Negl Trop Dis 2016;10(8):e0004961.

57. Cortegiani A, Misseri G, Ippolito M, et al. Procalcitonin levels in candidemia versus bacteremia: a systematic review. Crit Care 2019;23(1):190.

58. Grace E, Turner RM. Use of procalcitonin in patients with various degrees of chronic kidney disease including renal replacement therapy. Clin Infect Dis 2014;59(12):1761–7.

59. Avrillon V, Locatelli-Sanchez M, Folliet L, et al. Lung cancer may increase serum procalcitonin level. Infect Disord Drug Targets 2015;15(1):57–63.

60. Chaftari AM, Hachem R, Reitzel R, et al. Role of Procalcitonin and Interleukin-6 in Predicting Cancer, and Its Progression Independent of Infection. PLoS One 2015; 10(7):e0130999.

61. Schneider R, Cohen MJ, Benenson S, et al. Procalcitonin in hemodialysis patients presenting with fever or chills to the emergency department. Intern Emerg Med 2020;15(2):257–62.

62. Tao M, Zheng D, Liang X, et al. Diagnostic value of procalcitonin for bacterial infections in patients undergoing hemodialysis: a systematic review and meta-analysis. Ren Fail 2022;44(1):81–93.

63. Level C, Chauveau P, Guisset O, et al. Mass transfer, clearance and plasma concentration of procalcitonin during continuous venovenous hemofiltration in patients with septic shock and acute oliguric renal failure. Crit Care 2003;7(6): R160–6.

64. Soulountsi V, Schizodimos T, Kotoulas SC. Deciphering the epidemiology of invasive candidiasis in the intensive care unit: is it possible? Infection 2021;49(6): 1107–31.

65. Clancy CJ, Nguyen MH. Diagnosing Invasive Candidiasis. J Clin Microbiol 2018; 56(5). https://doi.org/10.1128/JCM.01909-17.

66. Evans L, Rhodes A, Alhazzani W, et al. Surviving Sepsis Campaign: International Guidelines for Management of Sepsis and Septic Shock 2021. Crit Care Med 2021;49(11):e1063–143.
67. Tillett WS, Cambier MJ, McCormack JE. The Treatment of Lobar Pneumonia and Pneumococcal Empyema with Penicillin. Bull N Y Acad Med 1944;20(3):142–78.
68. Huang DT, Yealy DM, Filbin MR, et al. Procalcitonin-Guided Use of Antibiotics for Lower Respiratory Tract Infection. New Engl J Med 2018;379(3):236–49.
69. Seymann GB, Bevins N, Wu C, et al. Prevalence of Discordant Procalcitonin Use at an Academic Medical Center. Am J Clin Pathol 2021. https://doi.org/10.1093/ajcp/aqab201.
70. El Haddad H, Chaftari AM, Hachem R, et al. Biomarkers of Sepsis and Bloodstream Infections: The Role of Procalcitonin and Proadrenomedullin With Emphasis in Patients With Cancer. Clin Infect Dis 2018;67(6):971–7.
71. Park JE, Lee B, Yoon SJ, et al. Complementary Use of Presepsin with the Sepsis-3 Criteria Improved Identification of High-Risk Patients with Suspected Sepsis. Biomedicines 2021;(9):9. https://doi.org/10.3390/biomedicines9091076.
72. Que YA, Guessous I, Dupuis-Lozeron E, et al. Prognostication of Mortality in Critically Ill Patients With Severe Infections. Chest 2015;148(3):674–82.
73. van Houten CB, de Groot JAH, Klein A, et al. A host-protein based assay to differentiate between bacterial and viral infections in preschool children (OPPORTUNITY): a double-blind, multicentre, validation study. Lancet Infect Dis 2017;17(4):431–40.

UNITED STATES POSTAL SERVICE® Statement of Ownership, Management, and Circulation (All Periodicals Publications Except Requester Publications)

1. Publication Title	2. Publication Number	3. Filing Date
INFECTIOUS DISEASE CLINICS OF NORTH AMERICA	001 – 556	9/18/2022

4. Issue Frequency	5. Number of Issues Published Annually	6. Annual Subscription Price
MAR, JUN, SEP, DEC	4	$357.00

7. Complete Mailing Address of Known Office of Publication (Not printer) (Street, city, county, state, and ZIP+4®)

ELSEVIER INC.
230 Park Avenue, Suite 800
New York, NY 10169

Contact Person
Malathi Samayan
Telephone (Include area code)
91-44-4299-4507

8. Complete Mailing Address of Headquarters or General Business Office of Publisher (Not printer)

ELSEVIER INC.
230 Park Avenue, Suite 800
New York, NY 10169

9. Full Names and Complete Mailing Addresses of Publisher, Editor, and Managing Editor (Do not leave blank)

Publisher (Name and complete mailing address)

DOLORES MELONI, ELSEVIER INC.
1600 JOHN F KENNEDY BLVD. SUITE 1800
PHILADELPHIA, PA 19103-2899

Editor (Name and complete mailing address)

KERRY HOLLAND, ELSEVIER INC.
1600 JOHN F KENNEDY BLVD. SUITE 1800
PHILADELPHIA, PA 19103-2899

Managing Editor (Name and complete mailing address)

PATRICK MANLEY, ELSEVIER INC.
1600 JOHN F KENNEDY BLVD. SUITE 1800
PHILADELPHIA, PA 19103-2899

10. Owner (Do not leave blank. If the publication is owned by a corporation, give the name and address of the corporation immediately followed by the names and addresses of all stockholders owning or holding 1 percent or more of the total amount of stock. If not owned by a corporation, give the names and addresses of the individual owners. If owned by a partnership or other unincorporated firm, give its name and address as well as those of each individual owner. If the publication is published by a nonprofit organization, give its name and address.)

Full Name	Complete Mailing Address
WHOLLY OWNED SUBSIDIARY OF REED/ELSEVIER, US HOLDINGS	1600 JOHN F KENNEDY BLVD. SUITE 1800 PHILADELPHIA, PA 19103-2899

11. Known Bondholders, Mortgagees, and Other Security Holders Owning or Holding 1 Percent or More of Total Amount of Bonds, Mortgages, or Other Securities. If none, check box → ☐ None

Full Name	Complete Mailing Address
N/A	

12. Tax Status (For completion by nonprofit organizations authorized to mail at nonprofit rates) (Check one)
The purpose, function, and nonprofit status of this organization and the exempt status for federal income tax purposes:
☒ Has Not Changed During Preceding 12 Months
☐ Has Changed During Preceding 12 Months (Publisher must submit explanation of change with this statement)

PS Form 3526, July 2014 [Page 1 of 4 (see instructions page 4)] PSN: 7530-01-000-9931 PRIVACY NOTICE: See our privacy policy on www.usps.com.

13. Publication Title	14. Issue Date for Circulation Data Below
INFECTIOUS DISEASE CLINICS OF NORTH AMERICA	JUNE 2022

15. Extent and Nature of Circulation			Average No. Copies Each Issue During Preceding 12 Months	No. Copies of Single Issue Published Nearest to Filing Date
a. Total Number of Copies (Net press run)			246	216
b. Paid Circulation (By Mail and Outside the Mail)	(1)	Mailed Outside-County Paid Subscriptions Stated on PS Form 3541 (Include paid distribution above nominal rate, advertiser's proof copies, and exchange copies)	162	150
	(2)	Mailed In-County Paid Subscriptions Stated on PS Form 3541 (Include paid distribution above nominal rate, advertiser's proof copies, and exchange copies)	0	0
	(3)	Paid Distribution Outside the Mails Including Sales Through Dealers and Carriers, Street Vendors, Counter Sales, and Other Paid Distribution Outside USPS®	49	43
	(4)	Paid Distribution by Other Classes of Mail Through the USPS (e.g. First-Class Mail®)	0	0
c. Total Paid Distribution (Sum of 15b (1), (2), (3), and (4))			211	193
d. Free or Nominal Rate Distribution (By Mail and Outside the Mail)	(1)	Free or Nominal Rate Outside-County Copies Included on PS Form 3541	19	8
	(2)	Free or Nominal Rate In-County Copies Included on PS Form 3541	0	0
	(3)	Free or Nominal Rate Copies Mailed at Other Classes Through the USPS (e.g. First-Class Mail)	0	0
	(4)	Free or Nominal Rate Distribution Outside the Mail (Carriers or other means)	19	8
e. Total Free or Nominal Rate Distribution (Sum of 15d (1), (2), (3) and (4))			19	8
f. Total Distribution (Sum of 15c and 15e)			230	201
g. Copies not Distributed (See Instructions to Publishers #4 (page #3))			16	15
h. Total (Sum of 15f and g)			246	216
i. Percent Paid (15c divided by 15f times 100)			91.73%	96.01%

* If you are claiming electronic copies, go to line 16 on page 3. If you are not claiming electronic copies, skip to line 17 on page 3

16. Electronic Copy Circulation	Average No. Copies Each Issue During Preceding 12 Months	No. Copies of Single Issue Published Nearest to Filing Date
a. Paid Electronic Copies	►	
b. Total Paid Print Copies (Line 15c) + Paid Electronic Copies (Line 16a)	►	
c. Total Print Distribution (Line 15f) + Paid Electronic Copies (Line 16a)	►	
d. Percent Paid (Both Print & Electronic Copies) (16b divided by 16c × 100)	►	

☒ I certify that 50% of all my distributed copies (electronic and print) are paid above a nominal price.

17. Publication of Statement of Ownership

☒ If the publication is a general publication, publication of this statement is required. Will be printed
in the DECEMBER 2022 issue of this publication.

☐ Publication not required.

18. Signature and Title of Editor, Publisher, Business Manager, or Owner	Date
Malathi Samayan - Distribution Controller *Malathi Samayan*	9/18/2022

I certify that all information furnished on this form is true and complete. I understand that anyone who furnishes false or misleading information on this form or who omits material or information requested on the form may be subject to criminal sanctions (including fines and imprisonment) and/or civil sanctions (including civil penalties).

PS Form 3526, July 2014 (Page 3 of 4) PRIVACY NOTICE: See our privacy policy on www.usps.com

Printed and bound by CPI Group (UK) Ltd, Croydon, CR0 4YY

08/05/2025

01864719-0004